THE ENCYCLOPEDIA OF
ESSENTIAL OILS

*The Complete Guide to the Use of Aromatic Oils
in Aromatherapy, Herbalism, Health & Well-Being*

Julia Lawless

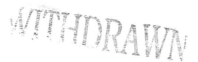
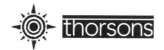

thorsons

Julia Lawless has been interested in aromatic oils since she was a child, when her mother, who was a biochemist, became involved in research in essential oils. In 1983 she took over the responsibility for the formulation of natural products using the oils for Aqua Oleum, the family business. She has studied the Western and Tibetan herbal medicine, and is a qualified aromatherapist and member of the Interanational Federation of Aromatherapists.

To my mother, Kerttu

Thorsons
An Imprint of HarperCollins*Publishers*
77–85 Fulham Palace Road,
Hammersmith, London W6 8JB

The website address is: www.thorsonselement.com

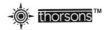

and *Thorsons* are trademarks
of HarperCollins*Publishers* Ltd

First published in Great Britain in 1992 by Element Books Limited
This edition published by Thorsons 2002

10

© Julia Lawless 1992
Cover illustration by Petula Stone
Botanical illustrations by Sarah Roche

Julia Lawless asserts the moral right to be
identified as the author of this work

A catalogue record of this book
is available from the British Library

ISBN-13 978-0-00-714518-8
ISBN-10 0-00-714518-7

Printed and bound in Great Britain by
Martins the Printers Ltd, Berwick upon Tweed

CONTENTS

PART II THE OILS   39

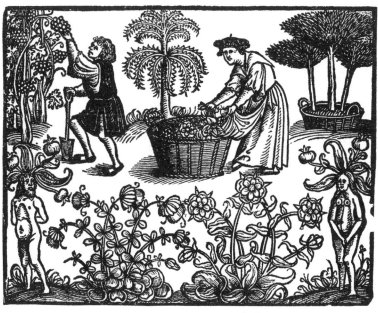

Woodcut from the title page of the *Grete Herball*, 1526

ACKNOWLEDGEMENTS

My own interest in essential oils and herbal remedies derives from the maternal side of my family who came from Finland, where home 'simples' retained popularity long after they had vanished from most parts of Britain. My Finnish grandmother knew a great deal about herbs and wild plants which she passed on to my mother, as she recalls:

> Mama's most important herb was parsley, which along with dill, marjoram, hops and others, were dried in bunches in the autumn, dangling at the ends of short lengths of cotton, all strung on a long length of thin rope stretching right across the kitchen stove. As scents are very evocative for remembering old things, I remember it so well – the strong and heady smell emanating from these herbs when they were hung up, and the stove was warm.

Later, as a biochemist, my mother became involved with the research of essential oils and plants, and helped inspire in me a fascination for herbs and the use of natural remedies. Without her early enthusiasm and guidance, I'm sure this book would never have been written.

I should like to sincerely thank the following people who have made the book possible by contributing their time and energy in various ways: Barbara Austin MNIMH of the Herbal Treatment Centre, Cheltenham, for her creative criticism and suggestions regarding the relationship between aromatherapy and medical herbalism; John Black and Roger Dyer for their valuable expertise and careful corrections concerning the production and chemistry of essential oils; Jill Harvey and John Hughes BAALA of the Gloucestershire County Library for helping sort through all the early herbals in the 'Hartland' collection; and Merilyn King RMN of Coney Hill Hospital, Gloucester, for her painstaking work on the medical terminology and usage.

I would also like to thank all my friends who have been so encouraging, especially my father for all his help; Judith Allan for her editorial notes; Cara Denman for her guidance; Jill Purce for her initial assistance; and last but not least my husband Alec, for his constant support, and our daughter Natasha, for putting up with me.

My appreciation also goes to the services of the British Library, the Chelsea Physic Garden, the Royal Horticultural Society and my local Minchinhampton Library in Gloucestershire. It is my hope that this book will contribute a little to the current knowledge about aromatic plants and essential oils, and help bridge the gap between their different areas of application.

How to Use This Book

The Encyclopaedia of Essential Oils is divided into two parts:

Part I is a general introduction to aromatics, showing their changing role throughout history, from the ritual part they played in ancient civilizations, through medieval alchemy, to their modern day applications in aromatherapy, herbalism and perfumery.

Part II is a systematic survey of over 160 essential oils shown in alphabetical order according to the common name of the plants from which they are derived. Detailed information on each oil includes its botanical origins, herbal/folk tradition, odour characteristics, principal constituents and safety data, as well as its home and commercial uses.

This book can be approached in several ways:

1. It can be employed as a concise *reference guide* to a wide range of aromatic plants and oils, in the same way as a traditional herbal.
2. It can be used a *self-help manual*, showing how to use aromatherapy oils at home for the treatment of common complaints and to promote well-being.
3. It can be read from cover to cover as a *comprehensive textbook* on essential oils, shown in all their different aspects.

1. When using the book as a *reference guide* to essential oils, the name of the plant or oil may be found in the **Botanical Index** at the back of the book, where it is listed under:

    a) its common name: for example, frankincense;
    b) its Latin or botanical term: *Boswellia carteri;*
    c) its essential oil trade name: olibanum;
    d) or by its folk names: gum thus.

Other varieties, such as Indian frankincense (*Boswellia serrata*), may be found in the **Botanical Classification** section under their common family name 'Burseraceae', along with related species such as elemi, linaloe, myrrh and opopanax. Less common essential oils, such as blackcurrant (which is used mainly by the food industry), do not appear in the main body of the book, but are included in the **Botanical Classification** section under their common family name, in this case 'Grossulariaceae'.

2. When using the book as a *self-help manual* on aromatherapy, it is best to consult the **Therapeutic Index** at the end of the book, where common complaints are grouped according to different parts of the body:

    ☐ Skin Care
    ☐ Circulation, Muscles and Joints
    ☐ Respiratory System
    ☐ Digestive System
    ☐ Genito-urinary and Endocrine Systems
    ☐ Immune System
    ☐ Nervous System

If for example, we have been working long hours at a desk and have developed a painful cramp in our neck, we should turn to the section on **Circulation, Muscles and Joints** where we find the heading 'Muscular Cramp and Stiffness'. Of the essential oils which are listed, those shown in italics are generally considered to be the most useful and/or readily available, in this case allspice, lavender, marjoram, rosemary and black pepper.

The choice of which oil to use depends on what is to hand, and on assessing the quality of each oil by consulting their entry in Part II of the book. Special attention should be paid to the Safety Data on each oil: both allspice and black pepper are known to be skin irritants if used in high concentration; rosemary and marjoram should be avoided during pregnancy; rosemary should not be used by epileptics at all. On the basis of our assessment, we may choose to use lavender, marjoram and a little black pepper which would make an excellent blend. Some of the principles behind blending oils can be found in Chapter 5, **Creative Blending**.

The various methods of application are indicated by the letters **M**, massage; **C**, compress; **B**, bath etc. Turn to Chapter 4, **How to Use Essential Oils at Home**, where you will find instructions on how to make up a massage oil or compress, and how many drops of oil to use in a bath. Further information on how essential oils work in specific cases can be found in Chapter 3, **The Body – Actions and Applications.**

3. Used as a *comprehensive textbook*, *The Encyclopaedia of Essential Oils* provides a wealth of information about the essential oils themselves in all their various aspects, including their perfumery and flavouring applications. It shows the development of aromatics through history and the relationship between essential oils and other herbal products. It defines different kinds of aromatic materials and their methods of extraction, giving up-to-date areas of production. In addition, it includes information on their chemistry, pharmacology and safety levels. The 'Actions' ascribed to each plant refer either to the properties of the whole herb, or to parts of it, or to the essential oil. Difficult technical terms, mainly of a botanical or medical nature, are explained in the **General Glossary** at the end of the book.

However, since the therapeutic guidelines presented in the text are aimed primarily at the lay person without medical qualifications, the section dealing with the aromatherapy application of essential oils at home is limited to the treatment of common complaints only. Although there is a great deal of research being carried out at present into the potential uses of essential oils in the treatment of diseases such as cancer, AIDS and psychological disorders, these discussions fall beyond the scope of this book. References to the medical and folk use of particular plants in herbal medicine and their actions are intended to provide background information only, and are not intended as a guide for self-treatment.

PART I
AN INTRODUCTION TO AROMATICS

1. HISTORICAL ROOTS

Natural Plant Origins

When we peel an orange, walk through a rose garden or rub a sprig of lavender between our fingers, we are all aware of the special scent of that plant. But what exactly is it that we can smell? Generally speaking, it is essential oils which give spices and herbs their specific scent and flavour, flowers and fruit their perfume. The essential oil in the orange peel is not difficult to identify; it is found in such profusion that it actually squirts out when we peel it. The minute droplets of oil which are contained in tiny pockets or glandular cells in the outer peel are very volatile, that is, they easily evaporate, infusing the air with their characteristic aroma.

But not all plants contain essential or volatile oils in such profusion. The aromatic content in the flowers of the rose is so very small that it takes one ton of petals to produce 300g of rose oil. It is not fully understood why some plants contain essential oils and others not. It is clear that the aromatic quality of the oils plays a role in the attraction or repulsion of certain insects or animals. It has also been suggested that they play an important part in the transpiration and life processes of the plant itself, and as a protection against disease. They have been described as the 'hormone' or 'life-blood' of a plant, due to their highly concentrated and essential nature.

Aromatic oils can be found in all the various parts of a plant, including the seeds, bark, root, leaves, flowers, wood, balsam and resin. The bitter orange tree, for example, yields orange oil from the fruit peel, petitgrain from the

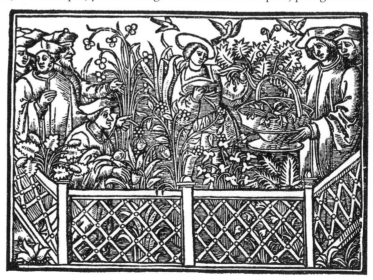

A Herbalists Garden; *Le Jardin de Santé*, 1539

leaves and twigs, and neroli oil from the orange blossoms. The clove tree produces different types of essential oil from its buds, stalks and leaves, whereas the Scotch pine yields distinct oils from its needles, wood and resin. The wide range of aromatic materials obtained from natural sources and the art of their extraction and use has developed slowly over the course of time, but its origins reach back to the very heart of the earliest civilizations.

Ancient Civilizations

Aromatic plants and oils have been used for thousands of years, as incense, perfumes and cosmetics and for their medical and culinary applications. Their ritual use constituted an integral part of the tradition in most early cultures, where their religious and therapeutic roles became inextricably intertwined. This type of practice is still in evidence: for example, in the East, sprigs of juniper are burnt in Tibetan temples as a form of purification; in the West, frankincense is used during the Roman Catholic mass.

> In the ancient civilizations, perfumes were used as an expression of the animist and cosmic conceptions, responding above all to the exigencies of a cult ... associated at first with theophanies and incantations, the perfumes made by *fumigation, libation* and *ablution*, grew directly out of the ritual, and became an element in the art of therapy.[1]

The Vedic literature of India dating from around 2000 BC, lists over 700 substances including cinnamon, spikenard, ginger, myrrh, coriander and sandalwood. But aromatics were considered to be more than just perfumes; in the Indo-Aryan tongue, 'atar' means *smoke, wind, odour* and *essence,* and the *Rig Veda* codifies their use for both liturgical and therapeutic purposes. The manner in which it is written reflects a spiritual and philosophical outlook, in which humanity is seen as a part of nature, and the handling of herbs as a sacred task: 'Simples, you who have existed for so long, even before the Gods were born, I want to understand your seven hundred secrets! ... Come, you wise plants, heal this patient for me'.[2] Their understanding of plant lore developed into the traditional Indian or Ayurvedic system of medicine, which has enjoyed an unbroken transmission up to the present day.

The Chinese also have an ancient herbal tradition which accompanies the practice of acupuncture, the earliest records being in the *Yellow Emperor's Book of Internal Medicine* dating from more than 2000 years BC. Among the remedies are several aromatics such as opium and ginger which, apart from their therapeutic applications, are known to have been utilized for religious purposes since the earliest times, as in the Li-ki and Tcheou-Li ceremonies. Borneo camphor is still used extensively in China today for ritual purposes.

But perhaps the most famous and richest associations concerning the first aromatic materials are those surrounding the ancient Egyptian civilization. Papyrus manuscripts dating back to the reign of Khufu, around 2800 BC, record the use of many medicinal herbs, while another papyrus written about 2000 BC speaks of 'fine oils and choice perfumes, and the incense of temples, whereby every god is gladdened'.[3] Aromatic gums and oils such as cedar and myrrh were employed in the embalming process, the remains of which are still detectable thousands of years later, along with traces of scented unguents and oils such as styrax and frankincense contained in a number of ornate jars and cosmetic pots found in the tombs. The complete iconography covering the process of preparation for such oils, balsams and fermented liqueurs was preserved in stone inscriptions by the people of the Nile valley. The Egyptians were, in fact, experts of cosmetology and renowned for their herbal preparations and ointments. One such remedy was known as 'kyphi'; a mixture of sixteen different ingredients which could be used as an incense, a perfume or taken internally as a medicine. It was said to be antiseptic, balsamic, soothing and an antidote to poison which, according to Plutarch, could lull one to sleep, allay anxieties and brighten dreams.

Treasures from the East

Natural aromatics and perfume materials constituted one of the earliest trade items of the ancient world, being rare and highly prized. When the Jewish people began their exodus from Egypt to Israel around 1240 BC, they took with them many precious gums and oils together with knowledge of their use. On their journey, according to the Book of Exodus, the Lord transmitted to Moses the formula for a special anointing oil, which included myrrh, cinnamon, calamus, cassia and olive oil among its ingredients. This holy oil was used to consecrate Aaron and his sons into priesthood, which continued from generation to generation. Frankincense and myrrh, as treasures from the East, were offered to Jesus at his birth.

The Phoenician merchants also exported their scented oils and gums to the Arabian peninsula and gradually throughout the Mediterranean region, particularly Greece and Rome. They introduced the West to the riches of the Orient: they brought camphor from China, cinnamon from India, gums from Arabia and rose from Syria, always ensuring that they kept their trading routes a closely guarded secret .

The Greeks especially learnt a great deal from the Egyptians; Herodotus

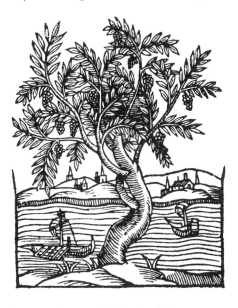

'Lentisco del Peru' (Mastic Tree) from Durante's *Herbario Nuovo*, 1585. Gums and oils were regarded as highly prized trade items throughout the Mediterranean region

and Democrates, who visited Egypt during the fifth century BC, were later to transmit what they had learnt about perfumery and natural therapeutics. Herodotus was the first to record the method of distillation of turpentine, in about 425 BC, as well as furnishing the first information about perfumes and numerous other details regarding odorous materials. Dioscorides made a detailed study of the sources and uses of plants and aromatics employed by the Greeks and Romans which he compiled into a five volume materia medica, known as the *Herbarius*.

Hippocrates who was born in Greece about 460 BC and universally revered as the 'father of medicine', also prescribed perfumed fumigations and fomentations; indeed 'from Greek medical practice there is derived the term 'iatralypte', from the physician who cured by the use of aromatic unctions'.[4] One of the most famous of these Greek preparations, made from myrrh, cinnamon and cassia, was called 'megaleion' after its creator Megallus. Like the Egyptian 'kyphi', it could be used both as a perfume and as a remedy for skin inflammation and battle wounds.

The Romans were even more lavish in their use of perfumes and aromatic oils than the Greeks. They used three kinds of perfumes: 'ladysmata', solid unguents; 'stymmata', scented oils; and 'diapasmata', powdered perfumes. They were used to fragrance their hair, their bodies, their clothes and beds ; large amounts of scented oil were used for massage after bathing. With the fall of the Roman Empire and the advent of Christianity, many of the Roman physicians fled to Constantinople taking the books of Galen, Hippocrates and Dioscorides with them. These great Graeco-Roman works were translated into Persian, Arabic and other languages, and at the end of the Byzantine Empire, their knowledge passed on to the Arab world. Europe, meanwhile, entered the so-called Dark Ages.

Alchemy

Between the seventh and thirteenth centuries the Arabs produced many great men of science, among them Avicenna (AD 980–1037). This highly gifted physician and scholar wrote over a hundred books in his lifetime, one of which was devoted entirely to the flower most cherished by Islam, the rose. Among his discoveries, he has been credited with the invention of the refrigerated coil, a breakthrough in the art of distillation, which he used to produce pure essential oils and aromatic water. However, in 1975 Dr Paolo Rovesti led an archaeological expedition to Pakistan to investigate the ancient Indus Valley civilization. There, in the museum of Taxila at the foot of the Himalayas, he found a perfectly preserved distillation apparatus made of terracotta. The presence of perfume containers also exhibited in the museum dating from the same period, about 3000 BC, confirmed its use for the preparation of aromatic oils. This discovery suggests that the Arabs simply revived or improved upon a process that had been known for over 4000 years!

Rose water became one of the most popular scents and came to the West at the time of the Crusades, along with other exotic essences, and the method of distillation. By the thirteenth century, the 'perfumes of Arabia' were famous throughout Europe. During the Middle Ages, floors were strewn with aromatic plants and little herbal bouquets were carried as a protection against plague and other infectious diseases. Gradually the Europeans, lacking the gum-yielding trees of the Orient, began to experiment with their own native herbs such as lavender, sage and rosemary. By the sixteenth century lavender water and essential oils known as 'chymical oils' could be bought from the apothecary, and, following the invention of printing, the period 1470 to 1670 saw the publication of many herbals such as the *Grete Herball* published in 1526, some of which included illustrations of the retorts and stills used for the extraction of volatile oils.

In the hands of the philosophers, the art of distillation was employed in the practice of alchemy, the hermetic pursuit dedicated to the transformation of base metals into gold, the gross into the subtle. It was primarily a religious quest in which the various stages of the distillation process were equated with stages of an inner psychic transmutation, 'dissolution and coagulation': separation (black, lead), extraction (white, quicksilver), fusion (red, sulphur) and finally sublimation (gold or 'lapis'). In the same way that aromatic material could be distilled to produce a pure and potent essence, so could the human emotions be refined and concentrated to reveal their valuable fruit, or true nature. In this context, volatile oils can be equated with the purified human psyche or 'quintessence' of the alchemists, being an emanation of matter and manifestation of spirit, mediator between the two realms.

> Alchemy was the bridge across which the rich symbolism of the ancient world – Arab, Greek, Gnostic – was transported into our own era ... thus symbolism fell from the rarefied heights into the melting-pot, and began to be tested in a continuous, dynamic interaction with the findings of chemistry.[5]

The Scientific Revolution

Throughout the Renaissance period, aromatic materials filled the pharmacopoeias which for many centuries remained the main protection against epidemics. Over the next few centuries the medicinal properties and applications of increasing numbers of new essential oils were analysed and recorded by the pharmacists. The list included both well-established aromatics such as cedar, cinnamon, frankincense, juniper, rose, rosemary, lavender and sage, but also essences like artemisia, cajeput, chervil, orange flower, valerian and pine.

The perfumery and distillation industries attracted illustrious names of the day and in the northern countries of Europe, especially at Grasse in France, flourishing commercial enterprises sprang up. By the end of the seventeenth century, the profession of perfumery broke away from the allied fields, and a distinction was made between perfumes and the aromatics that had become the domain of the apothecary.

Alchemy gave way to technical chemistry, and with it went the interest in the inter-relatedness of matter and spirit, and the interdependence of medicine and psychology. There developed the idea of combating speculation with logic and deductive reason. With the scientific revolution of the early nineteenth century, chemists were able to identify for the first time the various constituents of the oils, and give them specific names such as 'geraniol', 'citronellol' and 'cineol'. In the *Yearbook of Pharmacy and Transactions of the British Pharmaceutical Conference* in 1907, we find for example:

> A pilea of undetermined botanical species has yielded a white essential oil with an odour of turpentine ... A small amount of pinene was detected but its other constituents have not yet been identified. This oil is of interest as being the first instance of an essential oil derived from the family Uricaceae.[6]

It is ironic that this enthusiastic research laid the ground for the development of the oils' synthetic counterparts, and the growth of the modern drug industry. Herbal medicine and aromatic remedies lost their credibility as methods of treatment went out of the hands of the individual and into those of professionals. By the middle of the twentieth century, the role of essential oils had been reduced almost entirely to their employment in perfumes, cosmetics and foodstuffs.

2. AROMATHERAPY AND HERBALISM

The Birth of Aromatherapy

The term 'aromatherapy' was first coined in 1928 by Gattefossé, a French chemist working in his family's perfumier business. He became fascinated with the therapeutic possibilities of the oils after discovering by accident that lavender was able to rapidly heal a severe burn on his hand and help prevent scarring. He also found that many of the essential oils were more effective in their totality than their synthetic substitutes or their isolated active ingredients. As early as 1904 Cuthbert Hall had shown that the anti-septic power of eucalyptus oil in its natural form was stronger than its isolated main active constituent, 'eucalyptol' or 'cineol'.

Another French doctor and scientist, Dr Jean Valnet, used essential oils as part of his programme by which he was able to successfully treat specific medical and psychiatric disorders, the results of which were published in 1964 as *Aromatherapie*.

The work of Valnet was studied by Madame Marguerite Maury who applied his research to her beauty therapy, in which she aimed to revitalize her clients by creating a 'strictly personal aromatic complex which she adapted to the subject's temperament and particular health problems. Hence, going far beyond any simple aesthetic objective, perfumed essences when correctly selected, represent many medicinal agents.'[7]

In some respects, the word 'aromatherapy' can be misleading because it suggests that it is a form of healing which works exclusively through our sense of smell, and on the emotions. This is not the case for, apart from its scent, each essential oil has an individual combination of constituents which interacts with the body's chemistry in a direct manner, which then in turn affects certain organs or systems as a whole. For example, when the oils are used externally in the form of a massage treatment, they are easily absorbed via the skin and transported throughout the body. This can be demonstrated by rubbing a clove of garlic on the soles of the feet; the volatile oil content will be taken into the blood and the odour will appear on the breath a little while later. It is interesting to note that different essential oils are absorbed through the skin at varying rates, for example:

Turpentine: 20 mins.
Eucalyptus and thyme: 20–40 mins.
Anise, bergamot and lemon: 40–60 mins.
Citronella, pine, lavender and geranium: 60–80 mins.
Coriander, rue and peppermint: 100–120 mins.

It is therefore important to recognize that essential oils have three distinct modes of action with regard to how they inter-relate with the human body: pharmacological, physiological and psychological. The pharmacological effect is concerned with the chemical changes which take place when an essential oil enters the bloodstream and reacts with the hormones and enzymes etc; the physiological mode is concerned with the way in which an essential oil affects the systems of the body, whether they are sedated or stimulated, etc; the psychological effect takes place when an essence is inhaled, and an individual responds to its odour. With relation to the first two points, aromatherapy has a great deal in common with the tradition of medical herbalism or phytotherapy – in other words, it is not simply the aroma which is important but also the chemical interaction between the oils and the body, and the physical changes which are brought about.

Herbal Medicine

The practice of aromatherapy could be seen as part of the larger field of herbal medicine, since the essential oil is only one of many ways in which a plant can be prepared as a remedy. Since all essential oils are derived directly from plants, it can be valuable to see them within a botanical context rather than as isolated products. In some ways the use of aromatic oils for therapeutic purposes benefits from being placed within a herbal context not only because it gives us further insight into their characteristics, but because the two forms of therapy are not synonymous, but complementary.

Although most plants which yield essential oils are also used in medical herbalism, it is important to distinguish the therapeutic qualities of a particular oil from those of the herb taken as a whole or prepared in another manner. German chamomile, for example, is used extensively in the form of a herbal preparation such as an infusion, tincture or decoction, apart from being utilized for its volatile oil. Chamazulene, a major constituent of the oil, helps to account for the herb's age-old reputation as a general relaxant and soothing skin care remedy, due to its pain-relieving, antispasmodic, wound-healing and anti-inflammatory activities. For the treatment of nervous conditions, insomnia and dermal irritation or disease, the essential oil is both useful and effective. But although the aromatic principle of the plant plays a central role in its overall character, the herb also contains a bitter component (anthemic acid), tannins (tannic acid), mucilage and a glycoside among other things. The overall effect of the herb is the result of the action of all its pharmacologically active constituents which in the case of chamomile or *Matricaria* includes the astringency of the tannins and the stimulation of the bitters. The volatile oil is, of course, less concentrated in

Growing and storing herbs: the woman is scenting the linen chest; from *Das Kerüterbuch oder Herbarius*, 1534

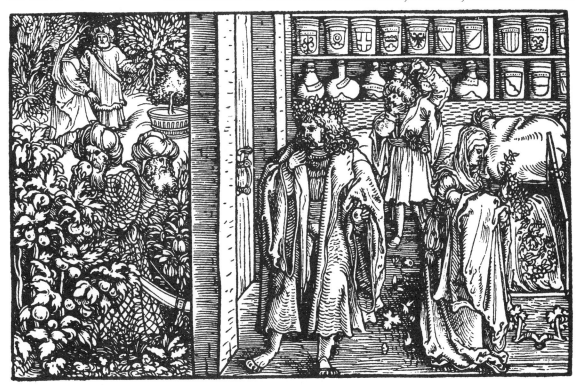

the form of an infusion, tincture or decoction, the potency of the oil is reduced (and inherently the safety margin increased), thus making the herbal preparation more suited to internal use.

Similarly with peppermint. Whilst the oil is eminently suited to the treatment of respiratory conditions as an inhalant, due in particular to its antispasmodic and antiseptic actions, for the longer term treatment of digestive disorders it is better to use extracts from the whole herb, where the action of the volatile oil is supported by the presence of bitters and tannins. In addition, in herbal medicine, the effect of one herb is usually supported and backed up by combining it with others.

Neither is it correct to assume that the essential oil is always the most active or therapeutically useful part of a plant. For example, although meadowsweet contains an essential oil outstanding in its antiseptic strength (according to Cavel,[8] 3.3cc of meadowsweet essence renders infertile 1000cc of microbic cultures in sewage, compared to 5.6cc of phenol per 1000cc), it also possesses several other valuable components, notably salicylic glycosides which are characterized by their excellent pain-relieving and anti-inflammatory qualities. Indeed, the familiar drug aspirin, being derived from salicylic acid, is named after this herb, its old country name being 'spiraea'.

The kernels of the (bitter and sweet) almond tree are used to produce a fixed oil commonly known as sweet almond oil, which has a great many cosmetic uses. The kernels from the bitter almond tree, which are used to produce the essential oil which gives marzipan its characteristic taste, also contain cyanide, the well-known poison, in its unrefined form. This shows that there can be a great difference in the properties of a plant, even the same part of a plant, depending upon how it has been prepared.

Therapeutic Guidelines

As a general rule which is in line with the present-day aromatherapy 'code of practice', it is best to use essential oils as external remedies only. This is mainly due to the high concentration of the oils and the potential irritation or damage that they can cause to the mucous membranes and delicate stomach lining in undiluted form. There even seems to be some kind of natural order in this scheme, in that volatile oils mix readily with oils and ointments suited to external application, which are absorbed readily through the skin and vaporize easily for inhalation. When inhaled, they can affect an individual's mood or feelings, and at the same time cause physiological changes in the body. Indeed, in a Japanese experiment carried out in 1963, it was found that the effects of essential oils on the digestive system were likely to be stronger if they were inhaled than if they were ingested.

Herbs, on the other hand, yield up many of their qualities to water and alcohol which are appropriate for internal use but, lacking the concentrated aromatic element, they do not have the same subtle effects on the mind and emotions.

These are only superficial guidelines, for there are always exceptions to the rule. Plantain, for example, is an excellent wound-healing herb valuable for external use, although it does not contain any essential oil. Nor can we ignore the fact that a great many aromatic oils are used for flavouring our food and beverages and are consumed daily in minute amounts. Peppermint oil, for example, is used in a wide variety of alcoholic and non-alcoholic beverages, confectionery and prepared savoury foods, although the highest average use does not exceed 0.104 per cent. The mint oils, which include spearmint and cornmint, are also used extensively by the pharmaceutical and cosmetic industries in products such as toothpaste, cough and cold remedies, and as fragrance components in soaps, creams, lotions, as well as colognes and perfumes. In addition, cornmint is frequently used as the starting material for the production of 'menthol' for use in the drug industry.

It can be seen that the use of essential oils covers a wide and varied spectrum. On the one hand they share the holistic qualities of natural plant remedies, although it is true that some herbalists view essential oils in much the same light as they regard synthetic drugs, being a 'part' of the whole, rather than the entire herb. On the other hand , they play an active role in the modern pharmaceutical industry, either in their entirety or in the form of isolated constituents such as 'phenol' or 'menthol'.

It is not the aim of this book to glorify natural remedies (some of which are in fact highly toxic) at the expense of scientific progress, nor to uphold the principles of our present-day drug-orientated culture, but simply to provide information about the oils themselves in their multifaceted nature.

Safety Precautions

Safety Data: Always check with specific SAFETY DATA before using a new oil, especially with regard to toxicity levels, phototoxicity, dermal irritation and sensitization.

Contra-indications: Take note of any contra-indications when using particular oils. For example, fennel, hyssop and sage should be avoided by epileptics; clary sage should not be used while drinking alcohol; hops should not be used by anyone suffering from depression.

High Blood Pressure: Avoid the following oils in cases of high blood pressure: hyssop, rosemary, sage (all types) and thyme.

Homoeopathy: Homoeopathic treatment is not compatible with the following oils: black pepper, camphor, eucalyptus and the mint oils.

Pregnancy: During pregnancy use essential oils in half the usual stated amount. Take note of those oils which are contra-indicated in pregnancy.

Babies and Children: Use with care, in accordance with age.
Babies (0-12 months) – use 1 drop of lavender, rose, chamomile or mandarin diluted in 1 tsp base oil for massage or bathing.
Infants (1-5 years) – use 2-3 drops of 'safe' essential oils (non-toxic and non irritant to the skin), diluted in 1 tsp base oil for massage or bathing.
Children (6-12 years) – use as for adults but in half the stated amount.
Teenagers (over 12 years) – use as directed for adults.

3. THE BODY – ACTIONS AND APPLICATIONS

How Essential Oils Work

The therapeutic potential of essential oils, like other plant-derived remedies, has yet to be fully realized. Although numerous medical herbs have been utilized since antiquity, many of which have been exploited to provide the biologically active compounds which form the basis for most of our modern drugs (such as quinine and cocaine), there is still a great deal to be learnt about their precise pharmacology. This is particularly true of aromatic oils, which by their very nature have such a concentrated yet multifaceted make-up. In addition, 'only a small proportion of the world flora has been examined for pharmacologically active compounds, but with the ever-increasing danger of plants becoming extinct, there is a real risk that many important plant sources may be lost'.[9]

Modern research has largely confirmed the traditionally held beliefs regarding the therapeutic uses of particular plants, although with time the terminology has changed. A herb such as basil, at one time described as a 'protection against evil', or 'good for the heart' whose scent 'taketh away sorrowfulness', may in modern usage be described as an excellent prophylactic, nerve tonic and antidepressant. Like herbal remedies, an essential oil can cover a wide field of activities; indeed the same herb or oil (such as lemon balm) can stimulate certain systems of the body while sedating or relaxing others. In order to gain a clearer understanding of the way essential oils work, and some of their particular areas of activity, it may be helpful to take an overall view of the systems of the human body.

The Skin

Skin problems are often the surface manifestation of a deeper condition, such as a build-up of toxins in the blood, hormonal imbalance or nervous and emotional difficulties. In this area the versatility of essential oils is particularly valuable because they are able to combat such complaints on a variety of levels. Since essential oils are soluble in oil and alcohol and impart their scent to water, they provide the ideal ingredient for cosmetics and general skin care as well as for the treatment of specific diseases.

Within this context the following activities are of particular benefit:

Antiseptics for cuts, insect bites, spots, etc; for example, thyme, sage, eucalyptus, tea tree, clove, lavender and lemon.
Anti-inflammatory oils for eczema, infected wounds, bumps, bruises, etc; for example, German and Roman chamomile, lavender and yarrow.
Fungicidal oils for athletes foot, candida, ringworm, etc; for example, lavender, tea tree, myrrh, patchouli and sweet marjoram.
Granulation stimulating or cicatrising(healing) agents for burns, cuts, scars, stretch marks, etc; for example, lavender, chamomile, rose, neroli, frankincense and geranium.
Deodorants for excessive perspiration, cleaning wounds, etc; for example, bergamot, lavender, thyme, juniper, cypress, Spanish sage, lemongrass.
Insect repellents and parasiticides for lice, fleas, scabies, ticks, mosquitos, ants, moths, etc; for example, spike lavender, garlic, geranium, citronella, eucalyptus, clove, camphor, Atlas cedarwood.

The Circulation, Muscles and Joints

Essential oils are easily absorbed via the skin and mucosa into the bloodstream, affecting the nature of the circulation as a whole. Oils with a rubefacient or warming effect not only cause a better local blood circulation, but also influence the inner organs. They bring a warmth and glow to the surface of the skin and can provide considerable pain relief through their analgesic or numbing effect. Such oils can relieve local inflammation by setting free mediators in the body which in turn cause the blood vessels to expand, so the blood is able to move more quickly and the swelling is reduced. Some oils like hyssop tend to have a balancing or regulating effect on the circulatory system as a whole, reducing the blood pressure if it is too high or stimulating the system if it is sluggish.

Hypotensives for high blood pressure, palpitations, stress, etc; for example, sweet marjoram, ylang ylang, lavender, lemon.
Hypertensives for poor circulation, chilblains, listlessness, etc; for example, rosemary, spike lavender, eucalyptus, peppermint, thyme.
Rubefacients for rheumatism of the joints, muscular stiffness, sciatica, lumbago, etc; for example, black pepper, juniper, rosemary, camphor, sweet marjoram.
Depurative or antitoxic agents for arthritis, gout, congestion, skin eruptions, etc; for example, juniper, lemon, fennel, lovage.
Lymphatic stimulants for cellulitis, obesity, water retention, etc; for example, grapefruit, lime, fennel, lemon, mandarin, white birch.
Circulatory tonics and astringents for swellings, inflammations, varicose veins, etc; for example, cypress, yarrow, lemon.

The Respiratory System

Nose, throat and lung infections are conditions which respond very well to treatment with essential oils. Inhalation is a very effective way of utilizing their properties, for 'although after arriving in the bronchi the main part will be exhaled directly by the lungs, they cause an increased bronchial secretion (a protective reaction) which is beneficial for many respiratory ailments'.[10] By inhalation they are absorbed into the blood circulation even faster than by oral application. In addition, most essential oils which are absorbed from the stomach are then excreted via the lungs, only a small part in the urine.

Expectorants for catarrh, sinusitis, coughs, bronchitis, etc; for example, eucalyptus, pine, thyme, myrrh, sandalwood, fennel.
Antispasmodics for colic, asthma, dry cough, whooping cough, etc; for example, hyssop, cypress, Atlas cedarwood, bergamot, chamomile, cajeput.
Balsamic agents for colds, chills, congestion, etc; for example, benzoin, frankincense, Tolu balsam, Peru balsam, myrrh.
Antiseptics for 'flu, colds, sore throat, tonsillitis, gingivitis, etc; for example, thyme, sage, eucalyptus, hyssop, pine, cajeput, tea tree, borneol.

The Digestive System

Although it is not recommended that essential oils be taken orally, they can by external application effect certain changes in the digestive processes. However, whereas herbal medicine has many remedies at its disposal for a wide variety of stomach, gall bladder and liver complaints, such as dandelion, marshmallow, chamomile and meadowsweet, much of their effectiveness is based on a combination of aromatic components, together with bitters, tannins and mucilage, which are absent in the volatile oil alone. The external application of essential oils in problems of the digestive system though effective, is consequently somewhat limited compared to the internal use of herbal remedies.

Antispasmodics for spasm, pain, indigestion, etc; for example, chamomile, caraway, fennel, orange, peppermint, lemon balm, aniseed, cinnamon.
Carminatives and stomachics for flatulent dyspepsia, aerophagia, nausea, etc; for example, angelica, basil, fennel, chamomile, peppermint, mandarin.
Cholagogues for increasing the flow of bile and stimulating the gall bladder; for example, caraway, lavender, peppermint and borneol.
Hepatics for liver congestion, jaundice, etc; for example, lemon, lime, rosemary, peppermint.
Aperitifs for loss of appetite, anorexia, etc; for example, aniseed, angelica, orange, ginger, garlic.

The Genito-urinary and Endocrine Systems

Like the digestive system, the reproductive organs can be affected by absorption via the skin into the bloodstream, as well as through hormonal changes. Some essential oils such as rose and jasmine have an affinity for the reproductive system having a general strengthening effect as well as helping to combat specific complaints like menstrual problems, genital infections and sexual difficulties. Other oils contain plant hormones which mimic the corresponding human hormones; oils such as hops, sage and fennel have been found to contain a form of oestrogen that influences the menstrual cycle, lactation and secondary sexual characteristics. Oestrogen also helps maintain a healthy circulation, good muscle and skin tone and strong bones in both men and women.

Other essential oils are known to influence the levels of hormone secretion of other glands, including the thyroid gland (which governs growth and metabolism), the adrenal medulla (which deals with stress reactions) and the adrenal cortex (which governs several processes including the production of oestrogen and androgen, the male sex hormone).

Antispasmodics for menstrual cramp (dysmenorrhoea), labour pains, etc; for example, sweet marjoram, chamomile, clary sage, jasmine, lavender.
Emmenagogues for scanty periods, lack of periods (amenorrhoea), etc; for example, chamomile, fennel, hyssop, juniper, sweet marjoram, peppermint.
Uterine tonics and regulators for pregnancy, excess menstruation (menorrhagia), PMT, etc; for example, clary sage, jasmine, rose, myrrh, frankincense, lemon balm.
Antiseptic and bactericidal agents for leucorrhoea, vaginal pruritis, thrush, etc; for example, bergamot, chamomile, myrrh, rose, tea tree.
Galactagogues for increasing milk flow; for example, fennel, jasmine, anise, lemongrass (sage, mint and parsley reduce it).
Aphrodisiacs for impotence and frigidity, etc; for example, black pepper, cardomon, clary sage, neroli, jasmine, rose, sandalwood, patchouli, ylang ylang.
Anaphrodisiacs for reducing sexual desire; for example, sweet marjoram, camphor.
Adrenal stimulants for anxiety, stress-related conditions, etc; for example, basil, geranium, rosemary, borneol, sage, pine, savory.

With regard to the kidneys, bladder and urinary system in general, it is difficult to bring about results simply by using essential oils. According to recent research, 'the diuretic effects of essential oils are virtually non-existent'.[12] In addition, the traditional diuretic agents such as juniper, lovage and parsley seed are considered unsuitable as essential oils for internal use due to toxicity levels and possible kidney damage; herb teas of fennel, dandelion or chamomile provide a milder alternative. Bathing and using a douche can help control urinary infections, especially when they are associated with nervous or stress-related symptoms.

Urinary antiseptics for cystitis, urethritis, etc; for example, bergamot, chamomile, tea tree, sandalwood.

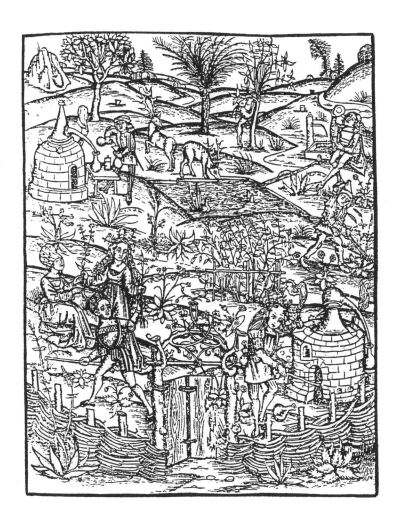

'Lerne the hygh and mervelous vertue of herbes ... use the effectes with reverence, and give thankes to the maker celestyall'; from Braunsweig's *The Vertuose Boke of Distyllacyon of the Waters of all Maner of Herbes*, 1527

The Immune System

Virtually all essential oils have bactericidal properties and by promoting the production of white blood cells, they can help prevent and treat infectious illness. It is these properties that gave aromatic herbs and oils such high repute with regard to infections such as malaria and typhoid in the tropics and epidemics of plague in the Middle Ages. 'People who use essential oils all the time ... mostly have a high level of resistance to illness, catching fewer colds, etc, than average and recovering quickly if they do.'[10]

Bactericidal and antiviral agents (prophylactics) for protection against colds, 'flu, etc; for example, tea tree, cajeput, niaouli, basil, lavender, eucalyptus, bergamot, camphor, clove, rosemary.

Febrifuge agents for reducing fever and temperature, etc; for example, angelica, basil, peppermint, thyme, sage, lemon, eucalyptus, tea tree.
Sudorifics and diaphoretics for promoting sweating, eliminating toxins, etc; for example, rosemary, thyme, hyssop, chamomile.

The Nervous System

Recent research shows that the properties of many oils correspond to the traditionally held views: chamomile, bergamot, sandalwood, lavender and sweet marjoram were found to have a sedative effect on the central nervous system; jasmine, peppermint, basil, clove and ylang ylang were found to have a stimulating effect. Neroli was found to be stimulating and lemon to be sedating, contrary to popular belief. Some oils are known to be 'adaptogens', that is, they have a balancing or normalizing effect on the systems of the body: geranium and rosewood were either sedative or stimulating according to each situation and individual.

Words like 'relaxing' and 'uplifting' often have more to do with odour description and emotional response rather than physiological effect – although the two are related. Consequently, oils such as bergamot, lemon balm or lemon can be sedating to the nervous system, but reviving to the 'spirit'. Conversely, oils such as jasmine, ylang ylang and neroli can be nerve stimulants yet soothing and relaxing on a more subtle emotional level.

Sedatives for nervous tension, stress, insomnia, etc; for example, chamomile, bergamot, sandalwood, lavender, sweet marjoram, lemon balm, hops, valerian, lemon.
Stimulants for convalescence, lack of strength, nervous fatigue, etc; for example, basil, jasmine, peppermint, ylang ylang, neroli, angelica, rosemary.
Nerve tonics (nervines) for strengthening the nervous system as a whole; for example, chamomile, clary sage, juniper, lavender, marjoram, rosemary.

The Mind

This area is perhaps the most discussed and least understood area of activity regarding essential oils. There is no doubt that throughout history aromatic oils have been used for their power to influence the emotions and states of mind: this is the basis for their employment as incense for religious and ritualistic purposes. It is already known that two olfactory nerve tracts run right into the limbic system (the part of the brain concerned with memory and emotion), which means that scents can evoke an immediate and powerful response which defies rational analysis.

Recent research at Warwick University, England, and Toho University, Japan, has aimed to put these traditionally held beliefs and applications into a scientific context. They came up with two types of reaction to odours which they called a 'hard-wired' response or a 'soft-wired' response: the first type is ingrained from before birth and is purely instinctual; the second is learned or acquired later on. The first type may be, for example, the scent of the mother's skin or a sexual signal; the second might be the fragrance of honeysuckle, reminiscent of a childhood garden.

But to what extent is the effect of a particular oil dependent upon its chemical or physiological make-up, and to what extent does it rely upon a belief or an association? In dealing with the psychological or emotional responses to the scent of a particular oil, this kind of classification becomes much more difficult: surely here it is more appropriate to consider the temperament of each individual within a given context, rather than predict a set reaction.

At the Psychology of Perfumery Conference 1991, it was generally agreed

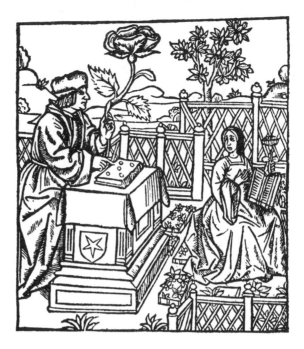

A discourse on the Virtues of the Rose; from Champier's *Rosa Gallica*, 1514

that 'while pharmacological effects may be very similar from one person to another, psychological effects are bound to be different.'[13] The effect of an odour on a human being was dependent on a variety of factors which include:

1. how the odour was applied,
2. how much was applied,
3. the circumstances in which it was applied,
4. the person to whom it was applied (age, sex, personality type),
5. what mood they were in to start with,
6. what previous associations they may have with the odour,
7. anosmia, or inability to smell (certain scents).

> We must, therefore, seek odoriferous substances which present affinities with the human being we intend to treat, those which will compensate for his deficiencies and those which will make his faculties blossom. It was by searching for this remedy that we encountered the *individual prescription* (IP), which on all points represents the identity of the individual.[14]

When we begin to consider individual needs, essential oils start to demonstrate the versatility of their nature . The rose is a good example; a flower which has been associated with beauty, love, and spiritual depth in folklore and religious texts (especially Sufi) but which also has a long tradition of usage for physical conditions such as skin problems, regulating the female cycle, promoting the circulation, purifying the blood and as a heart tonic. When we smell the fragrance of the rose, it carries all these rich associations with it, affecting our mind and body simultaneously, where the effect is moulded by personal experience.

'The general trend of modern thought is strictly dualistic; psychic and somatic happenings are treated as mutually exclusive rather than inclusive.'[15] Trying to disentangle spirit from matter leads nowhere; as David Hoffman says, 'Mind and Matter are mutually enfolded projections of a higher reality which is neither matter nor consciousness.'[16]

4. HOW TO USE ESSENTIAL OILS AT HOME

Essential oils can be used simply and effectively at home in a variety of ways, both for their scent and for their cosmetic and medicinal qualities. They can be used as perfumes and to revive pot pourris; they can be added to the bath and used to make individual beauty preparations. They can also be employed in the treatment of minor first aid cases and to help prevent and relieve many common complaints such as headaches, colds, period pains and aching muscles (see Therapeutic Index p. 199). They should always be stored in a cool place in dark bottles to protect them from photo-oxidation with as little contact with air as possible, and kept out of reach of children.

Some home uses for many essential oils can be found in the main body of the book, but the following list suggests a few possible uses for individual essences and shows some of the ways in which they can be applied.

Massage

This is the method favoured by professional aromatherapists, who usually carry out a full body massage. Specific essential oils are chosen to suit the condition and temperament of the patient, and blended with a base oil, such as sweet almond oil or grapeseed oil.

The essential oil content in a blend should usually be between 1 per cent and 3 per cent depending on the type of disorder. As a general rule, physical ailments like rheumatism or indigestion demand a stronger concentration than the more emotional or nervous conditions. A rough guideline is to say that 20 drops of essential oil is equivalent to one millilitre, so to make a blend it is possible to use the following proportions:

Essential oil	Base oil
20 to 60 drops	100ml
7 to 25 drops	25ml
3 to 5 drops	1 tsp

Massage is a relaxing and nourishing experience in itself, not least because of the unspoken communication based on touch, but it also ensures that the oils are effectively absorbed through the skin and into the bloodstream. For general well-being it is beneficial to practise self-massage on specific areas of the body, especially concentrating on the feet and hands. It is also useful to rub those particular parts of the body that are causing discomfort; for example, peppermint (in dilution) can be rubbed on the stomach in a clockwise direction to ease indigestion; marjoram can help to relax the neck and shoulders if they are stiff.

Skin Oils and Lotions

The essential oils are prepared in much the same manner as they would be for a massage, except that the base oil should include the more nourishing oils such as jojoba, avocado or apricot kernel oil. The emphasis here is on treating the skin itself and dealing with particular problems. A gentle circular movement of the fingers is often enough for the oils to be absorbed; it is important not to drag on the skin, especially in the delicate areas of the neck and around the eyes. Rose and neroli are good for dry or mature complexions; geranium, bergamot and lemon can help combat acne and greasy skin.

A few drops of essential oil can also be mixed into a bland cream or lotion, or added to a basic face mask, which might include oatmeal, honey or clay together with the pulp of various fruits. In some conditions, such as cold sores (herpes) and athlete's foot, it is better to use an alcohol-based lotion rather than an oil or cream. This can be made by adding 6 drops of essential oil to 5ml of isopropyl alcohol or vodka. This mixture can be further diluted in a litre of boiled and cooled water for treating open cuts or sores, such as those caused by chickenpox or genital herpes.

Hot and Cold Compresses

This is a very effective way of using essential oils to relieve pain and reduce inflammation. A hot compress can be made by filling a bowl with very hot water, then adding 4 or 5 drops of essential oil. Dip a folded piece of cotton cloth, cotton wool or a flannel into the bowl, squeeze out the excess water and place the cloth on the affected area until it has cooled to blood heat, then repeat. Hot compresses are particularly useful for backache, rheumatism and arthritis, abscesses, earache and toothache.

Cold compresses are made in a similar way, using ice cold rather than hot water. This type of compress is useful for headaches (apply to forehead or back of neck), sprains, strains and other hot, swollen conditions.

Hair Care

The hair can also be enhanced by the use of a few drops of essential oils in the final hair rinse or added straight to a mild shampoo. An alcohol-based scalp rub can also be made by adding 5ml of an essential oil to 100ml of vodka – this method can be used to condition the hair or to get rid of unwanted parasites such as lice and fleas. An excellent conditioning treatment for different types of hair can be made by adding about 3 per cent (or 60 drops) of an essential oil to a nourishing base oil such as olive oil with jojoba or sweet almond oil, massaging it into the scalp, then wrapping the hair in warm towels for an hour or two. Oils such as rosemary, West Indian bay and chamomile all help to condition and encourage healthy hair growth; lavender can be used to repel lice and fleas; bergamot and tea tree can help control dandruff.

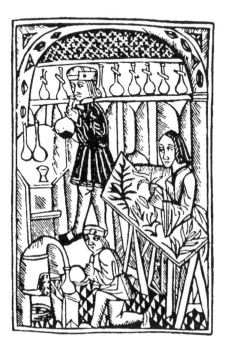

An Apothecary's shop where medicaments are being concocted from herbs and distilled oils; from a sixteenth century manuscript

Flower Waters

It is possible to make toilet or flower water at home by adding about 20 to 30 drops of essential oil to a 100ml bottle of spring or de-ionized water, leaving it for a few days in the dark and then filtering it using a coffee filter paper. Although essential oils do not dissolve in water they do impart their scent to it as well as their properties.

This method can be very helpful in the prevention and treatment of skin conditions such as acne, dermatitis and eczema, and to generally tone and cleanse the complexion. Almost any oil can be used, but the more traditional ones include rose, orange blossom, lavender and petitgrain; alternatively, blended flower waters can be made to suit specific complexions.

Baths

One of the easiest and most pleasurable ways of using essential oils is to add 5 to 10 drops of oil to the bath water when the tub is full. Aromatic bathing has traditionally been used as an enjoyable and sensual experience, especially by the Romans, but also to treat a wide range of complaints, including irritating skin conditions, muscular aches and pains, rheumatism and arthritis. An essence such as ylang ylang can be enjoyed as a euphoric aromatic experience in itself; chamomile or lavender can help to relieve stress-related complaints such as anxiety or insomnia; rosemary or pine can help soothe aching limbs. Take care to avoid those oils which may be irritating to the skin.

Vaporization

A delightful way to scent a room, free of the dust or smoke that can be caused by incense, is to use an oil burner, or aromatic diffuser. Alternatively, a few drops of oil can be placed on a light bulb ring or added to a small bowl of water placed on a radiator. Specific oils can be chosen to create different atmospheres: frankincense and cedarwood have been used traditionally in a ritual context, to create a peaceful and relaxed mood. Vaporized oils such as citronella or lemongrass also provide an excellent way of keeping insects at bay or clearing the air of unwanted smells like cigarette smoke.

At one time, the leaves of juniper and rosemary were burnt to help control epidemics and purify the air. Such oils can help keep the enviroment free of germs and inhibit the development of infections like the common cold or 'flu. An oil such as myrtle or eucalyptus can be used in the bedroom at night to help clear breathing difficulties or children's coughs. A few drops may also be put on the pillow or onto a handkerchief for use throughout the day.

Always ensure that the oil burner is in a safe place and out of reach of children or pets.

Steam Inhalation

This method is especially suited to sinus, throat and chest infections. Add about 5 drops of an oil such as peppermint or thyme to a bowl of hot water, cover the head and bowl with a towel and breathe deeply for a minute – then repeat. Sitting in a steaming hot bath is another way of inhaling a certain amount of essential oil, but obviously it is not so concentrated. This type of application can also act as a kind of facial sauna: oils like lemon or tea tree can help to unclog the pores and clear the complexion.

Douche

This can be useful to help combat common genito-urinary infections such as thrush, cystitis or pruritis. In the case of candida or thrush, add between 5 and 10 drops of tea tree to a litre of warm water and shake well. This mixture can either be used in a sitz bath, bidet or put into an enema/douche pot, which can be bought from some chemists. Certain oils such as lavender and cypress can also aid the healing process after childbirth.

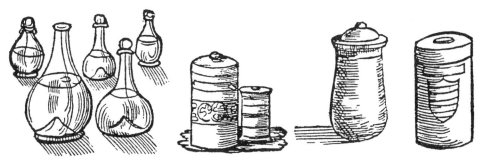

Olive oil, cosmetic and unguent jars; from Dioscorides's *De Materia Medica*, 1543

Neat Application

Generally speaking, essential oils are not applied to the skin in an undiluted form. However, there are some exceptions to the rule: lavender, for example, can be applied undiluted to burns, cuts and insect bites, tea tree to spots, and lemon to warts. Certain essential oils such as sandalwood, jasmine or rose make excellent perfumes, dabbed neat on the skin. Beware of those oils which are known to be phototoxic (discolour the skin when exposed to direct sunlight) such as bergamot; irritants such as red thyme; or skin sensitizers such as cinnamon bark. It can also be interesting to make an individual fragrance by blending a selection of oils – see Chapter 5. Certain oils may also be used to perfume linen and clothes or rejuvenate pot pourris: patchouli has been used for centuries in India to scent cloth.

Internal Use

Due to the high concentration of essential oils (and the high toxicity of a handful of essences) it is not recommended that they be taken at home in this manner. The International Federation of Aromatherapists also advises against this method of application. However, since essential oils are readily absorbed through the skin, they can affect the internal organs and systems of the body by external use. In a condition such as arthritis, for example, which indicates a build up of toxins in the joints, the use of dietary measures and herbal remedies can be greatly enhanced by the external application of oils such as juniper and white birch which help to purify the system as well as reduce pain and inflammation at the site of the swelling.

Essential Oils should not be used at home to treat serious medical or psychological problems.

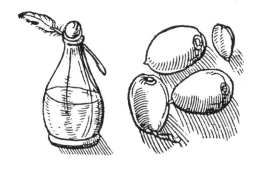

5. CREATIVE BLENDING

Therapeutic and Aesthetic Properties

Essential oils are blended principally for two reasons: for their medical effects or to create a perfume. When we are using pure essential oils, these are not two different categories but rather two ends of a scale. At one end of the scale we are dealing with the therapeutic action on a purely physical condition such as backache – at the other end, with an emotional or aesthetic response to a particular odour. But, of course, the individual who is suffering from lumbago also has a psychic or emotional disposition of which they may or may not be aware, which will naturally respond in a more subtle way to a particular blend of oils. Similarly, when we create a personal perfume which expresses the unique personality of an individual through fragrance, it has a generally remedial effect on the person as a whole.

Therefore, when we are blending oils, even if it is principally for their medicinal properties, it is always worth keeping the fragrance in mind. It is more pleasing to use a remedy that smells attractive to the individual concerned. Some scents can be quite incompatible – a predominantly floral blend, for example, would be unacceptable to the majority of men. How to choose the oils and combine them is very much a matter of personal choice, but there are some useful guidelines to keep in mind.

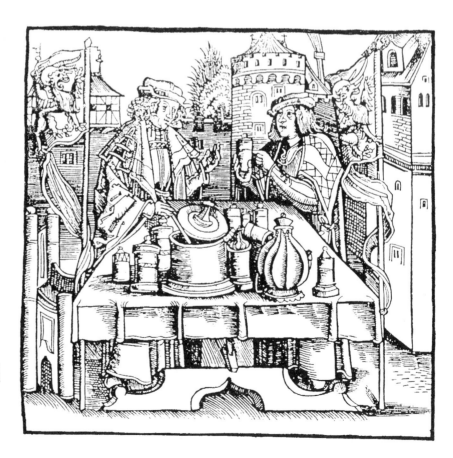

An engraving showing sixteenth century perfumers at work, with their chemical apparatus; from Brunschwig's *Liber de Arte Distillandi de Compositis*, 1512

Correct Proportions

For therapeutic purposes, essential oils are usually diluted before being applied to the skin. To make a massage or body oil the essential oil or oils should first be mixed with a light base oil such as grapeseed or sweet almond oil. (See also Chapter 4. How to Use Essential Oils at Home.) Other oils that could be used for the base include sunflower, hazelnut, safflower, peanut, soya or corn oil – mineral oils, however, are best avoided. The more nourishing and generally thicker oils which include jojoba, avocado, peach or apricot kernel, borage, olive, sesame, evening primrose and also some infused oils such as calendula or St Johns wort can also be included (up to about 10 per cent) in the treatment of specific conditions. A small quantity of wheatgerm oil (about 5 per cent) added to the blend will help to preserve it.

The essential oil content in a blend should usually be between 1 per cent and 3 per cent depending on the type of disorder; as a general rule, physical ailments demand a stronger concentration than the more emotional or nervous conditions. Some oils, such as the high quality florals including rose and jasmine, have more diffusive power than most other essences – this means that a very small percentage is all that is needed to have a powerful effect, or to influence the character of an entire blend.

Synergies

The proportions of each essential oil in a blend can also be vital to the effectiveness of the remedy as a whole (many aromatherapy books contain exact recipes for specific disorders). Some oils blended together have a mutually enhancing effect upon one another, so that the whole is greater than the sum of the parts: for example, the anti-inflammatory action of chamomile is supported by being mixed with lavender. When the blended oils are working harmoniously together, then the combination is called a 'synergy'. 'In order to create a good synergy, you must take into account not only the symptom to be treated but also the underlying cause of the disorder, the biological terrain, and the psychological or emotional factors involved.'[17]

This is very much the conclusion that Madame Maury reached when she prescribed an IP (or Individual Prescription) for her patients, in which the blended essences were matched not only to their physical requirements, but also to their circumstances and temperament.

In general, oils of the same botanical family blend well together. Also those which share common constituents usually mix well, such as the camphoraceous oils containing a good percentage of cineol, which includes all the members of the Myrtaceae group (eucalyptus, tea tree, cajeput, myrtle, etc.) but also many herbs including spike lavender, rosemary and Spanish sage. Most floral fragrances blend well together, as do the woods, balsams, citrus oils and spices, etc. Rosewood and linaloe combine well together, although they belong to different botanical families, since they both contain a high proportion of linalol and linalyl acetate.

Some oils such as rose, jasmine, oakmoss and lavender seem to enhance just about any blend, and can be found (mainly in an adulterated form) amongst the ingredients of most commercial perfumes – 'no perfume without rose'.

Some combinations, on the other hand, have an inhibiting power over one another. Essences with a predominance of aldehydes (such as citronella oil containing citronellal), those with mainly ketones (such as sage containing thujone) and those with high amounts of phenols (such as clove oil containing eugenol), when combined with each other tend to 'pull' in different directions. However, knowing the precise chemical make-up of each oil is not necessary for creating a good synergy; it is also a matter of getting to know the 'character' of each essential oil and trusting the intuition.

Fragrant Harmony

In the nineteenth century, a Frenchman called Piesse instigated a new approach to perfumery work by classifying odours according to the notes in a musical scale. He transposed the idea of musical harmony into the realm of fragrances where the corresponding notes to each scent formed perfectly balanced chords or harmonics when they were combined together.

The purist vision of Piesse has long since been discarded but continues to provide inspiration in perfumery work today since the oils are still divided into 'top', 'middle' and 'base' notes.

The top note has a fresh, light quality which is immediately apparent, due to the fast evaporation rate.
The middle note is the heart of the fragrance, which usually forms the bulk of the blend, whose scent emerges some time after the first impression.
The base note is a rich, heavy scent that emerges slowly and lingers. It also acts as a fixative to stop the lighter oils from dispersing too quickly.

Ylang ylang is said to be a well-balanced perfume oil in its own right. It could be described as having a very powerful sweet floral top note, a creamy-rich middle note, and a soft floral, slightly spicy base note.

For the sake of simplicity, each essential oil is also classified in this way according to its dominant character – although there are many different opinions on the matter! The following list provides nothing more than a general idea:

Top notes tea tree, eucalyptus, mandarin, lemon, basil
Middle notes geranium, lavender, marjoram, rosewood, rosemary
Base notes patchouli, rose, jasmine, benzoin, frankincense, myrrh

A well-balanced perfume is said to contain elements from each of these different categories, the quantities of each determining whether it is a heavy oriental-type scent or a light floral aroma. Although this theory is used primarily in fragrance work, the same principles can also be applied to aromatherapy and personalized remedies.

Personal Perfumes

Creating a perfume or an individual fragrance is like painting a picture or making a meal: it needs the correct balance of colours or flavours, neither too sparse nor too crowded; it also generally has a theme. A perfume should have a focus around which other fragrances unite. For example, if we want to create an oriental fragrance or a heart-warming, elevating type of blend, then woody or musky oils and balsams will play a central role. The exotic perfume 'Shalimar' by Guerlain contains a predominance of such oils, containing among its ingredients Peru balsam, benzoin, opopanax, vanilla, patchouli, rose, jasmine, orris and vetiver as well as rosewood, lemon, bergamot and mandarin.

Home perfumes need not be so complex: rose and benzoin (base notes), rosewood (middle note) and bergamot (top note) would together make a pleasing combination with an uplifting, warming quality. Rosewood is an oil which can be used to round off sharp edges, as well as providing a good bridge between citrus and floral or woody-balsamic notes. The overall character of a perfume also benefits from unusual or diverse combinations which can help to give personality to an otherwise 'flat' fragrance. A floral fragrance with a hint of spice such as clove or cinnamon can add depth and interest, but the percentage of such additions is critical because they can easily upset the balance.

A skilled perfumier can identify some 30,000 different odours, but to begin with it is best to become familiar with a few common oils and develop from there. By initially keeping to a maximum of three or four oils per blend it is possible to keep in touch with their individual scents and qualities, then slowly build up a personal vocabulary of odours.

Most commercial perfumes are diluted in alcohol; a typical eau de cologne contains no more than 3–5 per cent aromatic material, usually synthetic. Home-made perfumes are best made up simply of pure essences, which last longer and may be used neat on the skin or in the bath, etc.

Personal experimentation is the only way to really find out what works, for the unique quality of essential oils is that they possess an array of therapeutic possibilities complemented by a vast spectrum of fragrances which can be mixed in endless combinations! In the words of John Steele:

> Creative blending is an aesthetic alchemical process ... learning to 'listen through the nose'. To listen is to be receptive, to be empty. Every drop shifts the orchestration of olfactory vibrations, the 'song of the blend'. A blend is not made at once, rather it evolves, it organically grows and interacts not only with the essential oils, but also with the blender.[18]

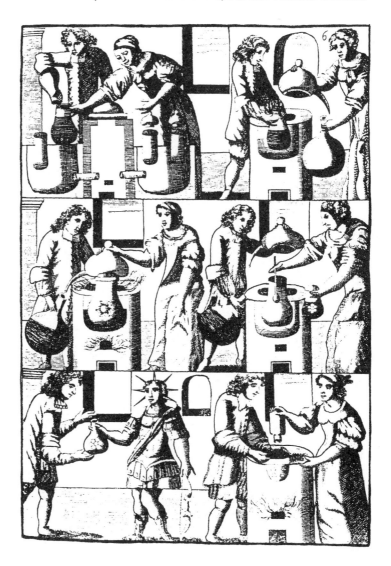

Various stages of the alchemical process, including the appearance of the golden flower; from *Mutus liber*, 1702

6. A GUIDE
TO AROMATIC MATERIALS

Habitat

Over thirty families of plants, with some ninety species, represent the main oil-producing group. The majority of spices (allspice, cardomon, clove, nutmeg, ginger, etc.) originate in tropical countries; conversely, the majority of herbs grow in temperate climates (bay, cumin, dill, marjoram, fennel, lavender, rosemary, thyme, etc.). The same plant grown in a different region and under different conditions can produce essential oils of widely diverse characteristics, which are known as 'chemotypes'. Common thyme (*Thymus vulgaris*), for example, produces several chemotypes depending on the conditions of its growth and dominant constituent, notably the citral or linalol types, the thuyanol type, and the thymol or carvacrol type. It is therefore important not only to know the botanical name of the plant from which an oil has been produced, but also its place of origin and main constituents. One of the main ways of defining the qualities of a particular oil and checking its purity is to ascertain the specific blend of components and look at its chemical character.

Chemistry

In general, essential oils consist of chemical compounds which have hydrogen, carbon and oxygen as their building blocks. These can be subdivided into two groups: the hydrocarbons which are made up almost exclusively of *terpenes* (monoterpenes, sesquiterpenes and diterpenes); and the oxygenated compounds, mainly *esters, aldehydes, ketones, alcohols, phenols* and *oxides*; acids, lactones, sulphur and nitrogen compounds are sometimes also present.

Terpenes

Common terpene hydrocarbons include limonene (antiviral, found in 90 per cent of citrus oils) and pinene (antiseptic, found in high proportions in pine and turpentine oils); also camphene, cadinene, caryophyllene, cedrene, dipentene, phellandrene, terpinene, sabinene, and myrcene among others. Some sesquiterpenes, such as chamazulene and farnesol (both found in chamomile oil), have been the object of great interest recently due to their outstanding anti-inflammatory and bactericidal properties.

Esters

Probably the most widespread group found in essential oils, which includes linalyl acetate (found in bergamot, clary sage and lavender), and geranyl acetate (found in sweet marjoram). They are characteristically fungicidal and sedative, often having a fruity aroma. Other esters include bornyl acetate, eugenyl acetate and lavendulyl acetate.

Aldehydes

Citral, citronellal and neral are important aldehydes found notably in lemon-scented oils such as melissa, lemongrass, lemon verbena, lemon-scented eucalyptus, citronella etc. Aldehydes in general have a sedative effect; citral has been found to have specifically antiseptic properties. Other aldehydes include benzaldehyde, cinnamic aldehyde, cuminic aldehyde and perillaldehyde.

Ketones

Some of the most common toxic constituents are ketones, such as thujone found in mugwort, tansy, sage and wormwood; and pulegone found in penny-royal and buchu – but this does not mean that *all* ketones are dangerous. Non-toxic ketones include jasmone found in jasmine, and fenchone in fennel oil. Generally considered to ease congestion and aid the flow of mucus, ketones are often found in plants which are used for upper respiratory complaints, such as hyssop and sage. Other ketones include camphor, carvone, menthone, methyl nonyl ketone and pinocamphone.

Alcohols

One of the most useful groups of compounds, tending to have good antiseptic and antiviral properties with an uplifting quality; they are also generally non-toxic. Some of the most common terpene alcohols include linalol (found in rosewood, linaloe and lavender), citronellol (found in rose, lemon eucalyptus and geranium) and geraniol (found in palmarosa); also borneol, menthol, nerol, terpineol, farnesol, vetiverol, benzyl alcohol and cedrol among others.

Phenols

These tend to have a bactericidal and strongly stimulating effect, but can be skin irritants. Common phenols include eugenol (found in clove and West Indian bay), thymol (found in thyme), carvacrol (found in oregano and savory); also methyl eugenol, methyl chavicol, anethole, safrole, myristicin and apiol among others.

Oxides

By far the most important oxide is cineol (or eucalyptol) which stands virtually in a class of its own. It has an expectorant effect, well known as the principal constituent of eucalyptus oil. It is also found in a wide range of other oils, especially those of a camphoraceous nature such as rosemary, bay laurel, tea tree and cajeput. Other oxides include linalol oxide found in hyssop (decumbent variety), ascaridol, bisabolol oxide and bisabolone oxide.

Methods of Extraction

In general, the term 'essential oil' is rather loosely applied to all aromatic products or extracts derived from natural sources, including concretes, resinoids and absolutes which contain a mixture of volatile and non-volatile components, such as wax or resin. This is not strictly accurate, since they are only partially composed of essential oils and are obtained by different methods of production, which include the use of solvents or more recently,

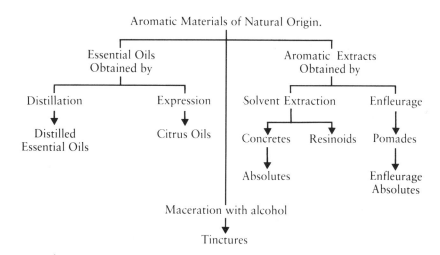

A chart showing the different ways in which aromatic material can be prepared

carbon dioxide extraction. However, it is always the essential oil content in a given product that accounts for its aromatic quality.

Some plant materials, especially flowers, are subject to deterioration and should be processed as soon as possible after harvesting; others, including seeds and roots, are either stored or transported for extraction, often to Europe or America. The method of extraction which is employed depends on the quality of the material which is being used, and the type of aromatic product that is required.

Essential Oils

An essential oil is extracted from the plant material by two main methods: by simple expression or pressure, as is the case with most of the citrus oils including lemon and bergamot, or by steam, water or dry distillation. The majority of oils such as lavender, myrrh, sandalwood and cinnamon are produced by steam distillation. This process only isolates the volatile and water-insoluble parts of a plant – many other (often valuable) constituents, such as tannins, mucilage and bitters are consequently excluded from the essential oil. Sometimes the resulting oil is redistilled or *rectified* to get rid of any remaining non-volatile matter; some essential oils are redistilled at different temperatures to obtain certain constituents and exclude others – as with camphor which is split into three fractions, white, yellow and brown.

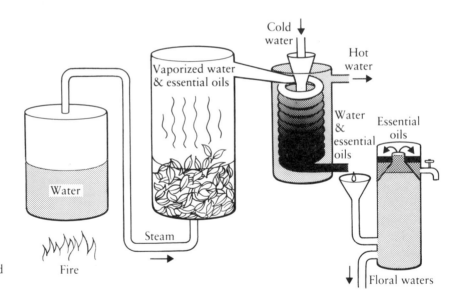

The process of steam distillation as it is practised today

Essential oils are usually liquid, but can also be solid (orris) or semi-solid according to temperature (rose). They dissolve in pure alcohol, fats and oils but not in water and, unlike the so-called 'fixed' plant oils (such as olive oil), they evaporate when exposed to air leaving no oily residue behind.

Concretes

Concretes are prepared almost exclusively from raw materials of vegetable origin, such as the bark, flower, leaf, herb or root. The aromatic plant material is subjected to extraction by hydrocarbon-type solvents, rather than distillation or expression. This is necessary when the essential oil is adversely affected by hot water and steam, as is the case with jasmine; it also produces a more true-to-nature fragrance. Some plants, such as lavender and clary sage, are either steam distilled to produce an essential oil or used to produce a concrete by solvent extraction. The remaining residue is usually solid and of a waxy non-crystalline consistency.

Most concretes contain about 50 per cent wax, 50 per cent volatile oil, such as jasmine; in rare cases, as with ylang ylang, the concrete is liquid and contains about 80 per cent essential oil, 20 per cent wax. The advantage of concretes is that they are more stable and concentrated than pure essential oils.

Resinoids

Resinoids are prepared from natural resinous material by extraction with a hydrocarbon solvent, such as petroleum ether or hexane. In contradistinction to concretes, the resinoids are prepared from dead organic material, whereas concretes are derived from previously live tissue. Typical resinous materials are balsams (Peru balsam or benzoin), resins (mastic and amber), oleoresins (copaiba balsam and turpentine) and oleo gum resins (frankincense and myrrh). Resinoids can be viscous liquids, semi-solid or solid, but are usually homogeneous masses of non-crystalline character. Occasionally the alcohol-soluble fraction of a resinoid is called an absolute.

Some resinous materials like frankincense and myrrh are used either to make an essential oil by steam distillation or a resin absolute by alcohol extraction directly from the crude oleo gum resin. Benzoin, on the other hand, is insufficiently volatile to produce an essential oil by distillation: liquid benzoin is often simply a benzoin resinoid dissolved in a suitable solvent or plasticizing diluent.

Like concretes, resinoids are employed in perfumery as fixatives to prolong the effect of the fragrance.

Absolutes

An absolute is obtained from the concrete by a second process of solvent extraction, using pure alcohol (ethanol) in which the unwanted wax is only slightly soluble. An absolute is usually subjected to repeated treatment with alcohol; even so, as is the case with orange flower absolute, a small proportion of the wax remains. Absolutes can be further processed by molecular distillation which removes every last trace of non-volatile matter. The alcohol is recovered by evaporation which requires a gentle vacuum towards the end of the process. Some absolutes, however, will still retain traces of ethyl alcohol, at about 2 per cent or less, and are not recommended for therapeutic work because of these impurities.

Absolutes are usually highly concentrated viscous liquids, but they can in some cases be solid or semi-solid (clary sage absolute). In recent years, much research has been devoted to the extraction of essential oils and aromatic materials using liquid carbon dioxide; oils produced in this manner are of excellent odour quality and are entirely free of unwanted solvent residues or non-volatile matter.

Pomades

True pomades are the products of a process known as enfleurage, which is virtually obsolete today. This was once the principal method for obtaining aromatic materials from flowers that continued to produce perfume long after they were cut. A glass plate was covered in a thin coating of specially prepared and odourless fat, called a *chassis*. The freshly cut flowers, such as jasmine or tuberose, were individually laid in the fat which became saturated with their volatile oils. The *chassis* would be frequently renewed with fresh material throughout the harvest. Eventually the fragrance-saturated fat, known as pomade, would be treated by extraction with alcohol to produce the pure absolute or perfume.

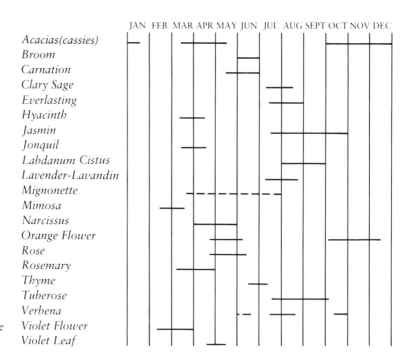

| | JAN | FEB | MAR | APR | MAY | JUN | JUL | AUG | SEPT | OCT | NOV | DEC |

Acacias(cassies)
Broom
Carnation
Clary Sage
Everlasting
Hyacinth
Jasmin
Jonquil
Labdanum Cistus
Lavender-Lavandin
Mignonette
Mimosa
Narcissus
Orange Flower
Rose
Rosemary
Thyme
Tuberose
Verbena
Violet Flower
Violet Leaf

Periods of the year for the treatment of various flowers once grown in Provence, France

Natural versus 'Nature Identical'

Many perfumes or oils, once obtained from flowers such as carnation, gardenia and lilac, are nowadays produced almost entirely synthetically. In the pharmaceutical industry these chemically constructed products are called 'nature identical'. The perfumery and flavouring industries require continuity in their products and naturally occurring substances are always subject to change, due to seasonal conditions. However, the so-called 'nature identical' products and the naturally occurring essential oils are of an entirely different character, which is reflected in their relative costs – the synthetic types being much cheaper to produce than the genuine ones.

Many aromatic oils, such as lavender or geranium, contain a relatively small number of major constituents, several minor constituents and also a very large number of trace elements. To reconstruct such a complex combination of components including all the trace elements, would be virtually impossible. Most 'nature identical' oils are said to be only about 96 per cent pure or accurate, yet it is the remaining 4 per cent, the trace elements, that often really define a particular fragrance. Such is the case with galbanum oil where the pyrazines, present at rather less than 0.1 per cent, are responsible for the powerful green odour of the oil.

It is also the specific combination of constituents in a real essential oil, including the trace elements, which give it value therapeutically. The reason for this might be that these minute amounts of trace elements have a synergistic or controlling effect on the main ones. For example, there are over 300 different constituents in rose, some of which have not yet been identified, which is why synthetic rose oil is unconvincing. 'Nature identical' oils cannot be used therapeutically as substitutes for the naturally occurring aromatic materials, not only because the subtle balance of constituents is lost but also because they lack the vital 'life force' of oils of natural origin.

PART II
THE OILS

A

AJOWAN
Trachyspermum copticum

FAMILY Apiaceae (Umbelliferae)

SYNONYMS *T. ammi, Ammi copticum, Carum ajowan, C. copticum, Ptychotis ajowan,* ajuan, omum.

GENERAL DESCRIPTION An annual herb with a greyish-brown seed, which resembles parsley in appearance.

DISTRIBUTION Chiefly India, also Afghanistan, Egypt, the West Indies and the Seychelle Islands.

OTHER SPECIES See Botanical Classification section.

HERBAL/FOLK TRADITION The seeds are used extensively in curry powders and as a general household remedy for intestinal problems. The tincture, essential oil and 'thymol' are used in Indian medicine, particularly for cholera.

ACTIONS Powerful antiseptic and germicide, carminative.

EXTRACTION Essential oil by steam distillation from the seed.

CHARACTERISTICS A yellow-orange or reddish liquid with a herbaceous-spicy medicinal odour, much like thyme.

PRINCIPAL CONSTITUENTS Thymol, pinene, cymene, dipentene, terpinene and carvacrol, among others.

SAFETY DATA Possible mucous membrane and dermal irritant. Due to high thymol level, should be avoided in pregnancy. Toxicity levels are unknown.

AROMATHERAPY/HOME USE Not recommended.

OTHER USES It has been used extensively for the isolation of thymol, but this has largely been replaced by synthetic thymol.

ALLSPICE
Pimenta dioica

FAMILY Myrtaceae

SYNONYMS *P. officinalis*, pimento, pimenta, Jamaica pepper.

GENERAL DESCRIPTION An evergreen tree which reaches about 10 metres high and begins to produce fruit in its third year. Each fruit contains two kidney-shaped green seeds which turn glossy black upon ripening.

DISTRIBUTION Indigenous to the West Indies and South America, it is cultivated extensively in Jamaica, Cuba and, to a lesser degree, in Central America. Imported berries are distilled in Europe and America.

OTHER SPECIES Four other varieties of pimento are found in Venezuela, Guyana and the West Indies which are used locally as spices.

HERBAL/FOLK TRADITION Used for flatulent indigestion and externally for neuralgic or rheumatic pain. Pimento water is used as a vehicle for medicines which ease dyspepsia and constipation since it helps prevent griping pains. It is used extensively as a domestic spice – allspice is so called because it tastes like a combination of cloves, juniper berries, cinnamon and pepper.

ACTIONS Anaesthetic, analgesic, anti-oxidant, antiseptic, carminative, muscle relaxant, rubefacient, stimulant, tonic.

EXTRACTION Essential oil by steam distillation from 1. the leaves, and 2. the fruit. The green unripe berries contain more oil than the ripe berries, but the largest percentage of oil is contained in the shell of the fruit. An oleoresin from the berries is also produced in small quantities.

CHARACTERISTICS 1. Pimenta leaf oil is a yellowish-red or brownish liquid with a powerful sweet-spicy scent, similar to cloves. 2. Pimenta berry oil is a pale yellow liquid with a sweet warm balsamic-spicy bodynote (middle note) and fresh, clean top note. It blends well with ginger, geranium, lavender, opopanax, labdanum, ylang ylang, patchouli, neroli, oriental and spicy bases.

PRINCIPAL CONSTITUENTS Mainly eugenol, less in the fruit (60–80 per cent) than in the leaves (up to 96 per cent), also methyl eugenol, cineol, phellandrene and caryophyllene among others.

SAFETY DATA Eugenol irritates the mucous membranes, and has been found to cause dermal irritation. Pimenta leaf and berry oil should therefore be used with care in low dilutions only.

AROMATHERAPY/HOME USE
CIRCULATION, MUSCLES AND JOINTS: Arthritis, fatigue, muscle cramp, rheumatism, stiffness etc.

'Used in tiny amounts ... in a massage oil for chest infections, for severe muscle spasm to restore mobility quickly, or where extreme cold is experienced.'[1]
RESPIRATORY SYSTEM: Chills, congested coughs, bronchitis.
DIGESTIVE SYSTEM: Cramp, flatulence, indigestion, nausea.
NERVOUS SYSTEM: Depression, nervous exhaustion, neuralgia, tension and stress.

OTHER USES Used in aromatic carminative medicines; as a fragrance component in cosmetics and perfumes, especially soaps, aftershaves, spicy and oriental fragrances. Both leaf and berry oil are used extensively for flavouring foods, especially savoury and frozen foods, as well as alcoholic and soft drinks.

ALMOND, BITTER
Prunus dulcis var. amara

FAMILY Rosaceae

SYNONYMS *P. amygdalus var. amara, Amygdalus communis var. amara, A. dulcis, P. communis.*

GENERAL DESCRIPTION The almond tree grows to a height of about 7 metres and is

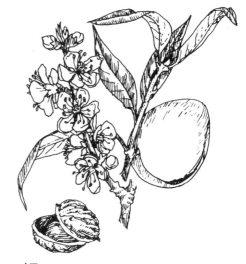

Almond Tree

popular as a garden tree due to its pinky-white blossom. It is botanically classified as a drupe.

DISTRIBUTION Native to Western Asia and North Africa, it is now extensively cultivated throughout the Mediterranean region, Israel and California.

OTHER SPECIES There are two main types of almond tree – bitter and sweet. The sweet almond does not produce any essential oil.

HERBAL/FOLK TRADITION A 'fixed' oil commonly known as 'sweet almond oil' is made by pressing the kernels from both the sweet and bitter almond trees. Unlike the essential oil, this fixed oil does not contain any benzaldehyde or prussic acid, and has many medical and cosmetic uses. It is used as a laxative, for bronchitis, coughs, heartburn and for disorders of the kidneys, bladder and biliary ducts. It helps relieve muscular aches and pains, softens the skin and premotes a clear complexion.

ACTIONS Anaesthetic, antispasmodic, narcotic, vermifuge (FFPA).

EXTRACTION Essential oil by steam distillation from the kernels. The nuts are first pressed and macerated in warm water for 12 to 24 hours before the oil is extracted. It is during this process that the prussic acid is formed; it is not present in the raw seed. Most commercial bitter almond oil is rectified to remove all prussic acid, i.e. free from prussic acid (FFPA).

CHARACTERISTICS Light colourless liquid with a characteristic 'marzipan' scent (FFPA).

PRINCIPAL CONSTITUENTS Benzaldehyde (95 per cent), prussic acid (3 per cent).

SAFETY DATA Prussic acid, also known as hydrocyanic acid or cyanide, is a well-known poison. Benzaldehyde is also moderately toxic.

AROMATHERAPY/HOME USE None. 'Should not be used in therapy either internally or externally.'[2]

OTHER USES Bitter almond oil is no longer used for internal medication. Rectified bitter almond oil is used for flavouring foods, mainly confectionery; the most common uses are 'almond essence' and marzipan. The oil (FFPA} is increasingly being replaced by synthetic benzaldehyde in food flavourings.

AMBRETTE SEED
Abelmoschus moschatus

FAMILY Malvaceae

SYNONYMS *Hibiscus abelmoschus,* musk seed, Egyptian alcee, target-leaved hibiscus, muskmallow.

GENERAL DESCRIPTION An evergreen shrub about 1.5 metres high, bearing large single yellow flowers with a purple centre. The capsules, in the form of five-cornered pyramids, contain the greyish-brown kidney-shaped seeds which have a musky odour.

DISTRIBUTION Indigenous to India; widely cultivated in tropical countries including Indonesia, Africa, Egypt, China, Madagascar, and the West Indies. Distillation of the oil is generally carried out in Europe and America.

OTHER SPECIES A variety, *H. esculentus,* is grown largely in Istanbul as a demulcent. Another variety is also found in Martinique, the seeds of which have a more delicate scent.

HERBAL/FOLK TRADITION Generally used as a stimulant and to ease indigestion, cramp and nervous dyspepsia. In Chinese medicine it is used to treat headache; in Egypt the seeds are used to sweeten the breath and are made into an emulsion with milk to be used for itch. The Arabs use the seeds to mix with coffee. Widely used as a domestic spice in the East.

ACTIONS Antispasmodic, aphrodisiac, carminative, nervine, stimulant, stomachic.

EXTRACTION Essential oil by steam distillation of the seeds. Liquid ambrette seed oil should be allowed to age for several months before it is used. A concrete and absolute are also produced by solvent extraction.

CHARACTERISTICS A pale yellowy-red liquid with a rich, sweet floral-musky odour, very tenacious. It blends well with rose, neroli, sandalwood, clary sage, cypress, patchouli, oriental and 'sophisticated' bases.

PRINCIPAL CONSTITUENTS Ambrettolide, ambrettolic acid, palmitic acid and farnesol.

SAFETY DATA Available information indicates the oil to be non-toxic, non-irritant and non-sensitizing.

AROMATHERAPY/HOME USE
CIRCULATION, MUSCLES AND JOINTS: Cramp, fatigue, muscular aches and pains, poor circulation.
NERVOUS SYSTEM: Anxiety, depression, nervous tension and stress-related conditions.

OTHER USES Employed by the cosmetic and perfumery industries in oriental-type scents and for the adulteration of musk; also used as a musk substitute. Used for flavouring alcoholic and soft drinks as well as some foodstuffs, especially confectionery.

AMYRIS
Amyris balsamifera

FAMILY Rutaceae

SYNONYMS *Schimmelia oleifera*, West Indian sandalwood, West Indian rosewood.

GENERAL DESCRIPTION A small bushy tree with compound leaves and white flowers which grows wild in thickets all over the island of Haiti.

DISTRIBUTION Mainly Haiti, it has now been introduced to tropical zones all over the world, e.g. Jamaica, South and Central America.

OTHER SPECIES Not to be confused with East Indian or Mysore sandalwood *(Santalum album),* to which it bears no relation.

HERBAL/FOLK TRADITION The locals call it 'candle wood' because of its high oil content; it burns like a candle. It is used as a torch by fishermen and traders. It also makes excellent furniture wood.

ACTIONS Antiseptic, balsamic, sedative.

EXTRACTION Essential oil by steam distillation from the broken-up wood and branches. Best if the wood is seasoned first. It provides a very plentiful yield.

CHARACTERISTICS A pale yellow, slightly viscous liquid with a musty, faintly woody scent, quickly fading away. It blends well with lavandin, citronella, oakmoss, sassafras, cedarwood and other wood oils.

PRINCIPAL CONSTITUENTS Caryophyllene, cadinene and cadinol.

SAFETY DATA Generally non-irritant; no other information available at present.

AROMATHERAPY/HOME USE Perfume.

OTHER USES As a cheap substitute for East Indian sandalwood in perfumes and cosmetics, although it does not have the same rich tenacity; chiefly employed as a fixative in soaps. Limited application in flavouring work, especially liqueurs.

ANGELICA
Angelica archangelica

FAMILY Apiaceae (Umbelliferae)

SYNONYMS *A. officinalis*, European angelica, garden angelica.

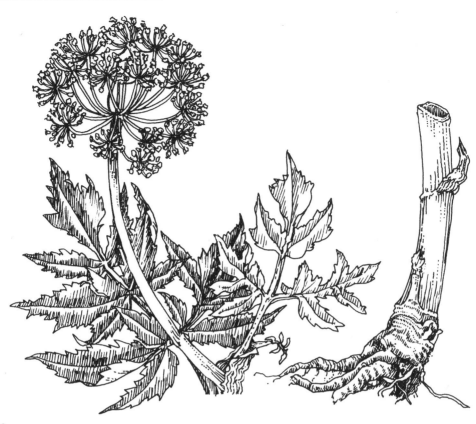

Angelica

GENERAL DESCRIPTION A large hairy plant with ferny leaves and umbels of white flowers. It has a strong aromatic scent and a large rhizome.

DISTRIBUTION Native to Europe and Siberia, cultivated mainly in Belgium, Hungary and Germany.

OTHER SPECIES There are over thirty different types of angelica but this is the most commonly used medicinally. See Botanical Classification section.

HERBAL/FOLK TRADITION This herb has been praised for its virtues since antiquity. It strengthens the heart, stimulates the circulation and the immune system in general. It has been used for centuries in Europe for bronchial ailments, colds, coughs, indigestion, wind and to stimulate the appetite. As a urinary antiseptic it is helpful in cystitis and is also used for rheumatic inflammation. The Chinese employ at least ten kinds of angelica, well known for promoting fertility, fortifying the spirit and for treating female disorders generally; it has a reputation second only to ginseng. It is current in the British Herbal Pharmacopoeia as a specific for bronchitis associated with vascular deficiency. Candied Angelica stalks are popular in France and Spain.

ACTIONS Antispasmodic, carminative, depurative, diaphoretic, digestive, diuretic, emmenagogue, expectorant, febrifuge, nervine, stimulant, stomachic, tonic. Reported to have bactericidal and fungicidal properties.

EXTRACTION Essential oil produced by steam distillation from the   1. roots and rhizomes, and,   2. fruit or seed. An absolute is also produced on a small scale, from the roots.

CHARACTERISTICS 1. A colourless or pale yellow oil which turns yellowy-brown with age, with a rich herbaceous-earthy bodynote.   2. The seed oil is a colourless liquid with a fresher, spicy top note. It blends well with patchouli, opopanax, costus, clary sage, oakmoss, vetiver and with citrus oils.

PRINCIPAL CONSTITUENTS Root and seed oil contain phellandrene, pinene, limonene, linalol and borneol; rich in coumarins including osthol, angelicin, bergapten and imperatorin; also contains plant acids.

SAFETY DATA Both root and seed oil are non-toxic and non-irritant. The root oil (not the seed oil) is phototoxic, probably due to higher levels of bergapten. Not to be used during pregnancy or by diabetics.

AROMATHERAPY/HOME USE
SKIN CARE: Dull and congested skin, irritated conditions, psoriasis.
CIRCULATION MUSCLES AND JOINTS: Accumulation of toxins, arthritis, gout, rheumatism, water retention.
RESPIRATORY SYSTEM: Bronchitis, coughs.
DIGESTIVE SYSTEM: Anaemia, anorexia, flatulence, indigestion.
NERVOUS SYSTEM: Fatigue, migraine, nervous tension and stress-related disorders.
IMMUNE SYSTEM: Colds.

OTHER USES Highly valued as a fragrance component in soaps, lotions and perfumes especially colognes, oriental and heavy chyprès fragrances. It is employed in some cosmetics for its soothing effect on skin complaints. Used extensively as a flavouring agent in most food categories, and in alcoholic and soft drinks, especially liqueurs.

ANISE, STAR
Illicium verum

FAMILY Illiciaceae

SYNONYMS Chinese anise, illicium, Chinese star anise.

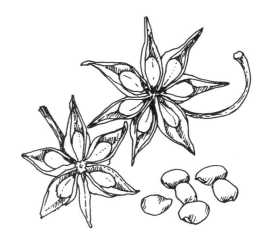

Star Anise

GENERAL DESCRIPTION Evergreen tree up to 12 metres high with a tall, slender white trunk. It bears fruit which consist of five to thirteen seed-bearing follicles attached to a central axis in the shape of a star.

DISTRIBUTION Native to south east China, also Vietnam, India and Japan. Mainly produced in China.

OTHER SPECIES Several other related species, e.g. Japanese star anise which is highly poisonous!

HERBAL/FOLK TRADITION Used in Chinese medicine for over 1300 years for its stimulating effect on the digestive system and for respiratory disorders such as bronchitis and unproductive coughs. In the East generally, it is used as a remedy for colic and rheumatism, and often chewed after meals to sweeten the breath and promote digestion. A common oriental domestic spice.

ACTIONS Antiseptic, carminative, expectorant, insect repellent, stimulant.

EXTRACTION Essential oil by steam distillation from the fruits, fresh or partially dried. An oil is also produced from the leaves in small quantities.

CHARACTERISTICS A pale yellow liquid with a warm, spicy, extremely sweet, liquorice-like scent. It blends well with rose, lavender, orange, pine and other spice oils, and has excellent masking properties.

PRINCIPAL CONSTITUENTS Trans-anethole (80–90 per cent).

SAFETY DATA Despite the anethole content, it does not appear to be a dermal irritant, unlike aniseed. In large doses it is narcotic and slows down the circulation; it can lead to cerebral disorders. Use in moderation only.

AROMATHERAPY/HOME USE
CIRCULATION, MUSCLES AND JOINTS: Muscular aches and pains, rheumatism.
RESPIRATORY SYSTEM: Bronchitis, coughs.
DIGESTIVE SYSTEM: Colic, cramp, flatulence, indigestion.
IMMUNE SYSTEM: Colds.

OTHER USES By the pharmaceutical industry in cough mixtures, lozenges, etc. and to mask undesirable odours and flavours in drugs. As a fragrance component in soaps, toothpaste and detergents as well as cosmetics and perfumes. Widely used for flavouring food, especially confectionery, alcoholic and soft drinks.

ANISEED
Pimpinella anisum

FAMILY Apiaceae (Umbelliferae)

SYNONYMS *Anisum officinalis, A. vulgare,* anise, sweet cumin.

GENERAL DESCRIPTION An annual herb, less than a metre high, with delicate leaves and white flowers.

DISTRIBUTION Native to Greece and Egypt, now widely cultivated mainly in India and China and to a lesser extent in Mexico and Spain.

OTHER SPECIES There are several different chemotypes of aniseed according to the country of origin. Not to be confused with star anise, which belongs to a different family altogether.

HERBAL/FOLK TRADITION Widely used as a domestic spice. The volatile oil content provides the basis for its medicinal applications: dry irritable coughs, bronchitis and whooping cough. The seed can be used in smoking mixtures. Aniseed tea is used for infant catarrh, also flatulence, colic and griping pains, also for painful periods and to promote breast milk. In Turkey a popular alcoholic drink, *raki*, is made from the seed.

ACTIONS Antiseptic, antispasmodic, carminative, diuretic, expectorant, galactagogue, stimulant, stomachic.

EXTRACTION Essential oil by steam distillation from the seeds.

CHARACTERISTICS Colourless to pale yellow liquid with a warm, spicy-sweet characteristic scent. Like star anise, it is a good masking agent.

PRINCIPAL CONSTITUENTS Trans-anethole (75–90 per cent).

SAFETY DATA Its major component, anethole, is known to cause dermatitis in some individuals – avoid in allergic and inflammatory skin conditions. In large doses it is narcotic and slows down the circulation; can lead to cerebral disorders. Use in moderation only.

AROMATHERAPY/HOME USE See *star anise.*

OTHER USES By the pharmaceutical industry in cough mixtures and lozenges and to mask undesirable flavours in drugs. Also used in dentifrices and as a fragrance component in soaps, toothpaste, detergents, cosmetics and perfumes, mostly of the industrial type. Employed in all major food categories.

ARNICA
Arnica montana

FAMILY Asteraceae (Compositae)

SYNONYMS *A. fulgens, A. sororia,* leopard's bane, wolf's bane.

GENERAL DESCRIPTION A perennial alpine herb with a creeping underground stem, giving rise to a rosette of pale oval leaves. The flowering erect stem is up to 60 cms high, bearing a single, bright yellow, daisy-like flower. The whole plant is very difficult to cultivate.

DISTRIBUTION Native to northern and central Europe; also found growing wild in the USSR, Scandinavia and northern India. The oil is produced mainly in France, Belgium and Germany.

OTHER SPECIES A related plant, *A. cordifolia,* and other species of arnica are used in America, where it is known as 'mountain tobacco'.

HERBAL/FOLK TRADITION This herb stimulates the peripheral blood supply when applied externally, and is considered one of the best remedies for bruises and sprains. It helps relieve rheumatic pain and other painful or inflammatory skin conditions, so long as the skin is not broken! It is never used internally due to toxicity levels.

ACTIONS Anti-inflammatory, stimulant, vulnerary.

EXTRACTION Essential oil by steam distillation of 1. flowers, and 2. root. The yield of essential oil is very small. An absolute, tincture and resinoid are also produced.

CHARACTERISTICS 1. A yellowy-orange liquid with a greenish-blue hint and a strong bitter-spicy scent reminiscent of radish. 2. Dark yellow or butter-brown oil more viscous than the flower oil, with a strong bitter scent.

PRINCIPAL CONSTITUENTS Thymohydroquinone dimethyl ether (80 per cent approx.), isobutyric ester of phlorol (20 per cent approx.) and other minor traces.

SAFETY DATA The essential oil is highly toxic and should never be used internally or on broken skin. However, the tincture or arnica ointment are valuable additions to the home medicine cabinet.

AROMATHERAPY/HOME USE None.

OTHER USES The tincture is mainly employed in pharmaceutical skin products. The oil from the flowers finds occasional use in herbaceous-type perfumes. It is also used to flavour certain liqueurs.

ASAFETIDA
Ferula asa-foetida

FAMILY Apiaceae (Umbelliferae)

SYNONYMS Asafoetida, gum asafetida, devil's dung, food of the gods, giant fennel.

GENERAL DESCRIPTION A large branching perennial herb up to 3 metres high, with a thick fleshy root system and pale yellow-green flowers.

DISTRIBUTION Native to Afghanistan, Iran and other regions of south west Asia.

OTHER SPECIES There are several other species of *Ferula* which yield the oleoresin known as 'asafetida', e.g. Tibetan asafetida, which is also used to a lesser extent in commerce.

HERBAL/FOLK TRADITION In Chinese medicine it has been used since the seventh century as a nerve stimulant in treating neurasthenia. It is also widely used in traditional Indian medicine, where it is believed to stimulate the brain. In general, it has the reputation for treating various ailments including asthma, bronchitis, convulsions, coughs, constipation, flatulence and hysteria. The foliage of the plant is used as a local vegetable. It is current in the British Herbal Pharmacopoeia as a specific for intestinal flatulent colic.

ACTIONS Antispasmodic, carminative, expectorant, hypotensive, stimulant. Animals are repelled by its odour.

EXTRACTION The oleoresin is obtained by making incisions into the root and above-ground parts of the plant. The milky juice is left to leak out and harden into dark reddish lumps, before being scraped off and collected. The essential oil is then obtained from the resin by steam distillation. An absolute, resinoid and tincture are also produced.

CHARACTERISTICS A yellowy-orange oil with a bitter acrid taste and a strong, tenacious odour resembling garlic. However, beneath this odour there is a sweet, balsamic note.

PRINCIPAL CONSTITUENTS Disulphides, notably 2-butyl propenyl disulphide with monoterpenes, free ferulic acid, valeric, traces of vanillin, among others.

SAFETY DATA Available information indicates the oil to be relatively non-toxic and non-irritant. However, it has the reputation for being the most adulterated 'drug' on the market. Before being sold, the oleoresin is often mixed with red clay or similar substitutes.

AROMATHERAPY/HOME USE
RESPIRATORY SYSTEM: 'There is evidence that the volatile oil is expelled through the lungs, therefore it is excellent for asthma, bronchitis, whooping cough etc.'[3]
NERVOUS SYSTEM: Fatigue, nervous exhaustion and stress- related conditions.

OTHER USES Now rarely used in pharmaceutical preparations; formerly used as a local stimulant for the mucous membranes. Occasionally used as a fixative and fragrance component in perfumes, especially rose bases and heavy oriental types. Employed in a wide variety of food categories, mainly condiments and sauces.

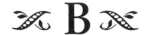

BALM, LEMON
Melissa officinalis

FAMILY Lamiaceae (Labiatae)

SYNONYMS Melissa, common balm, bee balm, sweet balm, heart's delight, honey plant.

GENERAL DESCRIPTION A sweet-scented herb about 60 cms high, soft and bushy, with bright green serrated leaves, square stems and tiny white or pink flowers.

DISTRIBUTION Native to the Mediterranean region, now common throughout Europe, Middle Asia, North America, North Africa and Siberia. Mainly cultivated in France, Spain, Germany and Russia.

OTHER SPECIES Several varieties, e.g. a variegated leaf type, common in gardens.

HERBAL/FOLK TRADITION One of the earliest known medicinal herbs – Paracelsus called it the 'Elixir of Life'. It was associated particularly with nervous disorders, the heart and the emotions. It was used for anxiety, melancholy, etc, and to strengthen and revive the vital spirit. Generally employed for digestive and respiratory complaints of nervous origin such as asthma, indigestion and flatulence. It also helps to regulate the menstrual cycle and promote fertility. Effective remedy for wasp and bee stings. In France the leaves are still used a great deal in pharmaceutical and herbal products. Current in the British Herbal Pharmacopoeia for flatulent dyspepsia, neurasthenia and depressive illness.

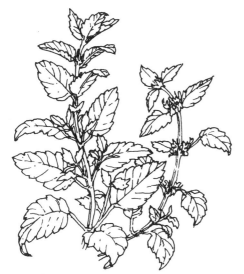

Lemon Balm

ACTIONS Antidepressant, antihistaminic, antispasmodic, bactericidal, carminative, cordial, diaphoretic, emmenagogue, febrifuge, hypertensive, insect-repellent, nervine, sedative, stomachic, sudorific, tonic, uterine, vermifuge.

EXTRACTION Essential oil by steam distillation from the leaves and flowering tops.

CHARACTERISTICS A pale yellow liquid with a light, fresh lemony fragrance. It blends well with lavender, geranium, floral and citrus oils.

PRINCIPAL CONSTITUENTS Citral, citronellol, eugenol, geraniol, linalyl acetate, among others.

SAFETY DATA Available information indicates non-toxic. Possible sensitization and dermal irritation: use in low dilutions only. Care must also be taken because this is one of the most frequently adulterated oils. Most commercial so-called 'melissa' contains some or all of the following: lemon, lemongrass or citronella.

AROMATHERAPY/HOME USE
SKIN CARE: Allergies, insect bites, insect repellent. 'Melissa in very low concentration is a very valuable oil indeed in treating eczema and other skin problems.'[4]
RESPIRATORY SYSTEM: Asthma, bronchitis, chronic coughs.

DIGESTIVE SYSTEM: Colic, indigestion, nausea.
GENITO-URINARY SYSTEM: Menstrual problems.
NERVOUS SYSTEM: Anxiety, depression, hypertension, insomnia, migraine, nervous tension, shock and vertigo.

OTHER USES Occasionally used in pharmaceutical preparations. Used extensively as a fragrance component in toiletries, cosmetics and perfumes. Employed in most major food categories including alcoholic and soft drinks.

BALSAM, CANADIAN
Abies balsamea

FAMILY Pinaceae

SYNONYMS *A. balsamifera, Pinus balsaamea,* balsam fir, balsam tree, American silver fir, balm of Gilead fir, Canada turpentine (oil).

GENERAL DESCRIPTION A tall, graceful evergreen tree up to 20 metres high, with a tapering trunk and numerous branches giving the tree an overall shape of a perfect cone. It forms blisters of oleoresin (the so-called 'balsam') on the trunk and branches, produced from special vesicles beneath the bark. The tree does not produce a 'true' balsam, since it does not contain benzoic or cinnamic acid in its esters; it is really an oleoresin, being a mixture of resin and essential oil.

DISTRIBUTION Native to North America, particularly Quebec, Nova Scotia and Maine.

OTHER SPECIES The hemlock spruce *(Tsuga canadensis)* also yields an exudation sold under the name of 'Canada balsam'. There are also many other species of fir which produce oils from their needles – see entry on silver fir and Botanical Classification section.
  NB Not to be confused with the genuine balsam of Gilead *(Commiphora opabalsamum),* of ancient repute.

HERBAL/FOLK TRADITION The oleoresin is used extensively by the American Indians for ritual purposes and as an external treatment for burns, sores, cuts and to relieve heart and chest pains. It is also used internally for coughs.

ACTIONS Antiseptic (genito-urinary, pulmonary), antitussive, astringent, cicatrisant, diuretic, expectorant, purgative, regulatory, sedative (nerve), tonic, vulnerary.

EXTRACTION 1. The oleoresin is collected by puncturing vesicles in the bark. 2. An essential oil is produced by steam distillation from the oleoresin, known as Canada balsam or Canada turpentine. (An essential oil is also produced by steam distillation from the leaf or needles, known as fir needle oil.)

CHARACTERISTICS 1. The oleoresin is a thick pale yellow or green honeylike mass which dries to crystal clear varnish, with a fresh sweet-balsamic, almost fruity odour. 2. A colourless mobile liquid with a sweet, soft-balsamic, pine-like scent. It blends well with pine, cedarwood, cypress, sandalwood, juniper, benzoin and other balsams.

PRINCIPAL CONSTITUENTS Consists almost entirely of monoterpenes, pinene, phellandrene, esters and alcohols.

SAFETY DATA Generally non-toxic, non-irritant, non-sensitizing. 'In large doses it is purgative and may cause nausea.'[39]

AROMATHERAPY/HOME USE
SKIN CARE: Burns, cuts, haemorrhoids, wounds.
RESPIRATORY SYSTEM: Asthma, bronchitis, catarrh, chronic coughs, sore throat.
GENITO-URINARY SYSTEM: Cystitis, genito-urinary infections.
NERVOUS SYSTEM: Depression, nervous tension, stress-related conditions – described as 'appeasing, sedative, elevating, grounding, opening'.[40]

OTHER USES The oil from the oleoresin is used in certain ointments and creams as an antiseptic and treatment for haemorrhoids.

Used in dentistry as an ingredient in root canal sealers. Also used as a fixative or fragrance component in soaps, detergents, cosmetics and perfumes. There is some low-level use in food products, alcoholic and soft drinks. The oleoresin is used as a medium in microscopy and as a cement in glassware.

BALSAM, COPAIBA
Copaifera officinalis

FAMILY Fabaceae (Leguminosae)

SYNONYMS Copahu balsam, copaiba, copaiva, Jesuit's balsam, Maracaibo balsam, para balsam.

GENERAL DESCRIPTION Wild-growing tropical tree up to 18 metres high, with thick foliage and many branches. The natural oleoresin occurs as a physiological product from various *Copaifera* species. Not a 'true' balsam.

DISTRIBUTION Native to north east and central South America. Mainly produced in Brazil; also Venezuela, Guyana, Surinam and Colombia.

OTHER SPECIES Several *Copaifera* speices yield an oleoresin: the Venezuelan type 'Maracaibo balsam' has a low oil content, the Brazilian type 'para balsam' has a high oil content. See also Botanical Classification section.

HERBAL/FOLK TRADITION Used for centuries in Europe in the treatment of chronic cystitis and bronchitis; also for treating piles, chronic diarrhoea and intestinal problems.

ACTIONS Batericidal, balsamic, disinfectant, diuretic, expectorant, stimulant.

EXTRACTION 1. The crude balsam is collected by drilling holes into the tree trunks; it is one of the most plentiful naturally occurring perfume materials. 2. An essential oil is obtained by dry distillation from the crude balsam. It is mainly the 'para balsams' with a high oil content (60–80 per cent), which are used for distillation.

CHARACTERISTICS 1. The crude balsam is a viscous, yellowy-brown or greenish-grey liquid which hardens upon exposure to air with a mild, woody, slightly spicy odour. It blends well with styrax, amyris, lavandin, cedarwood, lavender, oakmoss, woods and spices. 2. The oil is a pale yellow or greenish mobile liquid with a mild, sweet, balsamic-peppery odour. It blends well with cananga, ylang ylang, vanilla, jasmine, violet and other florals.

PRINCIPAL CONSTITUENTS Mainly caryophyllene.

SAFETY DATA Relatively non-toxic, non-irritant, possible sensitization. Large doses cause vomiting and diarrhoea.

AROMATHERAPY/HOME USE
DIGESTIVE SYSTEM: Intestinal infections, piles.
RESPIRATORY SYSTEM: Bronchitis, chills, colds, coughs, etc.
GENITO-URINARY SYSTEM: Cystitis.
NERVOUS SYSTEM: Stress-related conditons.

OTHER USES The oleoresin is used in pharmaceutical products especially cough medicines and iuretics. The oil and crude balsam are extensively used as a fixative and fragrance component in all types of perfumes, soaps, cosmetics and detergents. The crude is also used in porcelain painting.

BALSAM, PERU
Myroxylon balsamum var. pereirae

FAMILY Fabaceae (Leguminosae)

SYNONYMS *Toluifera pereira, Myrosperum pereira, Myroxylon pereirae,* Peruvian balsam, Indian balsam, black balsam.

GENERAL DESCRIPTION A large tropical tree up to 25 metres high, with a straight smooth trunk, beautiful foliage and very fragrant flowers. Every part of the tree contains a reinous juice, including the fibrous fruit. The balsam is a pathological product, obtained from the exposed lacerated wood, after strips of the bark have been removed. It is a 'true' balsam, which is collected in the form of a dark brown or amber semi-solid mass.

DISTRIBUTION Native to Central America; production mainly takes place in San Salvador.

OTHER SPECIES *Myroxylon frutescens* and guina-guina are close relations, as well as Tolu balsam.

HERBAL/FOLK TRADITION It stimulates the heart, increases blood pressure, and lessens mucous secretions; useful for respiratory disorders such as asthma, chronic coughs and bronchitis. Traditionally employed for rheumatic pain and skin problems including scabies, nappy rash, bedsores, prurigo, eczema, sore nipples and wounds; it also destroys the itch acarus and its eggs.

ACTIONS Anti-inflammatory, antiseptic, balsamic, expectorant, parasiticide, stimulant; promotes the growth of epithelial cells.

EXTRACTION A resin-free essential oil is produced from the crude balsam by high vacuum dry distillation. (A wood oil is also produced by steam distillation from the wood chippings, which is considered of inferior quality. A white balsam called 'myroxocarpin' is made from the fruit, and an extract called 'balsamito' from the young fruit.)

CHARACTERISTICS The oil is a pale amber or brown viscous liquid with a rich, sweet, balsamic, 'vanilla-like' scent. It blends well with ylang ylang, patchouli, petitgrain, sandalwood, rose, spices, floral and oriental bases.

PRINCIPAL CONSTITUENTS Benzoic and cinnamic acid esters such as benzyl benzoate, benzyl cinnamate and cinnamyl cinnamate as well as other traces. The crude balsam contains approximately 50–64 per cent oil, referred to as 'cinnamein', and 20–28 per cent resin.

SAFETY DATA Non-toxic, non-irritant; however the balsam (not the oil) is a common contact allergen, which may cause dermatitis. Those who have this sensitivity may also react to benzoin resinoid; this is called 'cross-sensitization'. The commercial oil is often a water-white liquid, being diluted with a solvent such as benzyl alcohol.

AROMATHERAPY/HOME USE
SKIN CARE: Dry and chapped skin, eczema, rashes, sores and wounds.
CIRCULATION, MUSCLES AND JOINTS: Low blood pressure, rheumatism.
RESPIRATORY SYSTEM: Asthma, bronchitis, coughs.
IMMUNE SYSTEM: Colds.
NERVOUS SYSTEM: Nervous tension, stress; like other balsams it has a warming, opening, comforting quality.

OTHER USES The balsam is extensively used in tropical medicinal preparations, and to some extent in pharmaceutical products, for example, cough syrup. Used as a fixative and fragrance component in soaps, detergents, creams, lotions and perfumes; the oil is often used in perfumery since this avoids any resin deposits or discolouration; used in most food categories, including alcoholic and soft drinks.

BALSAM, TOLU
Myroxylon balsamum var. balsamum

FAMILY Fabaceae (Leguminosae)

SYNONYMS *Toluifera balsamum, Balsamum tolutanum, B. americanum, Myrospermum toluiferum*, Thomas balsam, resin Tolu, opobalsam.

GENERAL DESCRIPTION A tall, graceful tropical tree, similar in appearance to the Peru balsam tree. The balsam is a pathological product, obtained by making V-shaped incisions into the bark and sap wood, often after the trunk has been beaten and scorched. It is a 'true' balsam.

DISTRIBUTION Native to South America, mainly Venezuela, Colombia and Cuba; also cultivated in the West Indies.

OTHER SPECIES There are many types of South American balsam-yielding trees, such as the Peru balsam – see entry.

HERBAL/FOLK TRADITION The balsam works primarily on the respiratory mucous membranes, and is good for chronic catarrh and non-inflammatory chest complaints, laryngitis and croup. It is still used as a flavour and mild expectorant in cough syrups and lozenges. As an ingredient in compound benzoin tincture and similar formulations, it is helpful in the treatment of cracked nipples, lips, cuts, bedsores, etc.

ACTIONS Antitussive, antiseptic, balsamic, expectorant, stimulant.

EXTRACTION The crude balsam is collected from the trees. It appears first in liquid form, then hardens and solidifies into an orange-brown brittle mass. An 'essential oil' is obtained from the crude by 1. steam distillation, or 2. dry distillation. (A resinoid and absolute are also produced for use primarily as fixatives.)

CHARACTERISTICS 1. A pale yellow-brown liquid with a sweet-floral scent and peppery undertone. 2. An amber-coloured liquid with a rich balsamic-floral scent, which slowly solidifies on cooling into a crystalline mass. Tolu balsam blends well with mimosa, ylang ylang, sandalwood, labdanum, neroli, patchouli, cedarwood and oriental, spicy and floral bases.

PRINCIPAL CONSTITUENTS The balsam contains approx. 80 per cent resin, 20 per cent oil, with cinnamic and benzoic acids, small amounts of terpenes, and traces of eugenol and vanillin.

SAFETY DATA Available information indicates it to be non-toxic, non-irritant, possible sensitization, see *Peru Balsam*.

AROMATHERAPY/HOME USE
SKIN CARE: Dry, chapped and cracked skin, eczema, rashes, scabies, sores, wounds.
RESPIRATORY SYSTEM: Bronchitis, catarrh, coughs, croup, laryngitis. 'It may be used as an inhalant by putting about a teaspoon into a steam bath.'[5]

OTHER USES As a fixative and fragrance component in colognes, cosmetics and perfumes (especially the dry distilled type). Some use in pharmaceutical preparations, e.g. cough syrups. Low levels used in many major food products, especially baked goods.

BASIL, EXOTIC
Ocimum basilicum

FAMILY Lamiaceae (Labiatae)

SYNONYMS Sweet basil, Comoran basil (oil), Reunion basil (oil).

GENERAL DESCRIPTION Botanically classified as identical from the French basil, though it is a larger plant with a harsher odour and different constituents.

DISTRIBUTION Mainly produced in the Comoro Islands, but it is also processed in Madagascar.

OTHER SPECIES The exotic basil is a dramatically different chemotype to the French basil and probably a seperate sub-species (possibly a form of *O. canum*), although this has not been specified. Essential oils are also produced in Morocco, Egypt, South Africa, Brazil and Indonesia from various chemotypes of the East Indian or shrubby basil *(O. gratissimum),* which contain a high percentage of either thymol or eugenol. The hairy or hoary basil *(O. canum),* originating in East Africa and found in India

and South America, is also used to extract oils rich in either methyl cinnamate or camphor, which are produced in West and East Africa, India, the West Indies and Indonesia. See also entry on French basil.

HERBAL/FOLK TRADITION See French Basil.

ACTIONS See Basil French.

EXTRACTION Essential oil by steam distillation from the leaves and flowering tops.

CHARACTERISTICS The Exotic type oil is yellow or pale green, with a slightly coarse sweet-herbaceous odour with a camphoraceous tinge. It's scent does not compare with the 'true' sweet basil oil.

PRINCIPAL CONSTITUENTS Mainly methyl chavicol (70-88 per cent), with small amounts of linalol, cineol, camphor, eugenol, limonene and citronellol.

SAFETY DATA Methyl chavicol is moderately toxic and irritating to the skin: 'the methyl chavicol content of Comoran basil is sufficient reason to discard it for therapeutic usage in favour of the French type.'[6] There has also been some recent concern over the possible carcinogenic effects of methyl chavicol. Basil should be avoided during pregnancy.

AROMATHERAPY/HOME USE None.

OTHER USE The oil is employed in high class fragrances, soaps and dental products; used extensively in major food categories especially meat products and savories.

BASIL, FRENCH
Ocimum basilicum

FAMILY Lamiaceae (Labiatae)

SYNOYNMS Common basil, joy-of-the-mountain, 'true' sweet basil, European basil.

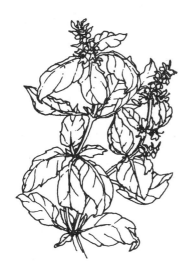

French Basil

GENERAL DESCRIPTION A tender annual herb, with very dark green, ovate leaves, greyish-green beneath, an erect square stem up to 60 cms high, bearing whorls of two-lipped greenish or pinky-white flowers. The whole plant has a powerful aromatic scent.

DISTRIBUTION Native to tropical Asia and Africa, it is now widely cultivated throughout Europe, the Mediterranean region, the Pacific Islands, North and South America. The European, French or 'true' sweet basil oil is produced in France, Italy, Egypt, Bulgaria, Hungary and the USA.

OTHER SPECIES There are many varieties of basil occurring all over the world, used both for their culinary and medicinal applications, such as bush basil *(O. minimum)*, holy basil *(O. sanctum)*, both from India, camphor basil *(O. kilimanjaricum)* from East Africa (also grown in India), and the fever plant *(O. viride)* from West Africa. However, there are two principal chemotypes most commonly used for the extraction of essential oil: the so-called 'French basil' and the 'exotic basil' – see separate entry.

HERBAL/FOLK TRADITION Widely used in Far Eastern medicine especially in the Ayurvedic tradition, where it is called *tulsi*. It is used for respiratory problems such as bronchitis, coughs, colds, asthma, 'flu and emphysema but is also used as an antidote to poisonous insect or snake bites. It has also been used against epidemics and fever, such as malaria. It improves blood circulation and the digestive system and in China it is used for stomach and kidney ailments.

In the West it is considered a 'cooling' herb, and is used for rheumatic pain, irritable skin conditions and for those of a nervous disposition. It is a popular culinary herb, especially in Italy and France.

ACTIONS Antidepressant, antiseptic, antispasmodic, carminative, cephalic, digestive, emmenagogue, expectorant, febrifuge, galactagogue, nervine, prophylactic, restorative, stimulant of adrenal cortex, stomachic, tonic.

EXTRACTION Essential oil by steam distillation from the flowering herb.

CHARACTERISTICS 'True' sweet basil oil is a colourless or pale yellow liquid with a light, fresh sweet-spicy scent and balsamic undertone. It blends well with bergamot, clary sage, lime, opopanax, oakmoss, citronella, geranium, hyssop and other 'green' notes.

PRINCIPAL CONSTITUENTS Linalol (40-45 per cent), methyl chavicol (23.8 per cent) and small amounts of eugenol, limonene and citronellol, among others.

SAFETY DATA Relatively non-toxic, non-irritant, possible sensitization in some individuals. Avoid during pregnancy.

AROMATHERAPY/HOME USE
SKIN CARE: Insect bites (mosquito, wasp), insect repellent.
CIRCULATION, MUSCLES AND JOINTS: Gout, muscular aches and pains, rheumatism.
RESPIRATORY SYSTEM: Bronchitis, coughs, earache, sinusitis.
DIGESTIVE SYSTEM: Dyspepsia, flatulence, nausea.
GENITO-URINARY SYSTEM: Cramps, scanty periods.
IMMUNE SYSTEM: Colds, fever, 'flu, infectious disease.

NERVOUS SYSTEM: Anxiety, depression, fatigue, insomnia, migraine, nervous tension: 'Oil of Basil is an excellent, indeed perhaps the best, aromatic nerve tonic. It clears the head, relieves intellectual fatigue, and gives the mind strength and clarity.'[7]

OTHER USES The oil is used in soaps, cosmetics and perfumery; it is also used extensively in major food categories, especially savouries.

BAY LAUREL
Laurus nobilis

FAMILY Lauraceae

SYNONYMS Sweet bay, laurel, Grecian laurel, true bay, Mediterranean bay, Roman laurel, noble laurel, laurel leaf (oil).

GENERAL DESCRIPTION An evergreen tree up to 20 metres high with dark green, glossy leaves and black berries; often cultivated as an ornamental shrub.

DISTRIBUTION Native to the Mediterranean region; extensively cultivated especially for its berries, in France, Spain, Italy, Morocco, Yugoslavia, China, Israel, Turkey and Russia. The oil is mainly produced in Yugoslavia.

OTHER SPECIES There are several related species, all of which are commonly called Bay : Californian bay *(Umbellularia california)*, West Indian bay *(Pimenta racemosa)* and the cherry laurel *(Prunus laurocerasus)*, which is poisonous.

HERBAL/FOLK TRADITION A popular culinary herb throughout Europe. The leaves were used by the ancient Greeks and Romans to crown their victors. Both leaf and berry were formerly used for a variety of afflictions including hysteria, colic, indigestion, loss of appetite, to promote menstruation and for fever. It is little used internally these days, due to its narcotic properties. A 'fixed' oil of bay, expressed from the berries, is still used for sprains, bruises, earache, etc.

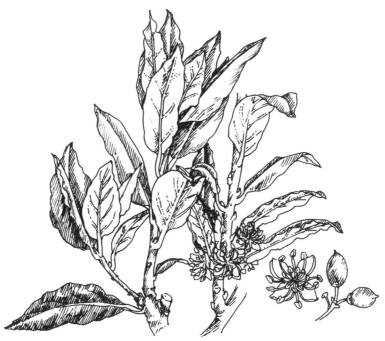

Bay Laurel

ACTIONS Antirheumatic, antiseptic, bactericidal, diaphoretic, digestive, diuretic, emmenagogue, fungicidal, hypotensive, sedative, stomachic.

EXTRACTION Essential oil by steam distillation from the dried leaf and branchlets. (An oil from the berries is produced in small quantities.)

CHARACTERISTICS A greenish-yellow liquid with a powerful, spicy-medicinal odour. It blends well with pine, cypress, juniper, clary sage, rosemary, olibanum, labdanum, lavender, citrus and spice oils.

PRINCIPAL CONSTITUENTS Cineol (30-50 per cent), pinene, linalol, terpineol acetate, and traces of methyl eugenol.

SAFETY DATA Relatively non-toxic and non-irritant; can cause dermatitis in some individuals. Use in moderation due to possible narcotic properties attributed to methyl eugenol. Should not be used during pregnancy.

AROMATHERAPY/HOME USE
DIGESTIVE SYSTEM: Dyspepsia, flatulence, loss of appetite.
GENITO-URINARY SYSTEM: Scanty periods.
IMMUNE SYSTEM: Colds, 'flu, tonsillitis and viral infections.

OTHER USES Used as a fragrance component in detergents, cosmetics, toiletries and perfumes, especially aftershaves. Extensively used in processed food of all types, as well as alcoholic and soft drinks.

BAY, WEST INDIAN
Pimenta racemosa

FAMILY Myrtaceae

SYNONYMS *Myrcia acris, Pimenta acris,* myrcia, bay, bay rum tree, wild cinnamon, bayberry, bay leaf (oil).

GENERAL DESCRIPTION A wild-growing tropical evergreen tree up to 8 metres high, with large leathery leaves and aromatic fruits.

DISTRIBUTION Native to the West Indies, particularly Dominica where the essential oil is produced.

OTHER SPECIES There are several other varieties, for example the anise-scented and lemon-scented bay, the oils of which have a totally different chemical composition. Not to be confused with bay laurel, the common household spice, nor with the North American bayberry or wax myrtle *(Myrcia cerifera)* well known for its wax yielding berries.

HERBAL/FOLK TRADITION The West Indian bay tree is often grown in groves together with the allspice or pimento bush, then the fruits of both are dried and powdered for the preparation of the household allspice. The so-called bay rum tree also provides the basic ingredient for the famous old hair tonic, which is made from the leaves by being distilled in rum. 'A hair application with both fragrant and tonic virtues ... useful for those who suffer from greasy hair and need a spirit-based, scalp-stimulating lotion to help them to control their locks!'[8]

ACTIONS Analgesic, anticonvulsant, antineuralgic, antirheumatic, antiseptic, astringent, expectorant, stimulant, tonic (for hair).

EXTRACTION Essential oil by water or steam distillation from the leaves. An oleoresin is also produced in small quantities.

CHARACTERISTICS A dark yellow mobile liquid with a fresh-spicy top note and a sweet-balsamic undertone. It blends well with lavander, lavandin, rosemary, geranium, ylang ylang, citrus and spice oils.

PRINCIPAL CONSTITUENTS Eugenol (up to 56 per cent), myrcene, chavicol and, in lesser amounts, methyl eugenol, linalol, limonene, among others.

SAFETY DATA Moderately toxic due to high eugenol content; also a mucous membrane irritant – use in moderation only. Unlike bay laurel, however, it does not appear to cause dermal irritation or sensitization.

AROMATHERAPY/HOME USE

SKIN CARE: Scalp stimulant, hair rinse for dandruff, greasy, lifeless hair, and premoting growth.

CIRCULATION, MUSCLES AND JOINTS: Muscular and articular aches and pains, neuralgia, poor circulation, rheumatism, sprains, strains.

IMMUNE SYSTEM: Colds, 'flu, infectious diseases.

OTHER USES Extensively used in fragrance work, in soaps, detergents, perfumes, aftershaves and hair lotions, including bay rum. Employed as a flavour ingredient in many major food categories, especially condiments, as well as alcoholic and soft drinks.

BENZOIN
Styrax benzoin

FAMILY Styracaceae

SYNONYMS Gum benzoin, gum benjamin, styrax benzoin.

GENERAL DESCRIPTION A large tropical tree up to 20 metres high with pale green citrus-like leaves, whitish underneath, bearing hard-shelled flattish fruit about the size of a nutmeg. The benzoin is a pathological product, formed when the trunk is cut; the tree exudes a balsamic resin which hardens upon exposure to air and sunlight.

DISTRIBUTION Native to tropical Asia; the two main regions of production are Sumatra, Java and Malaysia for 'Sumatra' benzoin, and Laos, Vietnam, Cambodia, China and Thailand for 'Siam' benzoin.

OTHER SPECIES There are many different varieties within the Styrax family which produce benzoin, but these are generally classified under either Sumatra benzoin (*S. paralleloneurus*) or Siam benzoin (*S. tonkinensis*) – see also Botanical Classification section.

HERBAL/FOLK TRADITION It has been used for thousands of years in the east as a medicine and incense; the fumigations were believed to drive away evil spirits. It was used by the Chinese herbalists for its heating and drying qualities, as a good urinary antiseptic and as an aid to digestion.

In the west, it is best known in the form of compound tincture of benzoin or Friars Balsam, used for respiratory complaints. Externally it is used for cuts and irritable skin conditions; internally it is used as a carminative for indigestion, etc. It also acts as a preservative of fats.

ACTIONS Anti-inflammatory, anti-oxidant, antiseptic, astringent, carminative, cordial, deodorant, diuretic, expectorant, sedative, styptic, vulnerary.

EXTRACTION The crude benzoin is collected from the trees directly. Benzoin resinoid, or 'resin absolute', is prepared from the crude using solvents, for example benzene and alcohol, which are then removed. Commercial benzoin is usually sold dissolved in ethyl glycol or a similar solvent. A 'true' absolute is also produced in small quantities.

CHARACTERISTICS 1. Sumatra crude benzoin occurs as greyish-brown brittle lumps with reddish streaks, with a styrax-like odour. There are several different qualities available; the so-called 'almond' grade is considered superior. 2. Siam benzoin comes in pebble or tear-shaped orange-brown pieces, with a sweet-balsamic vanilla-like scent, this type having a more refined odour than the Sumatra type.

Benzoin resinoid is produced from both the Siam and Sumatra types, or a mix of the two. It is an orange-brown viscous mass with an intensely rich sweet-balsamic odour. It blends well with sandalwood, rose, jasmine, copaiba balsam, frankincense, myrrh, cypress, juniper, lemon, coriander and other spice oils.

PRINCIPAL CONSTITUENTS 1. Sumatra Benzoin: mainly coniferyl cinnamate and sumaresinolic acid, with benzoic acid, cinnamic acid, and traces of styrene, vanillin and benzaldehyde. 2. Siam benzoin: mainly coniferyl benzoate (65-75 per cent), with benzoic acid, vanillin, siaresinolic acid and cinnamyl benzoate.

SAFETY DATA Non-toxic, non-irritant, possible sensitization. Compound benzoin tincture is 'regarded as moderately toxic, due probably to occasional contact dermatitis developed in some individuals... which contains, in addition to benzoin, aloe, storax, Tolu balsam and others.'[9]

AROMATHERAPY/HOME USE
SKIN CARE : Cuts, chapped skin, inflamed and irritated conditions.
CIRCULATION, MUSCLES AND JOINTS: Arthritis, gout, poor circulation, rheumatism.
RESPIRATORY SYSTEM: Asthma, bronchitis, chills, colic, coughs, laryngitis.
IMMUNE SYSTEM: 'Flu.
NERVOUS SYSTEM: Nervous tension and stress-related complaints. It warms and tones the heart and circulation, both physically and metaphorically: 'This essence creates a kind of euphoria; it interposes a padded zone between us and events.'[10]

OTHER USES Compound benzoin tincture is used in pharmaceuticals and in dentistry to treat gum inflammation. The resinoid and absolute are used extensively as fixatives and fragrance components in soaps, cosmetics, toiletries and perfumes, especially Siam benzoin. Both types are used in most food categories, including alcoholic and soft drinks.

BERGAMOT
Citrus bergamia

FAMILY Rutaceae

SYNONYM *Citrus aurantium subsp. bergamia.*

GENERAL DESCRIPTION A small tree, about 4.5 metres high with smooth oval leaves, bearing small round fruit which ripen from green to yellow, much like a miniature orange in appearance.

DISTRIBUTION Native to tropical Asia. Extensively cultivated in Calabria in southern Italy and also grown commercially on the Ivory Coast.

OTHER SPECIES Not to be confused with the herb bergamot or bee balm *(Monarda didyma).*

HERBAL/FOLK TRADITION Named after the Italian city of Bergamo in Lombardy, where the oil was first sold. The oil has been used in Italian folk medicine for many years, primarily for fever (including malaria) and worms; it does not feature in the folk tradition of any other countries. However, due to recent research in Italy, bergamot oil is now known to have a wide spectrum of applications, being particularly useful for mouth, skin, respiratory and urinary tract infections.

ACTIONS Analgesic, anthelmintic, antidepressant, antiseptic (pulmonary, genito-urinary), antispasmodic, antitoxic, carminative, digestive, diuretic, deodorant, febrifuge, laxative, parasiticide, rubefacient, stimulant, stomachic, tonic, vermifuge, vulnerary.

EXTRACTION Essential oil by cold expression of the peel of the nearly ripe fruit.
(A rectified or terpeneless oil is produced by vacuum distillation or solvent extraction.)

CHARACTERISTICS A light greenish-yellow liquid with a fresh sweet-fruity, slightly spicy-balsamic undertone. On ageing it turns a brownish-olive colour. It blends well with lavender, neroli, jasmine, cypress, geranium, lemon, chamomile, juniper, coriander and violet.

PRINCIPAL CONSTITUENTS Known to have about 300 compounds present in the expressed oil: mainly linalyl acetate (30-60 per cent), linalol (11-22 per cent) and other alcohols, sesquiterpenes, terpenes, alkanes and furocoumarins (including bergapten, 0.30-0.39 per cent).

SAFETY DATA Certain furocoumarins, notably bergapten, have been found to be phototoxic on human skin; that is, they cause sensitization and skin pigmentation when exposed to direct sunlight (in concentration and in dilution even after some time!). Extreme care must be taken when using the oil in dermal applications – otherwise a rectified or 'bergapten-free' oil should be substituted. Available information indicates it to be otherwise non-toxic and relatively non-irritant.

AROMATHERAPY/HOME USE
SKIN CARE: Acne, boils, cold sores, eczema, insect repellent and insect bites, oily complexion, psoriasis, scabies, spots, varicose ulcers, wounds.
RESPIRATORY SYSTEM: Halitosis, mouth infections, sore throat, tonsillitis.
DIGESTIVE SYSTEM: Flatulence, loss of appetite.
GENITO-URINARY SYSTEM: Cystitis, leucorrhoea, pruritis, thrush.
IMMUNE SYSTEM: Colds, fever, 'flu, infectious diseases.
NERVOUS SYSTEM: Anxiety, depression and stress-related conditions, having a refreshing and uplifting quality.

OTHER USES Extensively used as a fragrance and, to a degree, a fixative in cosmetics, toiletries, suntan lotions and perfumes – it is a classic ingredient of eau-de-cologne. Widely used in most major food categories and beverages, notably Earl Grey tea.

BIRCH, SWEET
Betula lenta

FAMILY Betulaceae

SYNONYMS *B. capinefolia*, cherry birch, southern birch, mahogany birch, mountain mahogany.

GENERAL DESCRIPTION A graceful tree about 25 metres high which has a pyramidal shape while young. It has bright green leaves and a dark reddish-brown aromatic bark, which is broken into plates or patches.

DISTRIBUTION Native to southern Canada and southeastern USA; produced mainly in Pennsylvania.

OTHER SPECIES There are numerous species of birch, spanning several continents, such as black birch *(B. nigra)* found in North America. Not to be confused with the European white birch *(B. alba)*, which produces birch tar oil used in chronic skin diseases.

HERBAL/FOLK TRADITION The cambium (the layer directly under the bark) is eaten in the spring, cut into strips like vermicelli. The bark, in the form of an infusion, is used as a general stimulant and to promote sweating. As a decoction or syrup, it is used as a tonic for dysentery and is said to be useful in genito-urinary irritation. The flavour of wintergreen and birch bark, in the form of a tea, was popular with the American Indians and European settlers. More recently, this has been translated into a preference for 'root beer' flavourings.

ACTIONS Analgesic, anti-inflammatory, antipyretic, antirheumatic, antiseptic, astringent, depurative, diuretic, rubefacient, tonic.

EXTRACTION Essential oil by steam distillation of the bark macerated in warm water.

CHARACTERISTICS Colourless, pale yellow or reddish tinted liquid with an intense, sweet-woody, wintergreen-like scent.

PRINCIPAL CONSTITUENTS Almost entirely methyl salicylate (98 per cent), produced during the maceration process. It is almost identical in composition to wintergreen oil.

SAFETY DATA Methyl salicylate, the major constituent, is not exactly toxic but very harmful in concentration. ' It can be absorbed through the skin, and fatal poisoning via this route has been reported.'[11] It is also classed as an enviromental hazard or marine pollutant.

AROMATHERAPY/HOME USE None.

OTHER USES Limited use as a counter-irritant in anti-arthritic and antineuralgic ointments and analgesic balms. Limited use as a fragrance component in cosmetics and perfumes; extensively used as a flavouring agent, especially 'root beer', chewing gum, toothpaste, etc. (usually very low-level use).

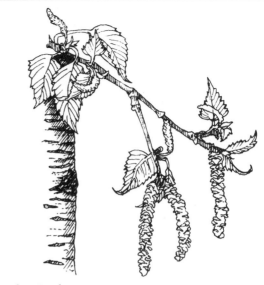

White Birch

BIRCH, WHITE
Betula alba

FAMILY Betulaceae

SYNONYMS *B. alba var. pubescens*, *B. odorata*, *B. pendula*, European white birch, silver birch.

GENERAL DESCRIPTION Decorative tree, up to 15-20 metres high, with slender branches, silvery-white bark broken into scales, and light green oval leaves. The male catkins are 2-5 cms long, the female up to 15 cms long.

DISTRIBUTION Native to the northern hemisphere; found throughout Eastern Europe, Russia, Germany, Sweden, Finland, the Baltic coast, northern China and Japan.

OTHER SPECIES Many cultivars exist of this species of birch. The paper birch (*B. papyrifera*) and *B. verrucosa* are also used for the production of birch bud oil and/or birch tar. NB Should not be confused with the oil from the sweet birch *(B. lenta)* which is potentially toxic.

HERBAL/FOLK TRADITION Birch buds were formerly used as a tonic in hair preparations. Birch tar is used in Europe for all types of chronic skin complaints: psoriasis, eczema, etc. In Scandinavia the young birch leaflets and twigs are bound into bundles and used in the sauna to tone the skin and promote the circulation. The sap is also tapped in the spring and drunk as a tonic. Buds, leaves and bark are used for 'rheumatic and arthritic conditions, especially where kidney functions appear to need support ... oedematous states; urinary infections and calculi.'[12]

ACTIONS Anti-inflammatory, antiseptic, cholagogue, diaphoretic, diuretic, febrifuge, tonic.

EXTRACTION 1. Essential oil by steam distillation from the leaf-buds. 2. Crude birch tar is extracted by slow destructive distillation from the bark; this is subsequently steam-distilled to yield a rectified birch tar oil.

CHARACTERISTICS 1. Pale yellow, viscous oil with a woody-green balsamic scent. It crystallizes at low temperatures. 2. The crude tar is an almost black, thick oily mass. The rectified oil is a brownish-yellow, clear oily liquid with a smoky, tar-like, 'Russian leather' odour. It blends well with other woody and balsamic oils.

PRINCIPAL CONSTITUENTS 1. Mainly betulenol and other sesquiterpenes. 2. In the tar oil: phenol, cresol, xylenol, guaiacol, creosol, pyrocatechol, pyrobetulin (which gives the 'leather' scent).

SAFETY DATA Non-toxic, non-irritant, non-sensitizing.

AROMATHERAPY/HOME USE
SKIN CARE: Dermatitis, dull or congested skin, eczema, hair care, psoriasis etc.
CIRCULATION, MUSCLES AND JOINTS: Accumulation of toxins, arthritis, cellulitis, muscular pain, obesity, oedema, poor circulation, rheumatism.

OTHER USES Birch bud oil is used primarily in hair tonics and shampoos, and in some cosmetics for its potential skin-healing effects. The crude tar is used in pharmaceutical preparations, ointments, lotions, etc. for dermatological diseases. It is also used in soap and leather manufacture – rectified birch tar oil provides the heart for many 'leather' type perfumes and aftershaves.

BOLDO LEAF
Peumus boldus

FAMILY Monimiaceae

SYNONYMS *Boldu boldus, Boldoa fragrans,* boldus, boldu.

GENERAL DESCRIPTION An evergreen shrub or small tree up to 6 metres high, with slender branches, sessile coarse leaves and bearing yellowish-green fruit; when dried the leaves turn a deep reddish-brown colour. The whole plant is aromatic.

DISTRIBUTION Native to Chile; naturalized in the Mediterranean region. Some essential oil is produced in Nepal and Vietnam.

OTHER SPECIES The Australian tree *Monimia rotundifolia* contains a similar oil, which has been used as a substitute. The oil of chenopodium or wormseed is also chemically related.

HERBAL/FOLK TRADITION The bark is used for tanning, the wood utilized in charcoal making and the fruit eaten by locals. In South America it has long been recognized as a valuable cure for gonorrhoea. In Western herbalism, the dried leaves are used for genito-urinary inflammation, gallstones, liver or gall bladder pain, cystitis and rheumatism. The dried leaves are current in the British Herbal Pharmacopoeia as a specific for cholelithiasis with pain.

ACTIONS Antiseptic, cholagogue, diaphoretic, diuretic, hepatic, sedative, tonic, urinary demulcent.

EXTRACTION Essential oil by steam distillation of the leaves.

CHARACTERISTICS A yellow liquid with a powerful spicy-camphoraceous, disagreeable odour.

PRINCIPAL CONSTITUENTS Cymene, ascaridole, cineol, linalol.

SAFETY DATA Extremely toxic. 'The oil has powerful therapeutic effects, and it can be considered harmful to the human organism even when used in very small doses ... should not be used in therapy, either internally or externally.'[13]

AROMATHERAPY/HOME USE None.

OTHER USES Used in pharmaceuticals in minute amounts for its therapeutic properties.

BORNEOL
Dryobalanops aromatica

FAMILY Dipterocarpaceae

SYNONYMS *D. camphora,* Borneo camphor, East Indian camphor, Baros camphor, Sumatra camphor, Malayan camphor.

GENERAL DESCRIPTION The camphora tree grows to a great height, a majestic tree often over 25 metres high, with a thick trunk up to 2 metres in diameter. Borneol is a natural exudation found beneath the bark in crevices and fissures of some mature trees (about 1 per cent); young trees produce only a clear yellow liquid known as 'liquid camphor'.

DISTRIBUTION Native to Borneo and Sumatra.

OTHER SPECIES To be distinguished from the Japanese or Formosa type of camphor, more commonly used in Europe, which is relatively toxic. See also Botanical Classification section.

HERBAL/FOLK TRADITION Borneol has long been regarded as a panacea by many Eastern civilizations, especially in ancient Persia, India and China. It was used as a powerful remedy against plague and other infectious diseases, stomach and bowel complaints. In China it was also used for embalming purposes. 'It is mentioned by Marco Polo in the thirteenth century and Camoens in 1571 who called it the "balsam of disease".'[14] It is valued for ceremonial purposes in the east generally, and in China particularly for funeral rites. Its odour repels insects and ants, and it is therefore highly regarded as timber for the construction of buildings.

ACTIONS Mildly analgesic, antidepressant, antiseptic, antispasmodic, antiviral, carminative, rubefacient, stimulant of the adrenal cortex, tonic (cardiac and general).

EXTRACTION The borneol is collected from the tree trunk in its crude crystalline form (the natives test each tree first by making incisions in the trunk to detect its presence). The so-called 'oil of borneol' is extracted by steam distillation of the wood.

CHARACTERISTICS Watery white to viscous black oil depending upon the amount of camphor which it contains, with a distinctive, sassafras-like, camphoraceous odour.

PRINCIPAL CONSTITUENTS The crude is made up of mainly d-borneol which is an alcohol, not a ketone (like Japanese camphor). The oil contains approx. 35 per cent terpenes: pinene, camphene, dipentene; 10 per cent alcohols: d-borneol, terpineol; 20 per cent sesquiterpenes, and 35 per cent resin.

SAFETY DATA Non-toxic, non-sensitizing, dermal irritant in concentration.

AROMATHERAPY/HOME USE
SKIN CARE: Cuts, bruises, insect repellent, CIRCULATION, MUSCLES AND JOINTS: Debility, poor circulation, rheumatism, sprains. RESPIRATORY SYSTEM: Bronchitis, coughs. IMMUNE SYSTEM: Colds, fever, 'flu and other infectious diseases. NERVOUS SYSTEM: Nervous exhaustion, stress-related conditions, neuralgia.

OTHER USES It is used to scent soap in the East but is still relatively unknown in the West in pharmaceutical and perfumery work. In China and Japan it is used for making varnish and ink; also as a dilutant for artists' colours. Mainly used for ritual purposes in the East.

BORONIA
Boronia megastigma

FAMILY Rutaceae

SYNONYM Brown boronia.

GENERAL DESCRIPTION A bushy evergreen shrub, up to 2 metres high, which bears an abundance of fragrant, nodding flowers with an unusual colouring – the petals are brown on the outside, yellow on the inside. Often grown as an ornamental shrub in gardens.

DISTRIBUTION Native to Western Australia; grows wild all over west and south west Australia.

OTHER SPECIES There are over fifteen species of boronia found in Western Australia; *B. megastigma* is one of the most common and the only one used for its perfume; other types smell of sarsaparilla, lemons or roses! Boronia is botanically related to the citrus tree.

HERBAL/FOLK TRADITION 'A botanist in the Victorian era suggested this species would be suitable for graveyard planting because of its dark flowers!'[15]

ACTIONS Aromatic.

EXTRACTION A concrete and absolute by the enfleurage method or petroleum-ether extraction, from the flowers. An essential oil is also produced in small quantities by steam distillation.

CHARACTERISTICS The concrete is a dark green butterlike mass with a beautiful warm, woody-sweet fragrance; the absolute is a green viscous liquid with a fresh, fruity-spicy scent and a rich, tenacious, floral undertone. It blends well with clary sage, sandalwood, bergamot, violet, helichrysum, costus, mimosa and other florals.

PRINCIPAL CONSTITUENTS Notably ionone; also eugenol, triacontane, phenols, ethyl alcohol and ethyl formate, among others.

SAFETY DATA Prohibitively expensive and therefore often adulterated.

AROMATHERAPY/HOME USE Perfume.

OTHER USES The absolute is used in high-class perfumery work, especially florals. Used in specialized flavour work, especially rich fruit products.

BROOM, SPANISH
Spartium junceum

FAMILY Fabaceae (Leguminosae).

SYNONYMS *Genista juncea*, genista, weavers broom, broom (absolute), gênet (absolute).

GENERAL DESCRIPTION A decorative plant,

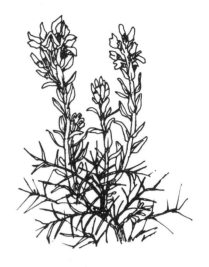

Broom

often cultivated as an ornamental shrub, up to 3 metres high with upright woody branches and tough flexible stems. It has bright green leaves and large, yellow, pea-like fragrant flowers, also bearing its seeds in pods or legumes.

DISTRIBUTION Native to southern Europe, especially southern Spain and southern France; mainly cultivated in Spain, France, Italy and USA (as a garden shrub). The absolute is produced in Southern France.

OTHER SPECIES Closely related to dyer's greenweed *(Genista tinctoria)* and the common or green broom *(Sarothamnus scoparius* or *Cytisus scoparius)*. There are also several other related species of broom, which are rich in their folk tradition.

HERBAL/FOLK TRADITION The twigs and bark have been used since ancient times to produce a strong fibre which can be made into cord or a coarse cloth. The branches were also used for thatching, basketwork, fencing and, of course, for making brooms. Spanish broom has similar therapeutic properties to the common broom, which is still current in the British Herbal Pharmocopoeia for cardiac dropsy, myocardial weakness, tachycardia and profuse menstruation. However, the Spanish broom is said to be five to six times more active than the common broom, and even that must be used with caution by professional herbalists due to the strength of the active ingredients: 'A number of cases of poisoning have occurred from the substitution of the dried flowers of *Spartium* for those of true Broom.'[16]

ACTIONS Antihaemorrhagic, cardioactive, diuretic, cathartic, emmenagogue, narcotic, vasoconstrictor.

EXTRACTION An absolute is obtained by solvent extraction from the dried flowers.

CHARACTERISTICS A dark brown, viscous liquid with an intensely sweet, floral, hay-like scent with a herbaceous undertone. It blends well with rose, tuberose, cassie, mimosa, violet, vetiver, and herbaceous-type fragrances.

PRINCIPAL CONSTITUENTS The absolute contains capryllic acid, phenols, aliphatics, terpenes, esters, scoparin and sparteine, as well as wax, etc.

SAFETY DATA Sparteine, which is contained in the flowers as the main active constituent, is toxic. In large doses, it causes vomiting, renal irritation, weakens the heart, depresses the nerve cells and lowers the blood pressure, and in extreme cases causes death.

AROMATHERAPY/HOME USE None.

OTHER USES Used in soaps, cosmetics and high-class perfumery; also as a flavour ingredient in sweet rich 'preserves', alcoholic and soft drinks.

BUCHU
Agothosma betulina

FAMILY Rutaceae

SYNOYNMS *Barosma betulina,* short buchu, mountain buchu, bookoo, buku, bucco.

GENERAL DESCRIPTION A small shrub with simple wrinkled leaves about 1-2 cms long;

other much smaller leaves are also present which are bright green with finely serrated margins. It has delicate stems bearing five-petalled white flowers. The whole plant has a strong, aromatic, blackcurrant-like odour.

DISTRIBUTION Native to the Cape of Good Hope in South Africa, it now grows wild all over South Africa. Dried leaves are exported to Holland, England and America.

OTHER SPECIES There are more than twelve so-called *Barosma* species in South Africa – the 'true' buchus are *B. crenulata* (contains high amounts of pulegone, a toxic constituent), *B. serratifolia* and *B. betulina.*

HERBAL/FOLK TRADITION The leaves are used locally for antiseptic purposes and to ward off insects. In western herbalism, the leaves are used for infections of the genito-urinary system, such as cystitis, urethritis and prostatitis. Current in British Herbal Pharmocopoeia 1983.

ACTIONS Antiseptic (especially urinary), diuretic, insecticide.

EXTRACTION Essential oil by steam distillation from the dried leaves.

CHARACTERISTICS Dark yellowy-brown oil with a penetrating minty-camphoraceous odour.

PRINCIPAL CONSTITUENTS Diosphenol (25-40 per cent), limonene and menthone, among others.

SAFETY DATA Should not be used during pregnancy. The toxicity of buchu is unknown but since *B. betulina* yields oils high in diophenols and *B. crenulata* yields oils high in pulegone, they should both be regarded as questionable at present.

AROMATHERAPY/HOME USE None.

OTHER USES A tincture, extract and oleoresin are produced for pharmaceutical use. Limited use in blackcurrant flavour and fragrance work, for example colognes and chyprè bases.

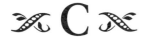

CABREUVA
Myrocarpus fastigiatus

FAMILY Fabaceae (Leguminosae)

SYNONYMS Cabureicica, 'Baume de Perou brun'.

GENERAL DESCRIPTION A graceful, tall tropical tree, 12-15 metres high, with a very hard wood, extremely resistant to moisture and mould growth. It yields a balsam when the trunk is damaged, like many other South American trees.

DISTRIBUTION Found in Brazil, Paraguay, Chile and north Argentina.

OTHER SPECIES Many varieties of *Myrocarpus* yield cabreuva oil, such as *M. frondosus*. It is also botanically related to the trees which yield copaiba, Peru and Tolu balsam.

HERBAL/FOLK TRADITION The wood is highly appreciated for carving and furniture making. It is used by the natives to heal wounds, ulcers and obviate scars. It was once listed in old European pharmocopoeias for its antiseptic qualities.

ACTIONS Antiseptic, balsamic, cicatrisant.

EXTRACTION Essential oil by steam distillation from wood chippings (waste from the timber mills).

CHARACTERISTICS A pale yellow, viscous liquid with a sweet, woody-floral scent, very delicate but having great tenacity. It blends well with rose, cassie, mimosa, cedarwood, rich woody and oriental bases.

PRINCIPAL CONSTITUENTS Mainly nerolidol (80 per cent approx.), farnesol, bisabolol, among others.

SAFETY DATA Non-toxic, non-irritant, non-sensitizing.

AROMATHERAPY/HOME USE
SKIN CARE: Cuts, scars, wounds.
RESPIRATORY SYSTEM: Chills, coughs.
IMMUNE SYSTEM: Colds.

OTHER USES Fragrance component and fixative in soaps and high-class perfumes, especially floral, woody or oriental types. Previously used for the isolation of nerolidol, now produced synthetically.

CADE
Juniperus oxycedrus

FAMILY Cupressaceae

SYNONYMS Juniper tar, prickly cedar, medlar tree, prickly juniper.

GENERAL DESCRIPTION A large evergreen shrub up to 4 metres high, with long dark needles and brownish-black berries about the size of hazelnuts.

DISTRIBUTION Native to southern France; now common throughout Europe and North Africa. The tar is produced mainly in Spain and Yugoslavia.

OTHER SPECIES There are many varieties of juniper which are used commercially apart from the prickly juniper: *J. communis* produces juniper oil, *J. virginiana* produces Virginian cedarwood oil, and in Yugoslavia an oil is produced from the fruits and twigs of *J. smreka*.

HERBAL/FOLK TRADITION Used in the treatment of cutaneous diseases, such as chronic eczema, parasites, scalp disease, hair loss, etc. especially in France and other continental countries. It is also used as an antiseptic wound dressing and for toothache.

ACTIONS Analgesic, antimicrobial, antipruritic, antiseptic, disinfectant, parasiticide, vermifuge.

EXTRACTION The crude oil or tar is obtained by destructive distillation from the branches and heartwood (usually in the form of shavings or chips). A rectified oil is produced from the crude by steam or vacuum distillation. In addition, an oil is occasionally produced from the berries by steam distillation.

CHARACTERISTICS The rectified oil is an orange-brown, oily liquid with a woody, smoky, leatherlike odour. It blends well with thyme, origanum, clove, cassia, tea tree, pine and medicinal-type bases.

PRINCIPAL CONSTITUENTS Cadinene, cadinol, p-cresol, guaiacol, among others.

SAFETY DATA Non-toxic, non-irritant, possible sensitization problems. Use with care, especially when treating inflammatory or allergic skin conditions. Turpentine (terebinth) oil makes a useful alternative, with less possibility of an allergic reaction.

AROMATHERAPY/HOME USE
SKIN CARE: Cuts, dandruff, dermatitis, eczema, spots, etc.

OTHER USES Extensively used in pharmaceutical work as a solvent for chemical drugs, in dermatological creams and ointments, as well as in veterinary medicine. Rectified cade is used in fragrance work, in soaps, lotions, creams and perfumes (especially leather and spice).

CAJEPUT
Melaleuca cajeputi

FAMILY Myrtaceae

SYNONYMS *M. minor,* cajuput, white tea tree, white wood, swamp tea tree, punk tree, paperbark tree.

GENERAL DESCRIPTION A tall evergreen tree up to 30 metres high, with thick pointed leaves and white flowers. The flexible trunk has a whitish spongy bark which flakes off easily. In Malaysia it is called 'caju-puti', meaning 'white wood', due to the colour of the timber.

DISTRIBUTION It grows wild in Malaysia, Indonesia, the Philippines, Vietnam, Java, Australia and south eastern Asia.

OTHER SPECIES Several other varieties of *Melaleuca* are used to produce cajeput oil, such as *M. quinquenervia* – see Botanical Classification section. Closely related to other members of the *Melaleuca* group, notably eucalyptus, clove, niaouli and tea tree.

HERBAL/FOLK TRADITION Held in high regard in the East, it is used locally for colds, headaches, throat infections, toothache, sore and aching muscles, fever (cholera), rheumatism and various skin diseases. Only the oil is used in the Western herbal tradition, known for producing a sensation of warmth and quickening the pulse. It is used for chronic laryngitis and bronchitis, cystitis, rheumatism and to expel roundworm.

ACTIONS Mildly analgesic, antimicrobial, antineuralgic, antispasmodic, antiseptic (pulmonary, urinary, intestinal), anthelmintic, diaphoretic, carminative, expectorant, febrifuge, insecticide, sudorific, tonic.

EXTRACTION Essential oil by steam distillation from the fresh leaves and twigs.

CHARACTERISTICS A pale yellowy-green, mobile liquid (the green tinge derives from traces of copper found in the tree), with a penetrating, camphoraceous-medicinal odour. Compared with eucalyptus oil, it has a slightly milder fruity body note.

PRINCIPAL CONSTITUENTS Cineol (14-65 per cent depending on source), terpineol, terpinyl acetate, pinene, nerolidol and other traces.

SAFETY DATA Non-toxic, non-sensitizing, may irritate the skin in high concentration.

AROMATHERAPY/HOME USE
SKIN CARE: Insect bites, oily skin, spots.
CIRCULATION, MUSCLES AND JOINTS: Arthritis, muscular aches and pains, rheumatism.
RESPIRATORY SYSTEM: Asthma, bronchitis, catarrh, coughs, sinusitis, sore throat.
GENITOURINARY SYSTEM: Cystitis, urethritis, urinary infection.
IMMUNE SYSTEM: Colds, 'flu, viral infections.

OTHER USES Used in dentistry and pharmaceutical work as an antiseptic; in expectorant and tonic formulations, throat lozenges, gargles, etc. Used as a fragrance and freshening agent in soaps, cosmetics, detergents and perfumes. Occasionally employed as a flavour component in food products and soft drinks.

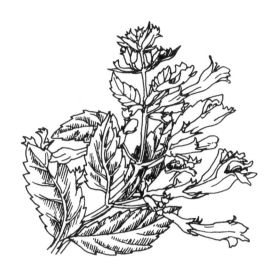

Calamintha

CALAMINTHA
Calamintha officinalis

FAMILY Lamiaceae (Labiatae)

SYNONYMS C. *clinopodium, Melissa calaminta,* calamint, common calamint, mill mountain, mountain balm, mountain mint, basil thyme, nepeta (oil), French marjoram (oil), wild basil (oil), catnip (oil).

GENERAL DESCRIPTION An erect, bushy, perennial plant not more than one metre high, with square stems, soft oval serrated leaves greyish-green beneath, and rather inconspicuous pale purple flowers. The whole plant has a strong aromatic scent which is attractive to cats.

DISTRIBUTION Native to Europe and parts of Asia (Himalayas), naturalized throughout North America and South Africa. Cultivated for its oil in the Mediterranean region, Yugoslavia, Poland and in the USA.

OTHER SPECIES There are numerous similar species found throughout the world, such as the lesser calamintha *(C. nepeta)* which has a stronger odour and is often used interchangeably with common calamint. It is also closely related to catmint or catnip *(Nepeta cataria)* also known as calamint, with which it shares similar properties. Not to be confused with winter and summer savory *(Satureja montana* and *S. hortensis).*

HERBAL/FOLK TRADITION It has a long history of use as a herbal remedy mainly for nervous and digestive complaints, also menstrual pain, colds, chills and cramp. Catmint is current in the British Herbal Pharmacopoeia as a specific for flatulent colic in children and for the common cold.

ACTIONS Anaesthetic (local), antirheumatic, antispasmodic, astringent, carminative, diaphoretic, emmenagogue, febrifuge, nervine, sedative, tonic.

EXTRACTION Essential oil by steam distillation from the flowering tops.

CHARACTERISTICS A pale yellow liquid with a herbaceous-woody, pungent odour, somewhat resembling pennyroyal.

PRINCIPAL CONSTITUENTS Citral, nerol, citronellol, limonene and geraniol, among others. The active ingredient that attracts cats is metatabilacetone (3-5 per cent). Constituents vary according to source.

SAFETY DATA Non-irritant, non-sensitizing; possible toxic effects in concentration. (The Chinese shrub *Actinidia polygama* also contains metatabilacetone, which is responsible for its hallucinogenic and narcotic effects.) Use in moderation. Avoid during pregnancy.

AROMATHERAPY/HOME USE
CIRCULATION, MUSCLES AND JOINTS: Chills, cold in the joints, muscular aches and pains, rheumatism.
DIGESTIVE SYSTEM: Colic, flatulence, nervous dyspepsia.
NERVOUS SYSTEM: Insomnia, nervous tension and stress-related conditions.

OTHER USES Used as a wild cat lure in the USA. Occasionally used in perfumery work.

CALAMUS
Acorus calamus var. angustatus

FAMILY Araceae

SYNONYMS *Calamus aromaticus*, sweet flag, sweet sedge, sweet root, sweet rush, sweet cane, sweet myrtle, myrtle grass, myrtle sedge, cinnamon sedge.

GENERAL DESCRIPTION A reed like aquatic plant about 1 metre high, with sword-shaped leaves and small greenish-yellow flowers. It grows on the margins of lakes and streams with the long-branched rhizome immersed in the mud. The whole plant is aromatic.

DISTRIBUTION Native to India; the oil is mainly produced in India and Russia and to a lesser extent in Europe (except Spain), Siberia, China, Yugoslavia and Poland (Polish and Yugoslavian oils have a uniform lasting scent).

OTHER SPECIES Not to be confused with the yellow flag iris which it resembles in appearance; they are botanically unrelated. There are several other varieties of aromatic sedge, mostly in the east, for example *Calamus odoratus* used in India as a medicine and perfume.

HERBAL/FOLK TRADITION The name derives from the Greek *calamos* meaning 'reed'. The properties of the herb are mainly due to the aromatic oil, contained largely in the root. It used to be highly esteemed as an aromatic stimulant and tonic for fever (typhoid), nervous complaints, vertigo, headaches, dysentery, etc. It is still current in the British Herbal Pharmacopoeia, for 'acute and chronic dyspepsia, gastritis, intestinal colic, anorexia, gastric ulcer.'[17] In Turkey and especially in India (where it is valued as a traditional medicine), it is sold as a candied rhizome for dyspepsia, bronchitis and coughs.

ACTIONS Anticonvulsant, antiseptic, bactericidal, carminative, diaphoretic, expectorant, hypotensive, insecticide, spasmolytic, stimulant, stomachic, tonic, vermifuge.

EXTRACTION Essential oil by steam distillation from the rhizomes (and sometimes the leaves).

CHARACTERISTICS A thick, pale yellow liquid with a strong, warm, woody-spicy fragrance; poor quality oils have a camphoraceous note. It blends well with cananga, cinnamon, labdanum, olibanum, patchouli, cedarwood, amyris, spice and oriental bases.

PRINCIPAL CONSTITUENTS Beta-asarone (amounts vary depending on source: the Indian oil contains up to 80 per cent, the Russian oil a maximum of 6 per cent), also calamene, calamol, calamenene, eugenol and shyobunones.

SAFETY DATA Oral toxin. The oil of calamus is reported to have carcinogenic properties.

AROMATHERAPY/HOME USE None. 'Should not be used in therapy, whether internally or externally.'[18]

OTHER USES Extensively used in cosmetic and perfumery work, in woody/oriental/leather perfumes and to scent hair powders and tooth powders in the same way as orris. Calamus and its derivatives (oil, extracts, etc.) are banned from use in foods.

CAMPHOR
Cinnamomum camphora

FAMILY Lauraceae

SYNOYNMS *Laurus camphora*, true camphor, hon-sho, laurel camphor, gum camphor, Japanese camphor, Formosa camphor.

GENERAL DESCRIPTION A tall, handsome, evergreen tree, up to 30 metres high, not unlike the linden. It has many branches bearing clusters of small white flowers followed by red berries. It produces a white crystalline substance, the crude camphor, from the wood of mature trees over fifty years old.

DISTRIBUTION Native to Japan and Taiwan principally, also China; cultivated in India, Ceylon, Egypt, Madagascar, southern Europe and America.

OTHER SPECIES There are many species of camphor: the ho-sho variety produces ho leaf and ho wood oil; the Chinese variety produces apopin oil; the Japan and Taiwan type, known as hon-sho or true camphor, produces two chemotypes: camphor-safrol (Japan) and camphor-linalol (Taiwan). All these are to be distinguished from the Borneo camphor or borneol which is of different botanical origin.

HERBAL/FOLK TRADITION A long-standing traditional preventative of infectious disease; a lump of camphor would be worn around the neck as a protection. In addition it was used for nervous and respiratory diseases in general, and for heart failure! However, in its crude form it is very poisonous in large doses, and has been removed from the British Pharmacopoeia.

ACTIONS Anti-inflammatory, antiseptic, antiviral, bactericidal, counter-irritant, diuretic, expectorant, stimulant, rubefacient, vermifuge.

EXTRACTION Crude camphor is collected from the trees in crystalline form. The essential

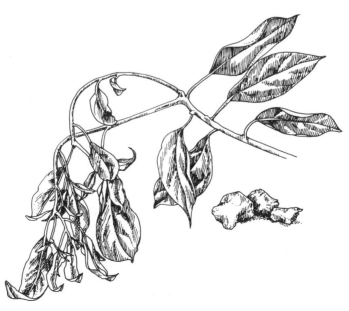

Camphor

oil is produced by steam distillation from the wood, root stumps and branches and then rectified under vacuum and filter pressed to produce three fractions, known as white, brown and yellow camphor.

CHARACTERISTICS White camphor is the lightest (lowest boiling) fraction, a colourless to pale yellow liquid with a sharp, pungent camphoraceous odour. Brown camphor is the middle fraction. Yellow camphor, a blue-green or yellowish liquid, is the heaviest.

PRINCIPAL CONSTITUENTS 1 White camphor contains mainly cineol, with pinene, terpineol, menthol, thymol and no safrol. 2. Brown camphor contains up to 80 per cent safrol and some terpineol. 3. Yellow camphor contains mainly safrol, sesquiterpenes and sesquiterpene alcohols.

SAFETY DATA Brown and yellow camphor (containing safrol) are toxic and carcinogenic and 'should not be used in therapy, either internally or externally.'[19] White camphor does not contain safrol and is relatively non-toxic, non-sensitizing and non-irritant. It is, however, an enviromental hazard or marine pollutant.

AROMATHERAPY/HOME USE White camphor may be used with care for:
SKIN CARE: Acne, inflammation, oily conditions, spots; also for insect prevention (flies, moths, etc).
CIRCULATION, MUSCLES AND JOINTS: Arthritis, muscular aches and pains, rheumatism, sprains, etc.
RESPIRATORY SYSTEM: Bronchitis, chills, coughs.
IMMUNE SYSTEM: Colds, fever, 'flu, infectious disease.

OTHER USES White and brown camphor are used as the starting material for the isolation of many perfumery chemicals, for example safrol and cineol. White camphor is used as a solvent in the paint and lacquer industry, and for the production of celluloid. Fractions of white oil are used as fragrance and masking agents in detergents, soaps, disinfectants and household products.

CANANGA
Cananga odorata

FAMILY Annonaceae

SYNONYM *C. odoratum var. macrophylla.*

GENERAL DESCRIPTION A tall tropical tree, up to 30 metres high, which flowers all year round. It bears large, fragrant, tender yellow flowers which are virtually identical to those of the ylang ylang.

DISTRIBUTION Native to tropical Asia: Java, Malaysia, the Philippines, the Moluccas.

OTHER SPECIES Very closely related to the tree which produces ylang ylang oil, *C. odorata var. genuina.* Cananga is considered an inferior product in perfumery work; being grown in different regions the oil has a different quality, heavier and less delicate than ylang ylang. However, cananga is truly a 'complete' oil whereas ylang ylang is made into several distillates.

HERBAL/FOLK TRADITION Used locally for infectious illnesses, for example malaria. The beautiful flowers are also used for decorative purposes at festivals.

ACTIONS Antiseptic, antidepressant, aphrodisiac, hypotensive, nervine, sedative, tonic.

EXTRACTION Essential oil by water distillation from the flowers.

CHARACTERISTICS Greenish-yellow or orange viscous liquid with a sweet, floral-balsamic tenacious scent. It blends well with calamus, birch tar, copaiba balsam, labdanum, neroli, oakmoss, jasmine, guaiacwood and oriental-type bases.

PRINCIPAL CONSTITUENTS Caryophyllene, benzyl acetate, benzyl alcohol, farnesol, terpineol, borneol, geranyl acetate, safrol, linalol, limonrne, methyl salicylate and over 100 minor components.

SAFETY DATA Non-toxic, non-irritant, possible sensitization especially in those with sensitive skin.

AROMATHERAPY/HOME USE
SKIN CARE: Insect bites, fragrance, general skin care.
NERVOUS SYSTEM: Anxiety, depression, nervous tension and stress-related complaints.

OTHER USES Fragrance component in soaps, detergents, cosmetics and perfumes, especially men's fragrances. Limited use as a flavour ingredient in some food products, alcoholic and soft drinks.

CARAWAY
Carum carvi

FAMILY Apiaceae (Umbelliferae)

SYNONYMS *Apium carvi*, carum, caraway fruits.

GENERAL DESCRIPTION A biennial herb up to 0.75 metres high with a much-branched stem, finely cut leaves and umbels of white flowers, with a thick and tapering root. The small seeds are curved with five distinct pale ridges.

DISTRIBUTION Native to Europe and western Asia, naturalized in North America. Now widely cultivated especially in Germany, Holland, Scandinavia and Russia.

OTHER SPECIES There are several varieties depending on origin – the English, Dutch and German types derive from Prussia, which are distinct from the Scandinavian variety. Those plants grown in northerly latitudes produce more oil.

HERBAL/FOLK TRADITION Used extensively as a domestic spice, especially in bread, cakes and cheeses. Traditional remedy for dyspepsia, intestinal colic, menstrual cramps, poor appetite, laryngitis and bronchitis. It promotes milk secretion and is considered specific for flatulent colic in children, according to the British Herbal Pharmacopoeia.

ACTIONS Antihistaminic, antimicrobial, antiseptic, aperitif, astringent, carminative, diuretic, emmenagogue, expectorant, galactagogue, larvicidal, stimulant, spasmolytic, stomachic, tonic, vermifuge.

EXTRACTION Essential oil by steam distillation from the dried ripe seed or fruit (approx. 2-8 per cent yield).

CHARACTERISTICS Crude caraway oil is a pale yellowish-brown liquid with a harsh, spicy odour. The redistilled oil is colourless to pale yellow, with a strong, warm, sweet-spicy odour, like rye bread. It blends well with jasmine, cinnamon, cassia and other spices; however, it is very overpowering.

PRINCIPAL CONSTITUENTS Mainly carvone (50-60 per cent) and limonene (40 per cent), with carveol, dihydrocarveol, dihydrocarvone, pinene, phellandrene, among others.

SAFETY DATA Non-toxic, non-sensitizing, may cause dermal irritation in concentration.

AROMATHERAPY/HOME USE
RESPIRATORY SYSTEM: Bronchitis, coughs, laryngitis.
DIGESTIVE SYSTEM: Dyspepsia, colic, flatulence, gastric spasm, nervous indigestion, poor appetite. See also sweet fennel and dill.
IMMUNE SYSTEM: Colds.

OTHER USES Used in carminative, stomachic and laxative preparations and as a flavour ingredient in pharmaceuticals; also to mask unpleasant tastes and odours. Fragrance component in toothpaste, mouthwash products, cosmetics and perfumes. Extensively used as a flavour ingredient in most major food categories, especially condiments. The German brandy 'Kummel' is made from the seeds.

CARDOMON
Elettaria cardamomum

FAMILY Zingiberaceae

SYNONYMS *Elettaria cardomomum var. cardomomum,* cardomom, cardamomi, cardomum, mysore cardomom.

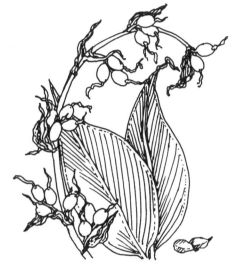

Cardomon

GENERAL DESCRIPTION A perennial, reed-like herb up to 4 metres high, with long, silky blade-shaped leaves. Its long sheathing stems bear small yellowish flowers with purple tips, followed by oblong red-brown seeds.

DISTRIBUTION Native to tropical Asia, especially southern India; cultivated extensively in India, Sri Lanka, Laos, Guatemala and El Salvador. The oil is produced principally in India, Europe, Sri Lanka and Guatemala.

OTHER SPECIES There are numerous related species found in the east, used as local spices and for medicinal purposes, such as round or Siam cardomon *(Amomum cardamomum)* found in India and China. An oil is also produced from wild cardomon *(E. cardamomum var. major).*

HERBAL/FOLK TRADITION Used extensively as a domestic spice, especially in India, Europe, Latin America and Middle Eastern countries. It has been used in traditional Chinese and Indian medicine for over 3000 years, especially for pulmonary disease, fever, digestive and urinary complaints. Hippocrates recommended it for sciatica, coughs, abdominal pains, spasms, nervous disorders, retention of urine and also for bites of venomous creatures.

Current in the British Herbal Pharmocopoeia as a specific for flatulent dyspepsia.

ACTIONS Antiseptic, antispasmodic, aphrodisiac, carminative, cephalic, digestive, diuretic, sialogogue, stimulant, stomachic, tonic (nerve).

EXTRACTION Essential oil by steam distillation from the dried ripe fruit (seeds). An oleoresin is also produced in small quantities.

CHARACTERISTICS A colourless to pale yellow liquid with a sweet-spicy, warming fragrance and a woody-balsamic undertone. It blends well with rose, olibanum, orange, bergamot, cinnamon, cloves, caraway, ylang ylang, labdanum, cedarwood, neroli and oriental bases in general.

PRINCIPAL CONSTITUENTS Terpinyl acetate and cineol (each may be present at up to 50 per cent), limonene, sabinene, linalol, linalyl acetate, pinene, zingiberene, among others.

SAFETY DATA Non-toxic, non-irritant, non-sensitizing.

AROMATHERAPY/HOME USE
DIGESTIVE SYSTEM: Anorexia, colic, cramp, dyspepsia, flatulence, griping pains, halitosis heartburn, indigestion, vomiting.
NERVOUS SYSTEM: Mental fatigue, nervous strain.

OTHER USES Employed in some carminative, stomachic and laxative preparations; also in the form of compound cardomon spirit to flavour pharmaceuticals. Extensively used as a fragrance component in soaps, cosmetics and perfumes, especially oriental types. Important flavour ingredient, particularly in curry and spice products.

CARROT SEED
Daucus carota

FAMILY Apiaceae (Umbelliferae)

SYNOYNMS Wild carrot, Queen Anne's lace, bird's nest.

GENERAL DESCRIPTION Annual or biennial herb, with a small, inedible, tough whitish root. It has a much-branched stem up to 1.5 metres high with hairy leaves and umbels of white lacy flowers.

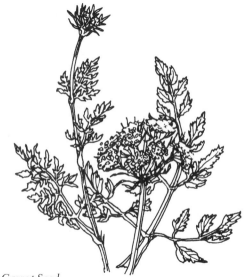

Carrot Seed

DISTRIBUTION Native to Europe, Asia and North Africa; naturalized in North America. The essential oil is mainly produced in France.

OTHER SPECIES An oil is also produced by solvent extraction from the red fleshy root of the common edible carrot *(D. carota subspecies sativus)* mainly for use as a food colouring.

HERBAL/FOLK TRADITION A highly nutritious plant, containing substantial amounts of Vitamins A, C, B_1 and B_2. The roots have a strong tonic action on the liver and gall bladder, good for the treatment of jaundice and other complaints. The seeds are used for the retention of urine, colic, kidney and digestive disorders, and to promote menstruation. In the Chinese tradition it is used to treat dysentery and to expel worms.

The dried leaves are current in the British Herbal Pharmacopoeia for calculus, gout, cystitis and lithuria.

ACTIONS Anthelmintic, antiseptic, carminative, depurative, diuretic, emmenagogue, hepatic, stimulant, tonic, vasodilatory and smooth muscle relaxant.

EXTRACTION Essential oil by steam distillation from the dried fruit (seeds).

CHARACTERISTICS A yellow or amber-coloured liquid with a warm, dry, woody-earthy odour. It blends well with costus, cassie, mimosa, cedarwood, geranium, citrus and spice oils.

PRINCIPAL CONSTITUENTS Pinene, carotol, daucol, limonene, bisabolene, elemene, geraniol, geranyl acetate, caryophyllene, among others.

SAFETY DATA Non-toxic, non-irritant, non-sensitizing.

AROMATHERAPY/HOME USE
SKIN CARE: Dermatitis, eczema, psoriasis, rashes, revitalizing and toning, mature complexions, wrinkles.
CIRCULATION, MUSCLES AND JOINTS: Accumulation of toxins, arthritis, gout, oedema, rheumatism.
DIGESTIVE SYSTEM: Anaemia, anorexia, colic, indigestion, liver congestion.
GENITO-URINARY AND ENDOCRINE SYSTEMS: Amenorrhoea, dysmenorrhoea, glandular problems, PMT.

OTHER USES Fragrance component in soaps, detergents, cosmetics and perfumes. Flavour ingredient in most major food categories, especially seasonings.

CASCARILLA BARK
Croton eluteria

FAMILY Euphorbiaceae

SYNONYMS Cascarilla, sweetwood bark, sweet bark, Bahama cascarilla, aromatic quinquina, false quinquina.

GENERAL DESCRIPTION A large shrub or small tree up to 12 metres high, with ovate silver-bronze leaves, pale yellowish-brown bark and small white fragrant flowers. It bears fruits and flowers all year round.

DISTRIBUTION Native to the West Indies, probably the Bahama Islands; found growing wild in Mexico, Colombia and Ecuador. The oil is mainly produced in the Bahamas and Cuba; some distillation takes place in America, France and England from the imported bark.

OTHER SPECIES An essential oil is also distilled locally from other *Croton* species. White, red and black cascarillas are also found in commerce.

HERBAL/FOLK TRADITION The bark is used as an aromatic bitter and tonic for dyspepsia, diarrhoea, dysentery, fever, debility, nausea, flatulence, vomiting and chronic bronchitis. The leaves are used as a digestive tea, and for flavouring tobacco. The bark also yields a good black dye.

ACTIONS Astringent, antimicrobial, antiseptic, carminative, digestive, expectorant, stomachic, tonic.

EXTRACTION Essential oil by steam distillation from the dried bark. (1.5-3 per cent yield).

CHARACTERISTICS A pale yellow, greenish or dark amber liquid with a spicy, aromatic, warm-woody odour. It blends well with nutmeg, pepper, pimento, sage, oakmoss, oriental and spicy bases.

PRINCIPAL CONSTITUENTS Cymene, diterpene, limonene, caryophyllene, terpineol and eugenol, among others.

SAFETY DATA Non-irritant, non-sensitizing, relatively non-toxic (possibly narcotic in large doses).

AROMATHERAPY/HOME USE
RESPIRATORY SYSTEM: Bronchitis, coughs
DIGESTIVE SYSTEM: Dyspepsia, flatulence, nausea.
IMMUNE SYSTEM: 'Flu.

OTHER USES Fragrance component in soaps, detergents, cosmetics and perfumes, especially men's fragrances. Flavour ingredient in most major food categories, soft drinks and alcoholic beverages, especially vermouths and bitters.

CASSIA
Cinnamomum cassia

FAMILY Lauraceae

SYNONYMS *C. aromaticum, Laurus cassia,* Chinese cinnamon, false cinnamon, cassia cinnamon, cassia lignea.

GENERAL DESCRIPTION A slender, evergreen tree up to 20 metres high, with leathery leaves and small white flowers. It is usually cut back to form bushes for commercial production.

DISTRIBUTION Native to the south eastern parts of China; found to a lesser extent in Vietnam and India (Cochin).

OTHER SPECIES Not to be confused with the Ceylon Cinnamon bark *(C. verum)* which is from a related species. There are also several other varieties from different regions used for essential oil production –See Botanical Classification section.

HERBAL/FOLK TRADITION Extensively used as local domestic spice. It is used medicinally in much the same way as Ceylon cinnamon, mainly for digestive complaints such as flatulent dyspepsia, colic, diarrhoea and nausea, as well as the common cold, rheumatism, kidney and reproductive complaints.
  The powdered bark is current in the British Herbal Pharmacopoeia as a specific for flatulent dyspepsia or colic with nausea.

ACTIONS Antidiarrhoeal, anti-emetic, anti-microbial, astringent, carminative, spasmolytic.

EXTRACTION Essential oil 1. by steam distillation from the leaves, and 2. by water distillation from the bark, leaves, twigs and stalks.

CHARACTERISTICS 1. Leaf oil is brownish-yellow (the rectified oil is pale yellow), with a sweet woody-spicy tenacious odour. 2. Bark oil is a dark brown liquid with a strong, spicy-warm, resinous odour.

PRINCIPAL CONSTITUENTS Leaf and Bark oil contain mainly cinnamic aldehyde (75-90 per cent) with some methyl eugenol, salicylaldehyde and methylsalicylaldehyde.

SAFETY DATA Dermal toxin, dermal irritant, dermal sensitizer, mucous membrane irritant.

AROMATHERAPY/HOME USE None. 'Should never be used on the skin (one of the most hazardous oils).'[28]

OTHER USES Some pharmaceutical applications due to bactericidal properties, such as mouthwashes, toothpastes, gargles; also tonic and carminative preparations. Extensively used in food flavouring, including alcoholic and soft drinks. Little used in perfumes and cosmetics, due to its dark colour.

CASSIE
Acacia farnesiana

FAMILY Mimosaceae

SYNONYMS *Cassia ancienne*, sweet acacia, huisache, popinac, opopanax.

GENERAL DESCRIPTION A bushy thorny shrub, much branched, up to 10 metres high. It has a very delicate appearance, similar to mimosa, with fragrant fluffy yellow flowers.

DISTRIBUTION Believed to be a native of the West Indies, now widely cultivated in tropical and semi-tropical regions throughout the world: mainly southern France and Egypt, also Lebanon, Morocco, Algeria and India.

OTHER SPECIES There are over 400 known species of acacia: other similar species are found in Central Africa, Zaire and Australia. Closely related to mimosa (*A. dealbata*) and Roman cassie (*A. cavenia*) which are also used for the production of essential oils. Not to be confused with opopanax or bisabol myrrh (*Commiphora erythrea*) although they share a common name.

HERBAL/FOLK TRADITION In India a local 'attar of cassie' is made as a perfume. The fresh flowers are used in baths for dry skin, and in the form of an infusion. In Venezuela the root is used for treating stomach cancer. In China it is used to treat rheumatoid arthritis and pulmonary tuberculosis.
  There are many types of acacia employed in herbal medicine, notably the Senegal acacia which yields a gummy exudation from the trunk known as gum arabic or gum acacia, mainly used as a demulcent.

ACTIONS Antirheumatic, antiseptic, antispasmodic, aphrodisiac, balsamic, insecticide.

EXTRACTION An absolute by solvent extraction from the flowers.

CHARACTERISTICS A dark yellow to brown viscous liquid with a warm, floral-spicy scent and rich balsamic undertone. It blends well with bergamot, costus, mimosa, frankincense, ylang ylang, orris and violet.

PRINCIPAL CONSTITUENTS The absolute contains about 25 per cent volatile constituents, mainly benzyl alcohol, methyl salicylate, farnesol, geraniol and linalol among others.

SAFETY DATA No available data on toxicity.

AROMATHERAPY/HOME USE Use with care for:
SKIN CARE: Dry, sensitive skin, perfume.

NERVOUS SYSTEM: Depression, frigidity, nervous exhaustion and stress-related conditions.

OTHER USES Used in high-class perfumes, especially oriental types. Used as a flavour ingredient in most food categories, especially fruit products, alcoholic and soft drinks.

CEDARWOOD, ATLAS
Cedrus atlantica

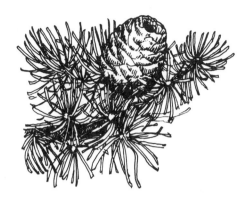

Cedarwood

FAMILY Pinaceae

SYNONYMS Atlantic cedar, Atlas cedar, African cedar, Moroccan cedarwood (oil), libanol (oil).

GENERAL DESCRIPTION Pyramid-shaped evergreen tree with a majestic stature, up to 40 metres high. The wood itself is hard and strongly aromatic, due to the high percentage of essential oil which it contains.

DISTRIBUTION Native to the Atlas mountains of Algeria; the oil is mainly produced in Morocco.

OTHER SPECIES Believed to have originated from the famous Lebanon cedars *(C. libani)*, which grow wild in Lebanon and on the island of Cyprus. It is also a close botanical relation to the Himalayan deodar cedarwood *(C. deodorata)*, which produces a very similar essential oil. (NB the oil is quite different from the Texas or Virginia cedarwood.)

HERBAL/FOLK TRADITION The oil from the Lebanon cedar was possibly the first to be extracted, it was used by the ancient Egyptians for embalming purposes, cosmetics and perfumery. The oil was one of the ingredients of 'mithridat', a renowned poison antidote that was used for centuries. The Lebanon cedar was prized as a building wood; its odour repelled ants, moths and other harmful insects, as does the oil from the Atlas cedar.

Traditionally, the oil was used in the East for bronchial and urinary tract infections, as a preservative and as an incense. It is still used as a temple incense by the Tibetans, and is employed in their traditional medicine.

ACTIONS Antiseptic, antiputrescent, antiseborrheic, aphrodisiac, astringent, diuretic, expectorant, fungicidal, mucolytic, sedative (nervous), stimulant (circulatory), tonic.

EXTRACTION Essential oil by steam distillation from the wood, stumps and sawdust. A resinoid and absolute are also produced in small quantities.

CHARACTERISTICS A yellow, orange or deep amber viscous oil with a warm, camphoraceous top note and sweet tenacious, woody-balsamic undertone. It blends well with rosewood, bergamot, boronia, cypress, calamus, cassie, costus, jasmine, juniper, neroli, mimosa, labdanum, olibanum, clary sage, vetiver, rosemary, ylang ylang, oriental and floral bases.

PRINCIPAL CONSTITUENTS Atlantone, caryophyllene, cedrol, cadinene, among others.

SAFETY DATA Non-toxic, non-irritant, non-sensitizing. Best avoided during pregnancy.

AROMATHERAPY/HOME USE
SKIN CARE: Acne, dandruff, dermatitis, eczema, fungal infections, greasy skin, hair loss, skin eruptions, ulcers.

CIRCULATION, MUSCLES AND JOINTS: Arthritis, rheumatism.
RESPIRATORY SYSTEM: Bronchitis, catarrh, congestion, coughs.
GENITO-URINARY SYSTEM: Cystitis, leucorrhoea, pruritis.
NERVOUS SYSTEM: Nervous tension and stress-related conditions.

OTHER USES Fragrance component and fixative in cosmetics and household products, soaps, detergents, etc, as well as in perfumes, especially men's fragrances.

CEDARWOOD, TEXAS
Juniperus ashei

FAMILY Cupressaceae

SYNONYMS *J. mexicana*, mountain cedar, Mexican cedar, rock cedar, Mexican juniper.

GENERAL DESCRIPTION A small, alpine evergreen tree up to 7 metres high with stiff green needles and an irregular shaped trunk and branches, which tend to be crooked or twisted. The wood also tends to crack easily, so it is not used for timber.

DISTRIBUTION Native to south western USA, Mexico and Central America; the oil is produced mainly in Texas.

OTHER SPECIES The name *J. mexicana* has erroneously been applied to many species; botanically related to the so-called Virginian cedarwood (*J. virginiana*) and the East African cedarwood (*J. procera*).

HERBAL/FOLK TRADITION In New Mexico the native Indians use cedarwood oil for skin rashes. It is also used for arthritis and rheumatism.

ACTIONS Antiseptic, antispasmodic, astringent, diuretic, expectorant, sedative (nervous), stimulant (circulatory).

EXTRACTION Essential oil by steam distillation from the heartwood and wood shavings, etc. (Unlike the Virginian cedar, the tree is felled especially for its essential oil.)

CHARACTERISTICS Crude – a dark orange to brownish viscous liquid with a smoky-woody, sweet tar-like odour. Rectified – a colourless or pale yellow liquid with a sweet, balsamic, 'pencil-wood' scent, similar to Virginian cedarwood but harsher. It blends well with patchouli, spruce, vetiver, pine and leather-type scents.

PRINCIPAL CONSTITUENTS Cedrene, cedrol (higher than the Virginian oil), thujopsene and sabinene, among others. Otherwise similar to Virginian cedarwood.

SAFETY DATA See *Virginian cedarwood*.

AROMATHERAPY/HOME USE See *Virginian cedarwood*.

OTHER USES See *Virginian cedarwood*.

CEDARWOOD, VIRGINIAN
Juniperus virginiana

FAMILY Cupressaceae

SYNONYMS Red cedar, eastern red cedar, southern red cedar, Bedford cedarwood (oil).

GENERAL DESCRIPTION A coniferous, slow-growing, evergreen tree up to 33 metres high with a narrow, dense and pyramidal crown, a reddish heartwood and brown cones. The tree can attain a majestic stature with a trunk diameter of over 1.5 metres.

DISTRIBUTION Native to North America, especially mountainous regions east of the Rocky Mountains.

OTHER SPECIES There are many cultivars of the red cedar; its European relative is the shrubby red cedar (*J. sabina*) also known as savin – see entry. It is also closely related to the East African cedarwood (*J. procera*).

HERBAL/FOLK TRADITION The North American Indians used it for respiratory infections, especially those involving an excess of catarrh. Decoctions of leaves, bark, twigs and fruit were used to treat a variety of ailments: menstrual delay, rheumatism, arthritis, skin rashes, venereal warts, gonorrhoea, pyelitis and kidney infections.

  It is an excellent insect and vermin repellent (mosquitoes, moths, woodworm, rats, etc.) and was once used with citronella as a commercial insecticide.

ACTIONS Abortifacient, antiseborrhoeic, antiseptic (pulmonary, genito-urinary), antispasmodic, astringent, balsamic, diuretic, emmenagogue, expectorant, insecticide, sedative (nervous), stimulant (circulatory).

EXTRACTION Essential oil by steam distillation from the timber waste, sawdust, shavings, etc. (At one time a superior oil was distilled from the red heartwood, from trees over twenty five years old.)

CHARACTERISTICS A pale yellow or orange oily liquid with a mild, sweet-balsamic, 'pencil-wood' scent. It blends well with sandalwood, rose, juniper, cypress, vetiver, patchouli and benzoin.

PRINCIPAL CONSTITUENTS Mainly cedrene (up to 80 per cent), cedrol (3-14 per cent), and cedrenol, among others.

SAFETY DATA Externally the oil is relatively non-toxic; can cause acute local irritation and possible sensitization in some individuals. Use in dilution only with care, in moderation. 'The oil is a powerful abortifacient ... use of the oil has been fatal.'[29] Avoid during pregnancy. Generally safer to use Atlas cedarwood.

AROMATHERAPY/HOME USE
SKIN CARE: Acne, dandruff, eczema, greasy hair, insect repellent, oily skin, psoriasis.
CIRCULATION, MUSCLES AND JOINTS: Arthritis, rheumatism.

RESPIRATORY SYSTEM: Bronchitis, catarrh, congestion, coughs, sinusitis.
GENITO-URINRY SYSTEM: Cystitis, leucorrhoea.
NERVOUS SYSTEM: Nervous tension and stress related disorders.

OTHER USES Extensively used in room sprays and household insect repellents. Employed as a fragrance component in soaps, cosmetics and perfumes. Used as the starting material for the isolation of cedrene.

CELERY SEED
Apium graveolens

FAMILY Apiaceae (Umbelliferae)

SYNONYM Celery fruit.

GENERAL DESCRIPTION A familiar biennial plant, 30-60 cms high, with a grooved, fleshy, erect stalk, shiny pinnate leaves and umbels of white flowers.

DISTRIBUTION Native to southern Europe; extensively cultivated as a domestic vegetable. The oil is principally produced in India, and also Holland, China, Hungary and the USA.

OTHER SPECIES There are many cultivated varieties, such as celeriac root (*A. graveolens var. rapaceum*) and the salad vegetable (*A. graveolens var. dulce*).

HERBAL/FOLK TRADITION Celery seed is widely used as a domestic spice. The seed is used in bladder and kidney complaints, digestive upsets and menstrual problems; the leaves are used in skin ailments. It is known to increase the elimination of uric acid and is useful for gout, neuralgia and rheumatoid arthritis. A remedy for hepatobiliary disorders, it has been found to have a regenerating effect on the liver.

  Current in the British Herbal Pharmacopoeia as a specific for rheumatoid arthritis with mental depression.

ACTIONS Anti-oxidative, antirheumatic, antiseptic (urinary), antispasmodic, aperitif, depurative, digestive, diuretic, carminative, cholagogue, emmenagogue, galactagogue, hepatic, nervine, sedative (nervous), stimulant (uterine), stomachic, tonic (digestive).

EXTRACTION Essential oil by steam distillation from the whole or crushed seeds. (An oil from the whole herb, an oleoresin and extract are also produced in small quantities.)

CHARACTERISTICS A pale yellow or orange oil with a spicy-warm, sweet, long-lasting odour. It blends well with lavender, pine, opopanax, lovage, tea tree, oakmoss, coriander and other spices.

PRINCIPAL CONSTITUENTS Limonene (60 per cent), apiol, selinene, santalol, sedanolide and sedanolic acid anhydride, among others.

SAFETY DATA Non-toxic, non-irritant, possible sensitization. Avoid during pregnancy.

AROMATHERAPY/HOME USE
CIRCULATION, MUSCLES AND JOINTS: Arthritis, build-up of toxins in the blood, gout, rheumatism.
DIGESTIVE SYSTEM: Dyspepsia, flatulence, indigestion, liver congestion, jaundice.
GENITO-URINARY AND ENDOCRINE SYSTEMS: Amenorrhoea, glandular problems, increases milk flow, cystitis.
NERVOUS SYSTEM: Neuralgia, sciatica.

OTHER USES Used in tonic, sedative and carminative preparations, and as a fragrance component in soaps, detergents, cosmetics and perfumes. Extensively used as a flavouring agent in foods, especially by the spice industry, and in alcoholic and soft drinks.

CHAMOMILE, GERMAN
Matricaria recutica

FAMILY Asteraceae (Compositae)

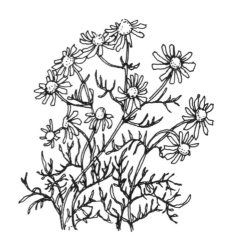

German Chamomile

SYNONYMS *M. chamomilla*, camomile, blue chamomile, matricaria, Hungarian chamomile, sweet false chamomile, single chamomile, chamomile blue (oil).

GENERAL DESCRIPTION An annual, strongly aromatic herb, up to 60 cms tall with a hairless, erect, branching stem. It has delicate feathery leaves and simple daisy-like white flowers on single stems. In appearance it is very similar to the corn chamomile (*Anthemis arvensis*) but can be distinguished from it because the latter is scentless.

DISTRIBUTION Native to Europe and north and west Asia; naturalized in North America and Australia. It is cultivated extensively, especially in Hungary and eastern Europe, where the oil is produced. It is no longer grown in Germany, despite the herbal name.

OTHER SPECIES There are many varieties of chamomile, such as the pineapple weed (*Chamaemelium suaveolens*) and the Roman chamomile (*C. nobile*), both of which are used to produce an essential oil.

HERBAL/FOLK TRADITION This herb has a long-standing medicinal tradition, especially in Europe for 'all states of tension and the visceral symptoms that can arise therefrom, such as nervous dyspepsia and nervous bowel, tension headaches, and sleeplessness; especially useful for all children's conditions, calming without depressing ...'[20]

An excellent skin care remedy, it has many of the same qualities as Roman chamomile, except that its anti-inflammatory properties are greater due to the higher percentage of azulene.

ACTIONS Analgesic, anti-allergenic, anti-inflammatory, antiphlogistic, antispasmodic, bactericidal, carlminative, cicatrisant, cholagogue, digestive, emmenagogue, febrifuge, fungicidal, hepatic, nerve sedative, stimulant of leucocyte production, stomachic, sudorific, vermifuge, vulnerary.

EXTRACTION Essential oil by steam distillation from the flower heads (up to 1.9 per cent yield). An absolute is also produced in small quantities, which is a deeper blue colour and has greater tenacity and fixative properties.

CHARACTERISTICS An inky-blue viscous liquid with a strong, sweetish warm-herbaceous odour. It blends well with geranium, lavender, patchouli, rose, benzoin, neroli, bergamot, marjoram, lemon, ylang ylang, jasmine, clary sage and labdanum.

PRINCIPAL CONSTITUENTS Chamazulene, farnesene, bisabolol oxide, en-yndicycloether, among others. (NB The chamazulene is not present in the fresh flower but is only produced during the process of distillation.)

SAFETY DATA Non-toxic, non-irritant; causes dermatitis in some individuals.

AROMATHERAPY/HOME USE
SKIN CARE: Acne, allergies, boils, burns, cuts, chilblains, dermatitis, earache, eczema, hair care, inflammations, insect bites, rashes, sensitive skin, teething pain, toothache, wounds.
CIRCULATION, MUSCLES AND JOINTS: Arthritis, inflamed joints, muscular pain, neuralgia, rheumatism, sprains.
DIGESTIVE SYSTEM: Dyspepsia, colic, indigestion, nausea.
GENITO-URINARY SYSTEM: Dysmenorrhoea, menopausal problems, menorrhagia.

NERVOUS SYSTEM: Headache, insomnia, nervous tension, migraine and stress-related complaints.

OTHER USES Used in pharmaceutical antiseptic ointments and in carminative, antispasmodic and tonic preparations. Extensively used in cosmetics, soaps, detergents, high-class perfumes and hair and bath products. Used as a flavour ingredient in most major food categories, including alcoholic and soft drinks.

CHAMOMILE, MAROC
Ormenis multicaulis

FAMILY Asteraceae (Compositae)

SYNONYMS O. *mixta*, *Anthemis mixta*, Moroccan chamomile.

GENERAL DESCRIPTION A handsome plant, 90 to 125 cms high with very hairy leaves and tubular yellow flowers, surrounded by white ligulets.

DISTRIBUTION Native to north west Africa and southern Spain, having probably evolved from the very common *Ormenis* species which grows all around the Mediterranean. Also found growing on the plains in Israel. The oil is distilled in Morocco.

OTHER SPECIES It is distantly related to the German and Roman chamomile botanically, although it does not resemble them physically.

HERBAL/FOLK TRADITION This is one of the more recent oils to appear on the market, and as such it does not have a long history of usage. The oil is often mistaken for a 'true' chamomile, though it should more correctly be called 'Ormenis oil' since: 'Chemically and olfactorily, the oil is distinctly different from the German or the Roman chamomile oils, and cannot be considered as a replacement for them.'[21]

ACTIONS Antispasmodic, cholagogue, emmenagogue, hepatic, sedative.

EXTRACTION Essential oil by steam distillation from the flowering tops.

CHARACTERISTICS Pale yellow to brownish yellow mobile liquid with a fresh-herbaceous top note and a sweet rich-balsamic undertone. It blends well with cypress, lavender, lavandin, vetiver, cedarwood, oakmoss, labdanum, olibanum and artemisia oils.

PRINCIPAL CONSTITUENTS Unknown.

SAFETY DATA Generally non-toxic and non-irritant – more specific safety data is unavailable at present.

AROMATHERAPY/HOME USE 'Sensitive skin, colic, colitis, headache, insomnia, irritability, migraine, amenorrhoea, dysmenorrhoea, menopause, liver and spleen congestion.'[22] Little is known about its therapeutic history and usage.

OTHER USES Employed extensively in perfumery work, especially in colognes, chyprès and fougere fragrance.

CHAMOMILE, ROMAN
Chamaemelum nobile

FAMILY Asteraceae (Compositae)

SYNONYMS *Anthemis nobilis*, camomile, English chamomile, garden chamomile, sweet chamomile, true chamomile.

GENERAL DESCRIPTION A small, stocky, perennial herb, up to 25 cms high, with a much-branched hairy stem, half spreading or creeping. It has feathery pinnate leaves, daisy-like white flowers which are larger than those of the German chamomile. The whole plant has an applelike scent.

DISTRIBUTION Native to southern and western Europe; naturalized in North America. Cultivated in England, Belgium, Hungary, United States, Italy and France.

OTHER SPECIES There are a great many varieties of chamomile found throughout the world, four of which are native to the British Isles, but the only one of these used therapeutically is the Roman chamomile (*C. nobile*).

HERBAL/FOLK TRADITION This herb has had a medical reputation in Europe and especially in the Mediterranean region for over 2000 years, and it is still in widespread use. It was employed by the ancient Egyptians and the Moors, and it was one of the Saxons' nine sacred herbs, which they called 'maythen'. It was also held to be the 'plant's physician', since it promoted the health of plants nearby.
It is current in the British Herbal Pharmacopoeia for the treatment of dyspepsia, nausea, anorexia, vomiting in pregnancy, dysmenorrhoea and specifically flatulent dyspepsia associated with mental stress.

ACTIONS Analgesic, anti-anaemic, antineuralgic, antiphlogistic, antiseptic, antispasmodic, bactericidal, carminative, cholagogue, cicatrisant, digestive, emmenagogue, febrifuge, hepatic, hypnotic, nerve sedative, stomachic, sudorific, tonic, vermifuge, vulnerary.

EXTRACTION Essential oil by steam distillation of the flower heads.

CHARACTERISTICS A pale blue liquid (turning yellow on keeping) with a warm, sweet, fruity-herbaceous scent. It blends well with bergamot, clary sage, oakmoss, jasmine, labdanum, neroli, rose, geranium and lavender.

PRINCIPAL CONSTITUENTS Mainly esters of angelic and tiglic acids (approx. 85 per cent), with pinene, farnesol, nerolidol, chamazulene, pinocarvone, cineol, among others.

SAFETY DATA Non-toxic, non-irritant; can cause dermatitis in some individuals.

AROMATHERAPY/HOME USE See *German chamomile*.

OTHER USES See *German chamomile*.

CHERVIL
Anthriscus cerefolium

FAMILY Apiaceae (Umbelliferae)

SYNONYMS *A. longirostris*, garden chervil, salad chervil.

GENERAL DESCRIPTION A delicate annual herb up to 30 cms high, with a slender, much branched stem, bright green, finely-divided, fern-like leaves, umbels of flat white flowerheads and long smooth seeds or fruits. The whole plant has a pleasing aromatic scent when bruised.

DISTRIBUTION Native to Europe and western Asia; naturalized in America, Australia and New Zealand. Widely cultivated, especially in southern Europe and America.

OTHER SPECIES A cultivated form of its wild relative, the wild chervil or garden-beaked parsley *(A. sylvestris)*, with which it shares similar properties and uses. Not to be confused with another common garden herb sweet cicely *(Myrrhis odorata)*, also known as sweet or smooth chervil.

HERBAL/FOLK TRADITION The name *chervil* comes from the Greek 'to rejoice', due to its delightful scent. The leaves are used as a domestic spice in salads, soups, omelettes, sauces and to flavour bread dough. In folk medicine it is used as a tea to ' tone up the blood and nerves. Good for poor memory and mental depression. Sweetens the entire digestive system.'[30]
The juice from the fresh herb is used to treat skin ailments such as eczema, abscesses and slow-healing wounds; also used for dropsy, arthritis and gout, among others.

ACTIONS Aperitif, antiseptic, carminative, cicatrisant, depurative, diaphoretic, digestive, diuretic, nervine, restorative, stimulant (metabolism), stomachic, tonic.

EXTRACTION Essential oil by steam distillation from seeds or fruit.

CHARACTERISTICS A pale yellow liquid with a sweet-herbaceous, anisic odour.

PRINCIPAL CONSTITUENTS Mainly methyl chavicol, also 1-allyl-2,4-dimethoxybenzene and anethole, among others.

SAFETY DATA Methyl chavicol and anethole are known to have toxic and irritant effects; methyl chavicol is reported to have possible carcinogenic effects. Since these constitute the major proportion of the essential oil, it is best avoided for therapeutic use.

AROMATHERAPY/HOME USE None.

OTHER USES Extensively employed as a flavour ingredient by the food industry, especially in meat products, as well as in alcoholic and soft drinks.

CINNAMON
Cinnamomum zeylanicum

FAMILY Lauraceae

SYNONYMS *C. verum*, *Laurus cinnamomum*, Ceylon cinnamon, Seychelles cinnamon, Madagascar cinnamon, true cinnamon, cinnamon leaf (oil), cinnamon bark (oil).

GENERAL DESCRIPTION A tropical evergreen tree up to 15 metres high, with strong branches and thick scabrous bark with young shoots speckled greeny-orange. It has shiny green, leathery leaves, small white flowers and oval bluish-white berries. The leaves have a spicy smell when bruised.

DISTRIBUTION Native to Sri Lanka, Madagascar, the Comoro Islands, South India, Burma and Indochina. It is also cultivated in India, Jamaica and Africa – each region tending to have its own particular species.

OTHER SPECIES Madagascar cinnamon is considered superior to the various other types of

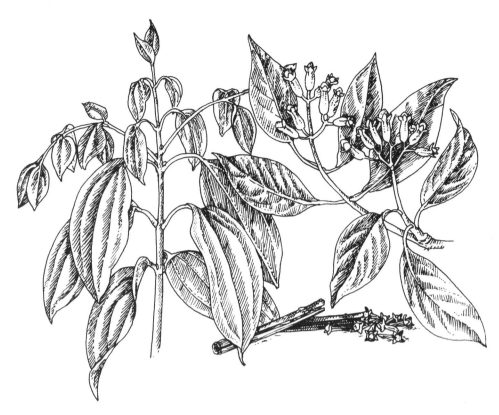

Cinnamon and Clove

cinnamon such as the Saigon cinnamon
(C. loureirii) and the Batavia Cinnamon
(C. burmanii). See also Botanical Classification
section.

HERBAL/FOLK TRADITION The inner bark
of the new shoots from the cinnamon tree are
gathered every two years and sold in the form of
sticks for use as a domestic spice. It has been
used for thousands of years in the east for a wide
range of complaints including colds, 'flu,
digestive and menstrual problems, rheumatism,
kidney troubles and as a general stimulant.
   Current in the British Herbal Pharmacopoeia
as a specific for flatulent colic and dyspepsia
with nausea.

ACTIONS Anthelmintic, antidiarrhoeal,
antidote (to poison), antimicrobial, antiseptic,
antispasmodic, antiputrescent, aphrodisiac,
astringent, carminative, digestive,
emmenagogue, haemostatic, orexigenic,
parasiticide, refrigerant, spasmolytic, stimulant

(circulatory, cardiac, respiratory), stomachic,
vermifuge.

EXTRACTION Essential oil by water or steam
distillation from the 1. leaves and twigs, and
2. dried inner bark.

CHARACTERISTICS 1. A yellow to brownish
liquid with a warm-spicy, somewhat harsh
odour. 2. A pale to dark yellow liquid with a
sweet, warm-spicy, dry, tenacious odour. It
blends well with olibanum, ylang ylang, orange,
mandarin, benzoin, Peru balsam and in oriental-
type mixtures.

PRINCIPAL CONSTITUENTS 1. Leaf –
eugenol (80–96 per cent), eugenol acetate,
cinnamaldehyde (3 per cent), benzyl benzoate,
linalol, safrol among others. 2. Bark -
cinnamaldehyde (40–50 per cent), eugenol
(4–10 per cent), benzaldehyde, cuminaldehyde,
pinene, cineol, phellandrene, furfurol, cymene,
linalol, among others.

SAFETY DATA 1. The leaf oil is relatively non-toxic, though possibly irritant due to cinnamaldehyde. Its major component, eugenol, causes irritation to the mucous membranes: use in moderation. 2. The bark oil is a dermal toxin, irritant and sensitizer; also irritant to the mucous membranes. 'Should never be used on the skin (one of the most hazardous oils).'[31]

AROMATHERAPY/HOME USE
Cinnamon bark oil – none.
Cinnamon leaf oil:
SKIN CARE: Lice, scabies, tooth and gum care, warts, wasp stings.
CIRCULATION, MUSCLES AND JOINTS: Poor circulation, rheumatism.
DIGESTIVE SYSTEM: Anorexia, colitis, diarrhoea, dyspepsia, intestinal infection, sluggish digestion, spasm.
GENITO-URINARY SYSTEM: Childbirth (stimulates contractions), frigidity, leucorrhoea, metrorrhagia, scanty periods.
IMMUNE SYSTEM: Chills, colds, 'flu, infectious diseases.
NERVOUS SYSTEM: Debility, nervous exhaustion and stress-related conditions.

OTHER USES Both bark and leaf oils are used for their fragrance and therapeutic actions in toothpastes, nasal sprays, mouthwashes, cough syrups and dental preparations. The leaf oil is used in soaps, cosmetics, toiletries and perfumes. Both are used extensively in food flavouring, especially in alcoholic and soft drinks, including Coca Cola.

CITRONELLA
Cymbopogon nardus

FAMILY Poaceae (Gramineae)

SYNONYMS *Andropogon nardus*, Sri Lanka citronella, Lenabatu citronella.

GENERAL DESCRIPTION A tall, aromatic, perennial grass, which has derived from the wild-growing 'managrass' found in Sri Lanka.

DISTRIBUTION Native to Sri Lanka, now extensively cultivated on the southernmost tip of the country.

OTHER SPECIES An important essential oil is also produced on a large scale from the Java or Maha Pengiri citronella *(C. winterianus)*. This variety is cultivated in the tropics worldwide, especially in Java, Vietnam, Africa, Argentina and Central America. There are many other related species of scented grasses.

HERBAL/FOLK TRADITION The leaves of citronella are used for their aromatic and medicinal value in many cultures, for fever, intestinal parasites, digestive and menstrual problems, as a stimulant and an insect repellent. It is used in Chinese traditional medicine for rheumatic pain.

ACTIONS Antiseptic, antispasmodic, bactericidal, deodorant, diaphoretic, diuretic, emmenagogue, febrifuge, fungicidal, insecticide, stomachic, tonic, vermifuge.

EXTRACTION Essential oil by steam distillation of the fresh, part-dried or dried grass. (The Java citronella yields twice as much oil as the Sri Lanka type.)

CHARACTERISTICS A yellowy-brown, mobile liquid with a fresh, powerful, lemony scent. The Java oil is colourless to pale yellow with a fresh, woody-sweet fragrance; it is considered of superior quality in perfumery work. It blends well with geranium, lemon, bergamot, orange, cedarwood and pine.

PRINCIPAL CONSTITUENTS Mainly geraniol(up to 45 per cent in the Java oil), citronellal (up to 50 per cent in the Java oil) with geranyl acetate, limonene and camphene, among others. The Sri Lanka variety contains more monoterpene hydrocarbons.

SAFETY DATA Non-toxic, non-irritant; may cause dermatitis in some individuals. Avoid during pregnancy.

AROMATHERAPY/HOME USE
SKIN CARE: Excessive perspiration, oily skin,

insect repellant. 'Mixed with cedarwood oil Virginia, it has been a popular remedy against mosquito attacks for many years prior to the appearance of DDT and other modern insecticides.'[23]

IMMUNE SYSTEM: Colds, 'flu, minor infections.
NERVOUS SYSTEM: Fatigue, headaches, migraine, neuralgia.

OTHER USES Extensively used in soaps, detergents, household goods and industrial perfumes. Employed in insect repellent formulations against moths, ants, fleas, etc, for use in the home and in the garden
   The Sri Lanka oil is used in most major food categories, including alcoholic and soft drinks. The Java oil is used as the starting material for the isolation of natural geraniol and citronellal.

CLOVE
Syzygium aromaticum

FAMILY Myrtaceae

SYNONYMS *Eugenia aromatica, E. caryophyllata, E. caryophyllus.*

GENERAL DESCRIPTION A slender evergreen tree with a smooth grey trunk, up to 12 metres high. It has large bright green leaves standing in pairs on short stalks. At the start of the rainy season long buds appear with a rosy-pink corolla at the tip; as the corolla fades the calyx slowly turns deep red. These are beaten from the tree and, when dried provide the cloves of commerce.

DISTRIBUTION Believed to be native to Indonesia; now cultivated worldwide, especially in the Philippines, the Molucca Islands and Madagascar. The main oil-producing countries are Madagascar, and Indonesia.

OTHER SPECIES The clove tree has been cultivated in plantations for over 2000 years. The original wild trees found in the Moluccas, produce an essential oil that contains no eugenol at all.

HERBAL/FOLK TRADITION Extensively used as a domestic spice worldwide. Tincture of cloves has been used for skin infections (scabies, athlete's foot); for digestive upsets; to dress the umbilical cord; for intestinal parasites; to ease the pain of childbirth (steeped in wine); and notably for toothache. The tea is used to relieve nausea.
   In Chinese medicine the oil is used for diarrhoea, hernia, bad breath and bronchitis as well as for those conditions mentioned above. In Indonesia, the 'Kretak' cigarette is popular, made from two parts tobacco and one part cloves.

ACTIONS Anthelmintic, antibiotic, anti-emetic, antihistaminic, antirheumatic, antineuralgic, anti-oxidant, antiseptic, antiviral, aphrodisiac, carminative, counter-irritant, expectorant, larvicidal, spasmolytic, stimulant, stomachic, vermifuge.

EXTRACTION Essential oil by water distillation from the 1. buds and 2. leaves, and by steam distillation from the 3. stalks or stems. A concrete, absolute and oleoresin are also produced from the buds in small quantities.

CHARACTERISTICS 1. Clove bud is a pale yellow liquid with a sweet-spicy odour and a fruity-fresh top note. The bud oil is favoured in perfumery work. It blends well with rose, lavender, vanillin, clary sage, bergamot, bay leaf, lavandin, allspice, ylang ylang and cananga. 2. Clove leaf is a dark brown oil with a crude, burnt-woody odour. 3. Clove stem oil is a pale yellow liquid with a strong spicy-woody odour.

PRINCIPAL CONSTITUENTS 1. Bud: 60–90 per cent eugenol, eugenyl acetate, caryophyllene and other minor constituents. 2. Leaf: 82–88 per cent eugenol with little or no eugenyl acetate, and other minor constituents. 3. Stem: 90–95 per cent eugenol, with other minor constituents.

SAFETY DATA All clove oils can cause skin and mucous membrane irritation; clove bud and stem oil may cause dermatitis in some individuals. Clove bud is the least toxic of the three oils due to the lower eugenol percentage. Use in moderation only in low dilution (less than 1 per cent).

AROMATHERAPY/HOME USE Only use clove bud oil, not the leaf or stem oil.

SKIN CARE: Acne, athlete's foot, bruises, burns, cuts, insect repellent (mosquito), toothache, ulcers, wounds.

CIRCULATION, MUSCLES AND JOINTS: Arthritis, rheumatism, sprains.

RESPIRATORY SYSTEM: Asthma, bronchitis.

DIGESTIVE SYSTEM: Colic, dyspepsia, nausea.

IMMUNE SYSTEM: Colds, 'flu, minor infections.

OTHER USES Used in dental preparations, and as a fragrance component in toothpastes, soaps, toiletries, cosmetics and perfumes. Extensively employed as a flavour ingredient in major food categories, alcoholic and soft drinks. Used in the production of printing ink, glue and varnish; clove leaf oil is used as the starting material for the isolation of eugenol.

CORIANDER
Coriandrum sativum

FAMILY Apiaceae (Umbelliferae)

SYNONYMS Coriander seed, Chinese parsley.

GENERAL DESCRIPTION A strongly aromatic annual herb about 1 metre high with bright green delicate leaves, umbels of lacelike white flowers, followed by a mass of green (turning brown) round seeds.

DISTRIBUTION Native to Europe and western Asia; naturalized in North America. Cultivated throughout the world, the oil is mainly produced in the USSR, Yugoslavia and Romania.

OTHER SPECIES Various chemotypes of the same species are found according to geographical location.

HERBAL/FOLK TRADITION A herb with a long history of use the seeds were found in the ancient Egyptian tomb of Rameses II. The seeds and leaves are widely used as a garnish and domestic spice, especially in curries. It has been used therapeutically, mainly in the form of an infusion for children's diarrhoea, digestive upsets, griping pains, anorexia and flatulence.

In Chinese medicine the whole herb is used for dysentery, piles, measles, nausea, toothache and for painful hernia.

ACTIONS Analgesic, aperitif, aphrodisiac, anti-oxidant, anti-rheumatic, antispasmodic, bactericidal, depurative, digestive, carminative, cytotoxic, fungicidal, larvicidal, lipolytic, revitalizing, stimulant (cardiac, circulatory, nervous system), stomachic.

EXTRACTION Essential oil by steam distillation from the crushed ripe seeds. (An essential oil is also produced by steam distillation from the fresh and dried leaves, which contains a high proportion of decyl aldehyde.)

CHARACTERISTICS A colourless to pale yellow liquid with a sweet, woody-spicy, slightly musky fragrance. It blends well with clary sage, bergamot, jasmine, olibanum, neroli, petitgrain, citronella, sandalwood, cypress, pine, ginger, cinnamon and other spice oils.

PRINCIPAL CONSTITUENTS Mainly linalol (55-75 per cent), decyl aldehyde, borneol, geraniol, carvone, anethole, among others; constituents; vary according to source.

SAFETY DATA Generally non-toxic, non-irritant, non-sensitizing. Stupefying in large doses – use in moderation.

AROMATHERAPY/HOME USE

CIRCULATION, MUSCLES AND JOINTS: Accumulation of fluids or toxins, arthritis, gout, muscular aches and pains, poor circulation, rheumatism, stiffness.

DIGESTIVE SYSTEM: Anorexia, colic, diarrhoea, dyspepsia, flatulence, nausea, piles, spasm.

IMMUNE SYSTEM: Colds, 'flu, infections (general), measles.

NERVOUS SYSTEM: Debility, migraine, neuralgia, nervous exhaustion.

OTHER USES Used as a flavouring agent in pharmaceutical preparations, especially digestive remedies. Used as a fragrance component in soaps, toiletries and perfumes. Employed by the food industry especially in meat products and to flavour liqueurs such as Chartreuse and Benedictine; also used for flavouring tobacco.

COSTUS
Saussurea costus

FAMILY Asteraceae (Compositae)

SYNONYMS *S. lappa, Aucklandia costus, Aplotaxis lappa, A. auriculata.*

GENERAL DESCRIPTION A large, erect, perennial plant up to 2 metres high with a thick tapering root and numerous almost black flowers.

DISTRIBUTION Native to northern India; cultivated in India and south west China. The oil is mainly produced in India.

OTHER SPECIES Closely related to elecampane *(Inula helenium)*, whose roots are also used to produce an essential oil.

HERBAL/FOLK TRADITION The root has been used for millennia in India and China for digestive complaints, respiratory conditions, as a stimulant and for infection including typhoid and cholera. It is also used as an incense.

ACTIONS Antiseptic, antispasmodic, antiviral, bactericidal, carminative, digestive, expectorant, febrifuge, hypotensive, stimulant, stomachic, tonic.

EXTRACTION The dried roots are macerated in warm water, then subjected to steam distillation followed by solvent extraction of the distilled water. (A concrete and absolute are also produced in small quantities.)

CHARACTERISTICS A pale yellow or brownish viscous liquid of soft, woody-musty, extremely tenacious odour. It blends well with patchouli, opopanax, ylang ylang, oriental and floral fragrances.

PRINCIPAL CONSTITUENTS Mainly sesquiterpene lactones, including dihydrocostus lactone and costunolide (together up to 50 per cent), other sesquiterpenes such as costols, caryophyllene and selinene, as well as costic and oleic acids, among others.

SAFETY DATA Non-toxic, non-irritant, possible sensitization in some individuals. Subject to frequent adulteration.

AROMATHERAPY/HOME USE
SKIN CARE: Perfume.
RESPIRATORY SYSTEM: Asthma, bronchitis, spasmodic cough.
DIGESTIVE SYSTEM: Flatulence, indigestion, spasm.
NERVOUS SYSTEM: Debility, nervous exhaustion and stress-related conditions.

OTHER USES Fixative and fragrance component in cosmetics and perfumes. Used as a flavour ingredient by the food industry, especially in confectionery, alcoholic and soft drinks.

CUBEBS
Piper cubeba

FAMILY Piperaceae

SYNONYMS *Cubeba officinalis,* cubeba, tailed pepper, cubeb berry, false pepper.

GENERAL DESCRIPTION An evergreen climbing vine up to 6 metres high with heart-shaped leaves. Altogether similar to the black pepper plant, except that the fruit or seeds of the cubeb retain their peduncle or stem – thus the name, tailed pepper.

DISTRIBUTION Native to Indonesia, cultivated throughout south east Africa, usually together with coffee crops. The oil is mainly produced at source in Indonesia.

OTHER SPECIES Closely related to the black pepper plant *(P. nigrum)* and to the South American matico *(P. augustifolium)*. There are also many other related species grown in Indonesia which are, often used for adulteration, such as false cubebs *(P. crassipes)*.

HERBAL/FOLK TRADITION The seeds are used locally as a domestic spice. It has been traditionally used for treating genito-urinary infections, such as gonorrhoea, cystitis, urethritis, abscess of the prostate gland and leucorrhoea. It is also used for digestive upsets and respiratory problems such as chronic bronchitis. The seeds have a local stimulating effect on the mucous membrane of the urinary and respiratory tracts, and the powder was found '90 per cent clinically effective in treating amoebic dysentery'.[32]

ACTIONS Antiseptic (pulmonary, genito-urinary), antispasmodic, antiviral, bactericidal, carminative, diuretic, expectorant, stimulant.

EXTRACTION Essential oil by steam distillation from the unripe but fully grown fruits or berries. (An oleoresin is also produced in small quantities.)

CHARACTERISTICS A pale greenish or bluish-yellow viscous liquid with a warm woody-spicy, slightly camphoraceous odour. It blends well with cananga, galbanum, lavender, rosemary, black pepper, allspice and other spices.

PRINCIPAL CONSTITUENTS Mainly sesquiterpenes and monoterpenes which include caryophyllene, cadinene, cubebene, sabinene, among others.

SAFETY DATA Non-toxic, non-irritant, non-sensitizing. Frequently subject to adulteration.

AROMATHERAPY/HOME USE
RESPIRATORY SYSTEM: Bronchitis, catarrh, congestion, chronic coughs, sinusitis, throat infections.

DIGESTIVE SYSTEM: Flatulence, indigestion, piles, sluggish digestion.
GENITO-URINARY SYSTEMS: Cystitis, leucorrhoea, urethritis.

OTHER USES Employed in diuretic and urinary antiseptic preparations and as a fragrance component in soaps, detergents, toiletries, cosmetics and perfumes. Used as a flavouring agent in most major food categories; also used for flavouring tobacco.

CUMIN
Cuminum cyminum

FAMILY Apiaceae (Umbelliferae)

SYNONYMS *C. odorum*, cummin, roman caraway.

GENERAL DESCRIPTION A small, delicate, annual herb about 50 cms high with a slender stem, dark green feathery leaves and small pink or white flowers followed by small oblong seeds.

DISTRIBUTION Native to upper Egypt, but from the earliest times cultivated in the Mediterranean region, especially Spain, France and Morocco; also in India and the USSR. The oil is mainly produced in India, Spain and France.

OTHER SPECIES Closely related to coriander *(Coriandrum sativum)*, with which it shares many properties.

HERBAL/FOLK TRADITION A traditional Middle Eastern spice, and one of the main ingredients of curry. Although it has gone out of use in Western herbalism it is still largely used in traditional Ayurvedic medicine, principally as a general stimulant but especially for digestive complaints such as colic, sluggish digestion and dyspepsia.

ACTIONS Anti-oxidant, antiseptic, antispasmodic, antitoxic, aphrodisiac, bactericidal, carminative, depurative, digestive, diuretic, emmenagogue, larvicidal, nervine, stimulant, tonic.

EXTRACTION Essential oil by steam distillation from the ripe seeds.

CHARACTERISTICS A pale yellow or greenish liquid with a warm, soft, spicy-musky scent. It blends well with lavender, lavandin, rosemary, galbanum, rosewood, cardomon and oriental-type fragrances.

PRINCIPAL CONSTITUENTS Mainly aldehydes (up to 60 per cent), including cuminaldehyde; monoterpene hydrocarbons (up to 52 per cent), including pinenes, terpinenes, cymene, phellandrene, myrcene and limonene; also farnesene and caryophyllene, among others.

SAFETY DATA Generally non-toxic, non-irritant and non-sensitizing; however the oil is phototoxic – do not expose treated skin to direct sunlight. Avoid during pregnancy.

AROMATHERAPY/HOME USE
CIRCULATION, MUSCLES AND JOINTS: Accumulation of fluids or toxins, poor circulation.
DIGESTIVE SYSTEM: Colic, dyspepsia, flatulence, indigestion, spasm.
NERVOUS SYSTEM: Debility, headaches, migraine, nervous exhaustion.

OTHER USES Used in veterinary medicine in digestive preparations. As a fragrance component in cosmetics and perfumes, and a flavour ingredient in many foods and drinks, especially meat products and condiments.

CYPRESS
Cupressus sempervirens

FAMILY Cupressaceae

SYNONYMS Italian cypress, Mediterranean cypress.

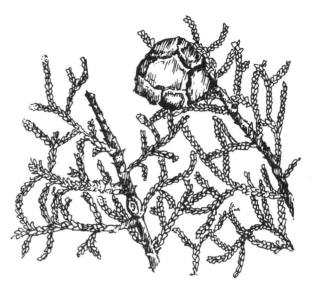

Cypress

GENERAL DESCRIPTION A tall evergreen tree with slender branches and a statuesque conical shape. It bears small flowers and round, brownish-grey cones or nuts.

DISTRIBUTION Native to the eastern Mediterranean; now grows wild in France, Italy, Corsica, Sardinia, Sicily, Spain, Portugal, North Africa, England and, to a lesser degree, the Balkan countries. Cultivation and distillation usually take place in France, also Spain and Morocco.

OTHER SPECIES There are many other species of cypress found throughout the world which are used to produce an essential oil, such as *C. lusitanica* found in Kenya. With regard to oil quality, however, *C. sempervirens* is considered superior.

HERBAL/FOLK TRADITION It was highly valued as a medicine and as an incense by ancient civilizations and it is still used as a purification incense by the Tibetans. It benefits the urinary system and is considered useful where there is excessive loss of fluid, such as heavy perspiration or menstrual loss and diarrhoea: 'The cones are ... very drying and binding, good to stop fluxes of all kinds.'[24]
  The Chinese consider the nuts very nutritious, beneficial for the liver and respiratory system and to check profuse perspiration.

ACTIONS Antirheumatic, antiseptic, antispasmodic, astringent, deodorant, diuretic, hepatic, styptic, sudorific, tonic, vasoconstrictive.

EXTRACTION Essential oil by steam distillation from the needles and twigs. An oil from the cones is available occasionally. (A concrete and absolute are also produced in small quantities.)

CHARACTERISTICS A pale yellow to greenish-olive mobile liquid with a smoky, sweet-balsamic tenacious odour. It blends well with cedarwood, pine, lavender, mandarin, clary sage, lemon, cardomon, Moroccan chamomile, ambrette seed, labdanum, juniper, benzoin, bergamot, orange, marjoram and sandalwood.

PRINCIPAL CONSTITUENTS Pinene, camphene, sylvestrene, cymene, sabinol, among others.

SAFETY DATA Non-toxic, non-irritant and non-sensitizing.

AROMATHERAPY/HOME USE
SKIN CARE: Haemorrhoids, oily and overhydrated skin, excessive perspiration, insect repellent, pyorrhoea (bleeding of the gums), varicose veins, wounds.
Circulation, Musles and Joints: Cellulitis, muscular cramp, oedema, poor circulation, rheumatism.
RESPIRATORY SYSTEM: Asthma, bronchitis, spasmodic coughing.
GENITO-URINARY SYSTEM: Dysmenorrhoea, menopausal problems, menorrhagia.
NERVOUS SYSTEM: Nervous tension and stress-related conditions.

OTHER USES Employed in some pharmaceutical products; used as a fragrance component in colognes, after-shaves and perfumes.

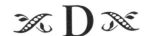

D

DEERTONGUE
Carphephorus odoratissimus

FAMILY Asteraceae (Compositae)

SYNONYMS *Trilisa odoratissima, Liatris odoratissima, Frasera speciosa,* hound's tongue, deer's tongue, Carolina vanilla, vanilla leaf, wild vanilla, vanilla trilisa, whart's tongue, liatrix (oleoresin or absolute).

GENERAL DESCRIPTION A herbaceous perennial plant distinguished by a naked receptacle and feathery pappus, with large, fleshy, dark green leaves, clasped at the base. When fresh, the leaves have little odour but when dried they acquire a vanilla-like odour, largely due to the coumarin that can be seen in crystals on the upper sides of the leaves.

DISTRIBUTION Native to eastern USA; gathered on the savannah land between North Carolina and Florida.

OTHER SPECIES There are several species of deertongue native to America, for example blazing star or prairie pine *(Liatris squarrosa),* and gayfeather *(L. spicata).* Not to be confused with the common vanilla *(Vanilla planifolia)* or with the European hound's tongue *(Cynoglossum officinale),* all of which have been used in herbal medicine.

HERBAL/FOLK TRADITION The roots have been used for their diuretic effects, and applied locally for sore throats and gonorrhoea. It has also been used as a tonic in treating malaria. In folklore the plant is associated with contraception and sterility in women.

ACTIONS Antiseptic, demulcent, diaphoretic, diuretic, febrifuge, stimulant, tonic.

EXTRACTION Oleoresin by solvent extraction from the dried leaves.

CHARACTERISTICS A dark green, heavy, viscous liquid with a rich, herbaceous, new-mown hay scent. It blends well with oakmoss, labdanum, lavandin, frankincense, clove, patchouli and oriental-type fragrances.

SPRINCIPAL CONSTITUENTS Mainly coumarin (1.6 per cent), with dihydrocoumarin and terpenes, aldehydes and ketones.

SAFETY DATA 'Coumarin has toxic properties including liver injury and haemorrhages.'[33] (There is also the possibility of dermal irritation and phototoxicity due to the lactones present.)

AROMATHERAPY/HOME USE None.

OTHER USES The oleoresin is used as a fixative and fragrance component in soaps, detergents and perfumery work. Used for flavouring tobacco and; also employed for the isolation of coumarin.

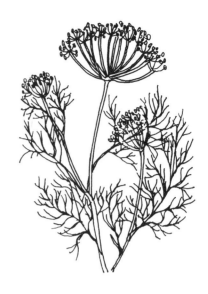

Dill

DILL
Anethum graveolens

FAMILY Apiaceae (Umbelliferae)

SYNONYMS *Peucedanum graveolens, Fructus anethi,* European dill, American dill.

GENERAL DESCRIPTION Annual or biennial herb up to 1 metre high with a smooth stem, feathery leaves and umbels of yellowish flowers followed by flat small seeds.

DISTRIBUTION Native to the Mediterranean and Black Sea regions; now cultivated worldwide, especially in Europe, USA, China and India. Dill seed oil is mainly produced in Europe (France, Hungary, Germany, England, Spain); dill weed oil in the USA.

OTHER SPECIES Indian dill or East Indian dill

(A. sowa) is widely cultivated in the east, especially in India and Japan. A commercial oil is produced from the seed which has a different chemical composition and contains 'dill apiol'.

HERBAL/FOLK TRADITION Used since the earliest times as a medicinal and culinary herb. In Germany and Scandinavia especially, it is used with fish and cucumber, and the seeds baked in bread. In the west and east it is used as a soothing digestive aid for indigestion, wind, colic etc. especially in children, for which it is still current in the British Herbal Pharmacopoeia.

ACTIONS Antispasmodic, bactericidal, carminative, digestive, emmenagogue, galactagogue, hypotensive, stimulant, stomachic.

EXTRACTION Essential oil by steam (sometimes water) distillation from 1. fruit or seed, 2. herb or weed (fresh or partially dried).

CHARACTERISTICS 1. A colourless to pale yellow mobile liquid with a light fresh warm-spicy scent. 2. A colourless or pale yellow mobile liquid with a powerful sweet-spicy aroma. It blends well with elemi, mint, caraway, nutmeg, spice and citrus oils.

PRINCIPAL CONSTITUENTS 1.Carvone (30–60 per cent), limonene, phellandrene, eugenol, pinene among others. 2. Carvone (much less), limonene, pinene, etc. as well as terpinene. There are several different chemotypes of dill, for example, phellandrene is present in the English and Spanish oils but not in the German.

SAFETY DATA Non-toxic, non-irritant, non-sensitizing.

AROMATHERAPY/HOME USE
DIGESTIVE SYSTEM: Colic, dyspepsia, flatulence, indigestion.
GENITO-URINARY AND ENDOCRINE SYSTEMS: Lack of periods; promotes milk flow in nursing mothers.

OTHER USES Used in some pharmaceutical digestive preparations such as 'dill water'. The weed oil is used as a fragrance component in detergents, cosmetics, perfumes and especially soaps. Both oils are used extensively in alcoholic, soft drinks and foodstuffs, especially pickles and condiments.

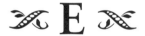

ELECAMPANE
Inula helenium

FAMILY Asteraceae (Compositae)

SYNONYMS *Helenium grandiflorum, Aster officinalis, A. helenium,* inula, scabwort, alant, horseheal, yellow starwort, elf dock, wild sunflower, velvet dock, 'essence d'aunee'.

GENERAL DESCRIPTION A handsome perennial herb up to 1.5 metres high, with a stout stem covered in soft hairs. It has oval pointed leaves which are velvety underneath, large, yellow, daisy-like flowers and large, fleshy rhizome roots.

DISTRIBUTION Native to Europe and Asia, naturalized in North America. Cultivated in Europe (Belgium, France, Germany) and Asia (China, India). The oil is mainly produced from imported roots in southern France.

OTHER SPECIES There are several varieties of *Inula*; the European and Asian species are slightly different having a harsher scent. Other varieties include golden samphire *(I. crithmoides)* and sweet inula *(I. graveolens* or *I. odora),* which share similar properties.

HERBAL/FOLK TRADITION A herb of ancient medical repute, which used to be candied and sold as a sweetmeat. It is used as an important spice, incense and medicine in the east. It is used in both western and eastern herbalism, mainly in the form of a tea for respiratory conditions such as asthma, bronchitis and whooping cough, disorders of the digestion, intestines and gall bladder and for skin disorders.

Current in the British Herbal Pharmacopoeia as a specific for irritating cough or bronchitis. Elecampane root is the richest source of inulin.

ACTIONS Alterative, anthelmintic, anti-inflammatory, antiseptic, antispasmodic, antitussive, astringent, bactericidal, diaphoretic, diuretic, expectorant, fungicidal, hyperglycaemic, hypotensive, stomachic, tonic.

EXTRACTION Essential oil by steam distillation from the dried roots and rhizomes. (An absolute and concrete are also produced in small quantities.)

CHARACTERISTICS A semi-solid or viscous dark yellow or brownish liquid with a dry, soft, woody, honey-like odour, often containing crystals. It blends well with cananga, cinnamon, labdanum, lavender, mimosa, frankincense, orris, tuberose, violet, cedarwood, patchouli, sandalwood, cypress, bergamot and oriental fragrances.

PRINCIPAL CONSTITUENTS Mainly sesquiterpene lactones, including alantolactone (or helenin), isolactone, dihydroisalantolactone, dihydralantolactone, alantic acid and azulene.

SAFETY DATA Non-toxic, non-irritant; however it is a severe dermal sensitizer. In clinical tests it caused 'extremely severe allergic reactions' in twenty-three out of twenty-five volunteers. On the basis of these results it is recommended that the oil 'should not used on the skin at all'.[34]

AROMATHERAPY/HOME USE None.

NB In *Phytoguide I*, sweet inula *(I. odora* or *I. graveolens)*, a deep green oil, is described as 'queen of mucolytic essential oils', having properties as diverse as:'anti-inflammatory, hyperthermic, sedative, cardio-regulative, diuretic and depurative'.[35] It is described as being an excellent oil for the cardiopulmonary zone including asthma, chronic bronchitis and unproductive coughs. This variety of *Inula* seems to avoid the sensitization problems of elecampane, at least when it is used as an inhalation or by aerosol treatment.

OTHER USES Alantolactone is used as an anthelmintic in Europe (it is also an excellent bactericide). The oil and absolute are used as fixatives and fragrance components in soaps, detergents, cosmetics and perfumes. Used as a flavour ingredient in alcoholic beverages, soft drinks and foodstuffs, especially desserts.

ELEMI
Canarium luzonicum

FAMILY Burseraceae

SYNONYMS *C. commune,* Manila elemi, elemi gum, elemi resin, elemi (oleoresin).

GENERAL DESCRIPTION A tropical tree up to 30 metres high which yields a resinous pathological exudation with a green pungent odour. Although it is called a gum, it is almost entirely made up of resin and essential oil.

DISTRIBUTION Native to the Philippine Islands and the Moluccas, where it is also cultivated. Distillation of the oil takes place at source.

OTHER SPECIES There are several other species of *Canarium* which grow wild or are cultivated in the Philippines, which also yield a 'gum'. It is also closely related to the trees yielding myrrh, frankincense and opopanax.

HERBAL/FOLK TRADITION The gum or oleoresin is used locally for skin care, respiratory complaints and as a general stimulant. Elemi was one of the aromatics used by the ancient Egyptians for the embalming process.

ACTIONS Antiseptic, balsamic, cicatrisant, expectorant, fortifying, regulatory, stimulant, stomachic, tonic.

EXTRACTION Essential oil by steam distillation from the gum. (A resinoid and resin absolute are also produced in small quantities.)

CHARACTERISTICS A colourless to pale yellow liquid with a light, fresh, balsamic-spicy, lemonlike odour. It blends well with myrrh, frankincense, labdanum, rosemary, lavender, lavandin, sage, cinnamon and other spices.

PRINCIPAL CONSTITUENTS The gum contains about 10–25 per cent essential oil of mainly phellandrene, dipentene, elemol, elemicin, terpineol, carvone and terpinolene among others.

SAFETY DATA Non-toxic, non-irritant, non-sensitizing.

AROMATHERAPY/HOME USE
SKIN CARE: Aged skin, infected cuts and

wounds, inflammations, rejuvenation, wrinkles – 'signifies drying and preservation'.[36]

RESPIRATORY SYSTEM: Bronchitis, catarrhal conditions, unproductive coughs.

NERVOUS SYSTEM: Nervous exhaustion and stress-related conditions.

OTHER USES Resinoid and oil are used primarily as fixatives but also as fragrance components in soaps, detergents, cosmetics and perfumes. Occasionally used as a flavouring ingredient in food products, alcoholic and soft drinks.

EUCALYPTUS, BLUE GUM
Eucalyptus globulus var. globulus

FAMILY Myrtaceae

SYNONYMS Gum tree, southern blue gum, Tasmanian blue gum, fever tree, stringy bark.

GENERAL DESCRIPTION A beautiful, tall, evergreen tree, up to 90 metres high. The young trees have bluish-green oval leaves while the mature trees develop long, narrow, yellowish leaves, creamy-white flowers and a smooth, pale grey bark often covered in a white powder.

DISTRIBUTION Native to Tasmania and Australia. Mainly cultivated in Spain and Portugal, also Brazil, California, Russia and China. Very little of this oil now comes from its native countries.

OTHER SPECIES There are over 700 different species of eucalyptus, of which at least 500 produce a type of essential oil. Many have been extracted simply for experimental purposes, and research is still being carried out with regard to the different constituents of each oil. In general, they can be divided into three categories. 1. The medicinal oils containing large amounts of cineol (or eucalyptol), such as the blue gum, but increasingly the blue malee *(E. polybractea)*, the narrow-leaved peppermint *(E. radiata var. australiana)* and the gully gum *(E. smithii)*.

2. The industrial oils containing mainly piperitone and phellandrene, such as the peppermint eucalyptus *(E. piperita)*, grey peppermint *(E. radiata var. phellandra)* and increasingly the broad-leaved peppermint *(E. dives var. Type)*. 3. The perfumery oils containing mainly citronellal, such as the lemon-scented eucalyptus *(E. citriodora)*. See also Botanical Classification section.

HERBAL/FOLK TRADITION A traditional household remedy in Australia, the leaves and oil are especially used for respiratory ailments such as bronchitis and croup, and the dried leaves are smoked like tobacco for asthma. It is also used for feverish conditions (malaria, typhoid, cholera, etc.) and skin problems like burns, ulcers and wounds. Aqueous extracts are used for aching joints, bacterial dysentery, ringworms, tuberculosis, etc. and employed for similar reasons in western and eastern medicine. The wood is also used for timber production in Spain.

ACTIONS Analgesic, antineuralgic, antirheumatic, antiseptic, antispasmodic, antiviral, balsamic, cicatrisant, decongestant, deodorant, depurative, diuretic, expectorant, febrifuge, hypoglycaemic, parasiticide, prophylactic, rubefacient, stimulant, vermifuge, vulnerary.

EXTRACTION Essential oil by steam distillation from the fresh or partially dried leaves and young twigs.

CHARACTERISTICS A colourless mobile liquid (yellows on ageing), with a somewhat harsh camphoraceous odour and woody-sweet undertone. It blends well with thyme, rosemary, lavender, marjoram, pine, cedarwood and lemon. (The narrow-leaved eucalyptus *(E. radiata var. australiana)* is often used in preference to the blue gum in aromatherapy work, being rich in cineol but with a sweeter and less harsh odour.)

PRINCIPAL CONSTITUENTS Cineol (70–85 per cent), pinene, limonene, cymene, phellandrene, terpinene, aromadendrene, among others.

SAFETY DATA Externally non-toxic, non-irritant (in dilution), non-sensitizing. 'When taken internally eucalyptus oil is toxic and as little as 3.5ml has been reported as fatal'.[37]

AROMATHERAPY/HOME USE
SKIN CARE: Burns, blisters, cuts, herpes, insect bites, insect repellent, lice, skin infections, wounds.
CIRCULATION, MUSCLES AND JOINTS: Muscular aches and pains, poor circulation, rheumatoid arthritis, sprains, etc.
RESPIRATORY SYSTEM: Asthma, bronchitis, catarrh, coughs, sinusitis, throat infections.
GENITO-URINARY SYSTEM: Cystitis, leucorrhoea.
IMMUNE SYSTEM: Chickenpox, colds, epidemics,'flu, measles.
NERVOUS SYSTEM: Debility, headaches, neuralgia.

OTHER USES The oil and cineol are largely employed in the preparation of liniments, inhalants, cough syrups, ointments, toothpaste and as pharmaceutical flavourings also used in veterinary practise and dentistry. Used as a fragrance component in soaps, detergents and toiletries – little used in perfumes. Used for the isolation of cineol and employed as a flavour ingredient in most major food categories.

EUCALYPTUS, LEMON-SCENTED
Eucalyptus citriodora

FAMILY Myrtaceae

SYNONYMS Lemon-scented gum, citron-scented gum, scented gum tree, spotted gum, 'boabo'.

GENERAL DESCRIPTION An attractive, tall, evergreen tree with a smooth dimpled bark, blotched in grey, cream and pink, cultivated as an ornamental. The trunk grows fast, straight and to considerable height, and is used for timber. The young leaves are oval, the mature leaves narrow and tapering.

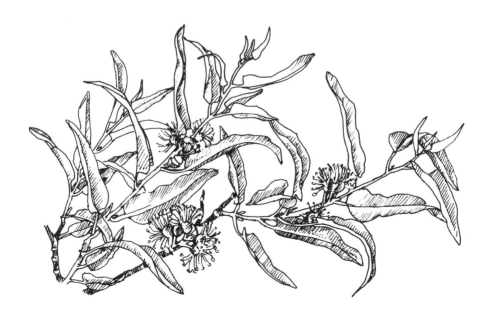

Eucalyptus, lemon-scented

DISTRIBUTION Native to Australia; cultivated mainly in Brazil and China.

OTHER SPECIES There are numerous other species of eucalyptus – see entry on eucalyptus blue gum. See also Botanical Classification section.

HERBAL/FOLK TRADITION Used traditionally for perfuming the linen cupboard by enclosing the dried leaves in a small cloth sachet. During the last century it was regarded as a good insect repellent, especially for cockroaches and silverfish.

ACTIONS Antiseptic, antiviral, bactericidal, deodorant, expectorant, fungicidal, insecticide.

EXTRACTION Essential oil by steam distillation from the leaves and twigs.

CHARACTERISTICS A colourless or pale yellow mobile liquid with a strong, fresh, citronella-like odour and sweet balsamic undertone.

PRINCIPAL CONSTITUENTS Citronellal (80–95 per cent), citronellol, geraniol and pinene, among others. (The gum or 'kino' contains the antibiotic substance 'citriodorol'.)

SAFETY DATA Non-toxic, non-irritant, possible sensitization in some individuals. Eucalyptus oil is toxic when taken internally, see eucalyptus blue gum entry.

AROMATHERAPY/HOME USE
SKIN CARE: Athlete's foot and other fungal infections (e.g. candida), cuts, dandruff, herpes, insect repellent, scabs, sores, wounds.
RESPIRATORY SYSTEM: Asthma, laryngitis, sore throat.
IMMUNE SYSTEM: Colds, fevers, infectious skin conditions such as chickenpox, infectious disease. 'The essential oil contained in the leaves appears to have bacteriostatic activity towards Staphylococcus aureus; this is due to synergism between the citronellol and citronellal present in the oil'.[38]

OTHER USES Used as a fragrance component (in place of *E. globulus*) in soaps, detergents and perfumes; also used in room sprays and insect repellents Employed for the isolation of natural citronellal.

EUCALYPTUS, BROAD-LEAVED PEPPERMINT
Eucalyptus dives var. Type

FAMILY Myrtaceae

SYNONYMS Broad-leaf peppermint, blue peppermint, menthol-scented gum.

GENERAL DESCRIPTION A robust, medium sized eucalyptus tree, with a short trunk, spreading branches and fibrous grey bark. The young leaves are blue and heart-shaped, the mature leaves are very aromatic, thick and tapering at both ends.

DISTRIBUTION Native to Tasmania and Australia, especially New South Wales and Victoria. Oil is also produced in South Africa.

OTHER SPECIES There are two types of broad-leaved peppermint although they look identical – one is rich in cineol *(E. dives var. C.)* and one is rich in 'piperitone' *(E. dives var. Type)*. It is also similar to the peppermint eucalyptus *(E. piperita)* and the grey or narrow-leaved peppermint *(E. radiata var. phellandra)*. See also entry on eucalyptus blue gum and Botanical Classification section.

HERBAL/FOLK TRADITION The aborigines used the burning leaves in the form of a fumigation for the relief of fever;'heat went out of sick man and into fire'.

ACTIONS See *Eucalyptus blue gum.*

EXTRACTION Essential oil by steam distillation from the leaves and twigs.

CHARACTERISTICS A colourless or pale yellow mobile liquid with a fresh, camphoraceous, spicy-minty odour.

PRINCIPAL CONSTITUENTS Piperitone (40–50 per cent), phellandrene (20-30 per cent), camphene, cymene, terpinene and thujene, among others. It is sold as Grades A, B or C according to the exact balance of constituents.

SAFETY DATA Non-toxic, non-irritant (in dilution), non-sensitizing. Eucalyptus oil is toxic if taken internally (see entry on eucalyptus blue gum).

AROMATHERAPY/HOME USE
SKIN CARE: Cuts, sores, ulcers etc.
CIRCULATION, MUSCLES AND JOINTS: Arthritis, muscular aches and pains, rheumatism, sports injuries, sprains, etc.
RESPIRATORY SYSTEM: Asthma, bronchitis, catarrh, coughs, throat and mouth infections, etc.
IMMUNE SYSTEM: Colds, fevers, 'flu, infectious illness, e.g. measles.
NERVOUS SYSTEM: Headaches, nervous exhaustion, neuralgia, sciatica.

OTHER USES Little used medicinally these days except in deodorants, disinfectants, mouthwashes, gargles and in veterinary practice. 'Piperitone' rich oils are used in solvents. Employed for the manufacture of thymol and menthol (from piperitone).

GENERAL DESCRIPTION Biennial or perennial herb up to 2 metres high, with feathery leaves and golden yellow flowers. There are two main varieties of fennel: bitter or common Fennel, slightly taller with less divided leaves occurring in a cultivated or wild form and sweet fennel (also known as Roman, garden or French fennel) which is always cultivated.

DISTRIBUTION Bitter fennel is native to the Mediterranean region, found growing wild in France, Spain, Portugal and North Africa (they produce the 'weed'oil). It is cultivated extensively worldwide, the main oil producers being Hungary, Bulgaria, Germany, France, Italy and India.
   Sweet fennel is thought to have originated on the island of Malta, having been introduced by monks or crusaders thousands of years ago. It is now grown principally in France, Italy and Greece.

OTHER SPECIES Bitter fennel (*F. vulgare var. amara*) and sweet fennel (*F. vulgare var. dulce*) are both closely related to the Florence fennel (*F. azoricum*), a smaller plant with a large cylindrical fleshy root which can be eaten as a vegetable. There are also many other cultivated varieties such as the German or Saxon fennel,

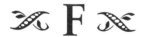

FENNEL
Foeniculum vulgare

FAMILY Apiaceae (Umbelliferae)

SYNONYMS *F. officinale, F. capillaceum, Anethum foeniculum,* fenkel.

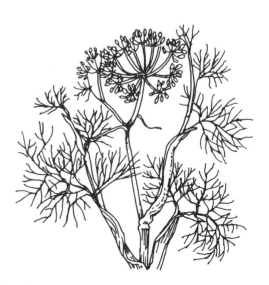

Fennel

the Russian, Indian and Japanese fennel, all of which produce slightly different oils.

HERBAL/FOLK TRADITION A herb of ancient medical repute, believed to convey longevity, courage and strength. It was also used to ward off evil spirits, strengthen the eyesight and to neutralize poisons. In eastern and western herbalism it is considered good for obstructions of the liver, spleen and gall bladder and for digestive complaints such as colic, indigestion, nausea and flatulence (an ingredient of children's 'gripe water').

It has traditionally been used for obesity, which may be due to a type of oestrogenic action, which also increases the milk of nursing mothers. Still current in the British Herbal Pharmacopoeia, used locally for conjunctivitis, blepharitis and pharyngitis.

ACTIONS Aperitif, anti-inflammatory, antimicrobial, antiseptic, antispasmodic, carminative, depurative, diuretic, emmenagogue, expectorant, galactagogue, laxative, orexigenic, stimulant (circulatory), splenic, stomachic, tonic, vermifuge.

EXTRACTION Essential oil by steam distillation. 1. Sweet fennel oil is obtained from crushed seeds, and 2. bitter fennel oil from crushed seeds or the whole herb (the wild 'weed').

CHARACTERISTICS 1. A colourless to pale yellow liquid with a very sweet, anise-like, slightly earthy-peppery scent. It blends well with geranium, lavender, rose and sandalwood. 2. The seed oil is a pale yellow liquid with a sharp, warm camphoraceous odour; the 'weed' oil is pale orange-brown with a sharp, peppery-camphoraceous odour.

PRINCIPAL CONSTITUENTS Anethole (50–60 per cent), limonene, phellandrene, pinene, anisic acid, anisic aldehyde, camphene, limonene, among others. In addition, bitter fennel oil contains 18–22 per cent fenchone, whereas the sweet fennel oil contains little or none.

SAFETY DATA Non-irritant, relatively non-toxic, narcotic in large doses; bitter fennel may cause sensitization in some individuals. Sweet fennel oil is preferred in aromatherapy and perfumery work, since it does not contain the harsh 'fenchone' note, and because it is non-sensitizing. Bitter fennel oil should not be used on the skin at all, although it is considered superior medicinally. Neither oil should be used by epileptics or during pregnancy. Use in moderation.

AROMATHERAPY/HOME USE Bitter fennel – none.
Sweet fennel:
SKIN CARE: Bruises, dull, oily, mature complexions, pyorrhoea.
CIRCULATION, MUSCLES AND JOINTS: Cellulitis, obesity, oedema, rheumatism.
RESPIRATORY SYSTEM: Asthma, bronchitis.
DIGESTIVE SYSTEM: Anorexia, colic, constipation, dyspepsia, flatulence, hiccough, nausea.
GENITO-URINARY SYSTEM: Amenorrhoea, insufficient milk (in nursing mothers), menopausal problems.

OTHER USES In pharmaceutical products it is known as 'codex' fennel oil, used in cough drops, lozenges, etc; also used in carminative and laxative preparations. Extensively used as a flavour ingredient in all major food categories, in soft drinks and especially in alcoholic drinks such as brandy and liqueurs. Fennel oil (mainly sweet) is used in soaps, toiletries and perfumes. It also provides a good masking agent for industrial products, room sprays, insecticides, etc.

FIR NEEDLE, SILVER
Abies alba

FAMILY Pinaceae

SYNONYMS *A. pectinata*, whitespruce, European silver fir, edeltanne, weisstanne, templin (cone oil), Strassburg or Vosges turpentine (oil), fir needle (oil).

GENERAL DESCRIPTION A relatively small coniferous tree, with a regular pyramidal shape and a silvery white bark, grown chiefly for timber and as Christmas trees.

DISTRIBUTION Native to north European mountainous regions; cultivated mainly in Switzerland, Poland, Germany, France, Austria and especially Yugoslavia.

OTHER SPECIES Oils that are distilled from the twigs and needles of various members of the coniferous families, *Abies, Larix, Picea, Pinus*, and *Tsuga*, are all commonly called fir needle oil – it is therefore important to know the specific botanical name. There are many other members of the fir or *Abies* family, notably the Canadian balsam *(A. balsamifera)* and the Siberian fir *(A. siberica)*, the most popular fir needle oil in Europe and the USA due to its fine fragrance. Others include the Japanese fir needle oil from *A.mayriana* or *A.sachalinensis*. See also entries on spruce, pines and the Botanical Classification section.

HERBAL/FOLK TRADITION It is highly esteemed on the Continent for its medicinal virtues and its fragrant scent. It is used mainly for respiratory complaints, fever, muscular and rheumatic pain.

ACTIONS Analgesic, antiseptic (pulmonary), antitussive, deodorant, expectorant, rubefacient, stimulant, tonic.

EXTRACTION Essential oil by steam distillation from the 1. needles and young twigs, and 2. fir cones, broken up pieces (templin oil)

CHARACTERISTICS 1. A colourless or pale yellow liquid of pleasing, rich, sweet-balsamic odour. 2. Similar to the needle oil, but with a more orange-like fragrance. It blends well with galbanum, labdanum, lavender, rosemary, lemon, pine and marjoram.

PRINCIPAL CONSTITUENTS 1. Santene, pinene, limonene, bornyl acetate, lauraldehyde among others. 2. Pinene, limonene, borneol, bornyl acetate, among others.

SAFETY DATA Non-toxic, non-irritant (except in high concentration), non-sensitizing.

AROMATHERAPY/HOME USE
CIRCULATION, MUSCLES AND JOINTS: Arthritis, muscular aches and pains, rheumatism.
RESPIRATORY SYSTEM: Bronchitis, coughs, sinusitis, etc.
IMMUNE SYSTEM: Colds, fever, 'flu.

OTHER USES Employed as an ingredient in some cough and cold remedies and rheumatic treatments. Used as a fragrance component in deodorants, room sprays, disinfectants, bath preparations, soaps and perfumes.

FRANKINCENSE
Boswellia carteri

FAMILY Burseraceae

SYNONYMS Olibanum, gum thus.

GENERAL DESCRIPTION A handsome small tree or shrub with abundant pinnate leaves and white or pale pink flowers. It yields a natural oleo gum resin which is collected by making incisions into the bark: at first, a milky-white liquid appears which then solidifies into tear-shaped amber to orange-brown lumps between the size of a pea and walnut.

DISTRIBUTION Native to the Red Sea region; grows wild throughout north east Africa. The gum is mainly produced in Somalia, Ethiopia,

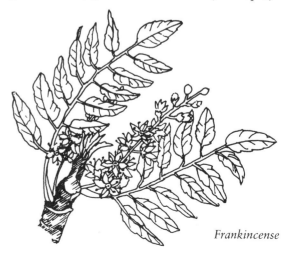

Frankincense

China and south Arabia, then distilled in Europe and, to a lesser extent, India.

OTHER SPECIES Other *Boswellia* species also yield olibanum gum, such as the Indian variety *B. serrata*. Constituents vary according to type and locality. See also Botanical Classification section.

HERBAL/FOLK TRADITION Used since antiquity as an incense in India, China and in the west by the Catholic Church. In ancient Egypt it was used in rejuvenating face masks, cosmetics and perfumes. It has been used medicinally in the east and west for a wide range of conditions including syphilis, rheumatism, respiratory and urinary tract infections, skin diseases, as well as digestive and nervous complaints.

ACTIONS Anti-inflammatory, antiseptic, astringent, carminative, cicatrisant, cytophylactic, digestive, diuretic, emmenagogue, expectorant, sedative, tonic, uterine, vulnerary.

EXTRACTION Essential oil by steam distillation from selected oleo gum resin (approx. 3–10 per cent oil to 60–70 per cent resin). An absolute is also produced, for use mainly as a fixative.

CHARACTERISTICS A pale yellow or greenish mobile liquid with a fresh, terpeney top note and a warm, rich, sweet-balsamic undertone. It blends well with sandalwood, pine, vetiver, geranium, lavender, mimosa, neroli, orange, bergamot, camphor, basil, pepper, cinnamon and other spices. It modifies the sweetness of citrus blends in an intriguing way.

PRINCIPAL CONSTITUENTS Mainly monoterpene hydrocarbons, notably pinene, dipentene, limonene, thujene, phellandrene, cymene, myrcene, terpinene; also octyl acetate, octanol, incensole, among others.

SAFETY DATA Non-toxic, non-irritant, non-sensitizing.

AROMATHERAPY/HOME USE
SKIN CARE: Blemishes, dry and mature complexions, scars, wounds, wrinkles.
RESPIRATORY SYSTEM: Asthma, bronchitis, catarrh, coughs, laryngitis.
GENITO-URINARY SYSTEM: Cystitis, dysmenorrhoea, leucorrhoea, metrorrhagia.
IMMUNE SYSTEM: Colds, 'flu.
NERVOUS SYSTEM: Anxiety, nervous tension and stress-related conditions – 'Frankincense has, among its physical properties, the ability to slow down and deepen the breath ... which is very conducive to prayer and meditation.'[25]

OTHER USES The gum and oil are used as fixatives and fragrance components in soaps, cosmetics and perfumes, especially oriental, spice and men's fragrances. Employed in some pharmaceuticals such as liniments and throat pastilles. Extensively used in the manufacture of incense. The oil is used in minute amounts in some foods (such as meat products), alcoholic and soft drinks.

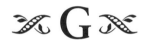

GALANGAL
Alpinia officinarum

FAMILY Zingiberaceae

SYNONYMS *Radix galanga minoris*, *Languas officinarum*, galanga, small galangal, Chinese ginger, ginger root, colic root, East Indian root.

GENERAL DESCRIPTION A reed-like plant reaching a height of about 1 metre, with irregularly branched rhizomes red or brown on the outside, light orange within.

DISTRIBUTION Native to south east China, especially the island of Hainan. Cultivated in China, Indonesia, Thailand and Japan.

OTHER SPECIES Similar species grow in Malaysia, Java, India, etc. It is closely related to ginger *(Zingiber officinale)* and to the large galanga *(Galanga officinalis)*. Not to be confused with the dried rhizomes of kaempferia galanga, known as 'kentjoer', which are used in Malaysia for medicinal purposes and for flavouring curry.

HERBAL/FOLK TRADITION It is used as a local spice, especially in curries; in India it is employed in perfumery. The root is current in the British Herbal Pharmacopoeia, indicated for dyspepsia, flatulence, colic, nausea and vomiting.

ACTIONS Antiseptic, bactericidal, carminative, diaphoretic, stimulant, stomachic.

EXTRACTION Essential oil by steam distillation from the rhizomes. (An oleoresin is also produced by solvent extraction.)

CHARACTERISTICS A greenish-yellow liquid with a fresh, spicy-camphoraceous odour. It blends well with chamomile maroc, sage, cinnamon, allspice, lavandin, pine needle, rosemary, patchouli, myrtle, opopanax and citrus oils.

PRINCIPAL CONSTITUENTS Pinene, cineol, eugenol and sesquiterpenes.

SAFETY DATA Safety data unavailable at present.

AROMATHERAPY/HOME USE (Possibly digestive upsets.)

OTHER USES Employed as a flavour ingredient, especially in spice and meat products. Occasionally used in perfumery work.

GALBANUM
Ferula galbaniflua

FAMILY Apiaceae (Umbelliferae)

SYNONYMS *F. gummosa*, galbanum gum, galbanum resin, 'bubonion'.

GENERAL DESCRIPTION A large perennial herb with a smooth stem, shiny leaflets and small flowers. It contains resin ducts which exude a milky juice, a natural oleoresin. The dried resinous exudation is collected by making incisions at the base of the stem.

DISTRIBUTION Native to the Middle East and western Asia; cultivated in Iran, Turkey, Afghanistan and Lebanon. Distillation usually takes place in Europe or the USA.

OTHER SPECIES There are two distinct types: Levant galbanum which is liquid or soft, and Persian galbanum which is solid or hard. Other *Ferula* species also yield galbanum gum, such as the muskroot; see also Botanical Classification section.

HERBAL/FOLK TRADITION It was used by the ancient civilizations as an incense, and in Egypt for cosmetics and in the embalming process. It is generally used in the east in a similar way to asafetida: for treating wounds, inflammations and skin disorders and also for respiratory, digestive and nervous complaints. Zalou root *(F. hermonic)* is used in Beirut as an aphrodisiac.

ACTIONS Analgesic, anti-inflammatory, antimicrobial, antiseptic, antispasmodic, aphrodisiac, balsamic, carminative, cicatrisant, digestive, diuretic, emmenagogue, expectorant, hypotensive, restorative, tonic.

EXTRACTION Essential oil by water or steam distillation from the oleoresin or gum – only the Levant or soft type is used for oil production. A partially deterpenized oil is produced, known as 'galbanol'. (A resinoid is also produced, mainly for use as a fixative.)

CHARACTERISTICS Crude – A dark amber or brown viscous liquid with a green-woody scent and a soft balsamic undertone. Oil – A colourless, or pale yellow or olive liquid with a fresh green topnote and woody-dry balsamic undertone. It blends well with hyacinth, violet, narcissus, lavender, geranium, oakmoss, opopanax, pine, fir, styrax and oriental bases.

PRINCIPAL CONSTITUENTS Pinene, cadinol, cadinene and myrcene, among others.

SAFETY DATA Non-toxic, non-irritant, non-sensitizing.

AROMATHERAPY/HOME USE
SKIN CARE: Abscesses, acne, boils, cuts, heals scar tissue, inflammations, tones the skin, mature skin, wrinkles, wounds – 'signifies drying and preservation'.[41]
CIRCULATION, MUSCLES AND JOINTS: Poor circulation, muscular aches and pains, rheumatism.
RESPIRATORY SYSTEM: Asthma, bronchitis, catarrh, chronic coughs.
DIGESTIVE SYSTEM: Cramp, flatulence, indigestion.
NERVOUS SYSTEM: Nervous tension and stress-related complaints.

OTHER USES The Persian gum used to be employed in pharmaceutical products. Both oil and resinoid are used as fixatives and fragrance components in soaps, detergents, creams, lotions and perfumes. Also used as a flavour ingredient in most major food categories, alcoholic and soft drinks.

GARDENIA
Gardenia jasminoides

FAMILY Rubiaceae

SYNONYMS *G. grandiflora, G. radicans, florida,* gardinia, Cape jasmine, common gardenia.

GENERAL DESCRIPTION A decorative bush, often grown for ornamental purposes, bearing fragrant white flowers.

DISTRIBUTION Native to the Far East, India and China. Efforts to produce the oil commercially have been largely unsuccessful.

OTHER SPECIES There are several varieties of gardenia depending on location, such as

G. citriodora or *G. calyculata* found in Japan and Indonesia.

HERBAL/FOLK TRADITION The flowers are used locally to flavour tea, much like jasmine.

ACTIONS Antiseptic, aphrodisiac.

EXTRACTION An absolute (and concrete) by solvent extraction from the fresh flowers.

CHARACTERISTICS A dark yellow, oily liquid with a sweet, rich, floral, jasmine-like scent. It blends well with ylang ylang, jasmine, tuberose, neroli, rose, spice and citrus oils.

PRINCIPAL CONSTITUENTS Mainly benzyl acetate, with phenyl acetate, linalol, linalyl acetate, terpineol and methyl anthranilate, among others – composition varies according to source.

SAFETY DATA Safety data unavailable at present. Almost all gardenia oil is now synthetically produced.

AROMATHERAPY/HOME USE Perfume.

OTHER USES Employed in high-class perfumery, especially oriental fragrances.

GARLIC
Allium sativum

FAMILY Amaryllidaceae or Liliaceae

SYNONYMS Common garlic, allium, poor man's treacle!

GENERAL DESCRIPTION A strongly scented perennial herb up to 1.2 metres high with long, flat, firm leaves and whitish flowering stems. The bulb is made up of several cloves pressed together within a thin white skin.

DISTRIBUTION It is said to have originated in south west Siberia and then spread to Europe and Central Asia. It is naturalized in North

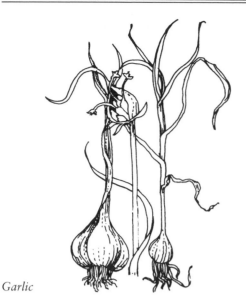

Garlic

America and cultivated worldwide. Major oil-producing countries include Egypt, Bulgaria, France, China, Germany and Japan.

OTHER SPECIES Closely related to the wild or wood garlic *(A. ursinum)* also known as 'ramsons'. There are also many other wild species with similar but less pronounced properties.

HERBAL/FOLK TRADITION It has been used for thousands of years for its medicinal virtues: for respiratory and urinary tract infections; digestive disorders and infestations; skin eruptions; heart disease, high blood pressure and arteriosclerosis, as well as epidemics and fever. It was used in the First World War for preventing gangrene and sepsis.

It has a high reputation in the East: in China it is used for diarrhoea, dysentery, tuberculosis, diphtheria, hepatitis, ringworm, typhoid and trachoma, among others. It is also held in high regard in the West: specific in the British Herbal Pharmacopoeia for chronic bronchitis. Its properties have been attested to by modern experimental and clinical research.

ACTIONS Amoebicidal, anthelmintic, antibiotic, antimicrobial, antiseptic, antitoxic, antitumour, antiviral, bactericidal, carminative, cholagogue, hypocholesterolemic, depurative, diaphoretic, diuretic, expectorant, febrifuge, fungicidal, hypoglycaemic, hypotensive,

insecticidal, larvicidal, promotes leucocytosis, stomachic, tonic.

EXTRACTION Essential oil by steam distillation from the fresh crushed bulbs.

CHARACTERISTICS A colourless to pale yellow mobile liquid with a strong, unpleasant, familiar garlic-like odour.

PRINCIPAL CONSTITUENTS Allicin, allylpropyl disulphide, diallyl disulphide, diallyl trisulphide, citral, geraniol, linalol, phellandrene, among others.

SAFETY DATA Generally non-toxic and non-irritant, although it has been known to irritate the stomach; may also cause sensitization in some individuals.

AROMATHERAPY/HOME USE Due to its unpleasant and pervasive smell, the oil is not often used externally. However, the capsules may be taken internally according to the instructions on the label for respiratory and gastro-intestinal infections, urinary tract infections such as cystitis, heart and circulatory problems, and to fight infectious diseases in general.

OTHER USES The oil is made into capsules and also included in many health food products mainly to help reduce high blood pressure and protect against heart disease. Extensively employed as a flavour ingredient in most major food categories, especially savouries.

GERANIUM
Pelargonium graveolens

FAMILY Geraniaceae

SYNONYMS Rose geranium, pelargonium.

GENERAL DESCRIPTION A perennial hairy shrub up to 1 metre high with pointed leaves, serrated at the edges and small pink flowers. The whole plant is aromatic.

DISTRIBUTION Native to South Africa; widely cultivated in Russia, Egypt, Congo, Japan, Central America and Europe (Spain, Italy and France). With regard to essential oil production, there are three main regions: Reunion (Bourbon), Egypt and Russia (also China).

OTHER SPECIES There are over 700 varieties of cultivated geranium and pelargonium, many of which are grown for ornamental purposes. There are several oil-producing species such as *P. odorantissimum* and *P. radens*, but *P. graveolens* is the main one commercially cultivated for its oil. See also Botanical Classification section.

HERBAL/FOLK TRADITION The British plant herb robert *(Geranium robertianum)* and the American cranesbill *(G. maculatum)* are the most widely used types in herbal medicine today, having been used since antiquity. They have many properties in common with the rose geranium, being used for conditions such as dysentery, haemorrhoids, inflammations, metrorrhagia and menorrhagia (excessive blood loss during menstruation). The root and herb of cranesbill is specifically indicated in the British Herbal Pharmacopoeia for diarrhoea and peptic ulcer.

ACTIONS Antidepressant, antihaemorrhagic, anti-inflammatory, antiseptic, astringent, cicatrisant, deodorant, diuretic, fungicidal, haemostatic, stimulant (adrenal cortex), styptic, tonic, vermifuge, vulnerary.

EXTRACTION Essential oil by steam distillation from the leaves, stalks and flowers. An absolute and concrete are also produced in Morocco.

CHARACTERISTICS The Bourbon oil is a greenish-olive liquid with a green, rosy-sweet, minty scent. The Bourbon oil is generally preferred in perfumery work; it blends well with lavender, patchouli, clove, rose, sandalwood, jasmine, juniper, neroli, bergamot and other citrus oils.

PRINCIPAL CONSTITUENTS Citronellol, geraniol, linalol, isomenthone, menthone, phellandrene, sabinene, limonene, among others. Constituents vary according to type and source.

SAFETY DATA Non-toxic, non-irritant, generally non-sensitizing; possible contact dermatitis in hypersensitive individuals, especially with the Bourbon type.

AROMATHERAPY/HOME USE
SKIN CARE: Acne, bruises, broken capillaries, burns, congested skin, cuts, dermatitis, eczema, haemorrhoids, lice, oily complexion, mature skin, mosquito repellent, ringworm, ulcers, wounds.
CIRCULATION, MUSCLES AND JOINTS: Cellulitis, engorgement of breasts, oedema, poor circulation.
RESPIRATORY SYSTEM: Sore throat, tonsillitis.
GENITO-URINARY AND ENDOCRINE SYSTEMS: Adrenocortical glands and menopausal problems, PMT.
NERVOUS SYSTEM: Nervous tension, neuralgia and stress-related conditions.

OTHER USES Used as a fragrance component in all kinds of cosmetic products: soaps, creams, perfumes, etc. Extensively employed as a flavouring agent in most major food categories, alcoholic and soft drinks.

GINGER
Zingiber officinale

FAMILY Zingiberaceae

SYNONYMS Common ginger, Jamaica ginger.

GENERAL DESCRIPTION An erect perennial herb up to 1 metre high with a thick, spreading, tuberous rhizome root, which is very pungent. Each year it sends up a green reedlike stalk with narrow spear-shaped leaves and white or yellow flowers on a spike direct from the root.

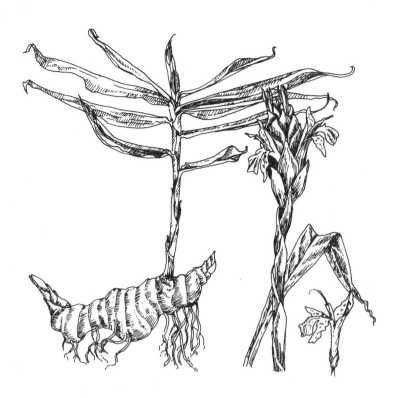

Ginger

DISTRIBUTION Native to southern Asia, extensively cultivated all over the tropics in Nigeria, the West Indies, India, China, Jamaica and Japan. Most oil is distilled in the UK, China and India.

OTHER SPECIES Several varieties according to location which are all used to produce oils with slight variations in their constitiuents; for example the African oil is generally darker. Another member of the same family, galangal *(Alpinia officinarum)*, is also known as ginger root or Chinese ginger.

HERBAL/FOLK TRADITION Ginger has been used as a domestic spice and as a remedy for thousands of years, especially in the East. Fresh ginger is used in China for many complaints including rheumatism, bacterial dysentery, toothache, malaria, and for cold and moist conditions such as excess mucus and diarrhoea.
   It is best known as a digestive aid, especially in the West: in the British Herbal

Pharmacopoeia it is specifically indicated for flatulent intestinal colic. Preserved and crystallized ginger is a popular sweet, in the East and West.

ACTIONS Analgesic, anti-oxidant, antiseptic, antispasmodic, antitussive, aperitif, aphrodisiac, bactericidal, carminative, cephalic, diaphoretic, expectorant, febrifuge, laxative, rubefacient, stimulant, stomachic, tonic.

EXTRACTION Essential oil by steam distillation from the unpeeled, dried, ground root. (An absolute and oleoresin are also produced for use in perfumery.)

CHARACTERISTICS A pale yellow, amber or greenish liquid with a warm, slightly green, fresh, woody-spicy scent. It blends well with sandalwood, vetiver, patchouli, frankincense, rosewood, cedarwood, coriander, rose, lime, neroli, orange and other citrus oils.

PRINCIPAL CONSTITUENTS Gingerin, gingenol, gingerone, zingiberine, linalol, camphene, phellandrene, citral, cineol, borneol, among others.

SAFETY DATA Non-toxic, non-irritant (except in high concentration), slightly phototoxic; may cause sensitization in some individuals.

AROMATHERAPY/HOME USE
CIRCULATION, MUSCLES AND JOINTS: Arthritis, fatigue, muscular aches and pains, poor circulation, rheumatism, sprains, strains etc.
RESPIRATORY SYSTEM: Catarrh, congestion, coughs, sinusitis, sore throat.
DIGESTIVE SYSTEM: Diarrhoea, colic, cramp, flatulence, indigestion, loss of appitite, nausea, travel sickness.
IMMUNE SYSTEM: Chills, colds, 'flu, fever, infectious disease.
NERVOUS SYSTEM: Debility, nervous exhaustion.

OTHER USES The oleoresin is used in digestive, carminative and laxative preparations; used as a fragrance component in cosmetics and perfumes, especially oriental and men's fragrances; extensively employed in all major food categories, alcoholic and soft drinks.

GRAPEFRUIT
Citrus x paradisi

FAMILY Rutaceae

SYNONYMS *C. racemosa, C. maxima var. racemosa*, shaddock (oil).

GENERAL DESCRIPTION A cultivated tree, often over 10 metres high with glossy leaves and large yellow fruits, believed to have derived from the shaddock *(C. grandis)*.

DISTRIBUTION Native to tropical Asia, and the West Indies; cultivated in California, Florida, Brazil and Israel. The oil is mainly produced in California.

OTHER SPECIES *C. paradisi* is a recent hybrid of *C. maxima* and *C. sinesis*. There are many different cultivars; for example, 'Duncan' is standard in Florida.

HERBAL/FOLK TRADITION It shares the nutritional qualities of other citrus species, being high in Vitamin C and a valuable protection against infectious illness.

ACTIONS Antiseptic, antitoxic, astringent, bactericidal, diuretic, depurative, stimulant (lymphatic, digestive), tonic.

EXTRACTION Essential oil by cold expression from the fresh peel. (Some oil is distilled from the peel and remains of the fruit after the juice has been utilized, but this is of inferior quality.)

CHARACTERISTICS A yellow or greenish mobile liquid with a fresh, sweet citrus aroma. It blends well with lemon, palmarosa, bergamot, neroli, rosemary, cypress, lavender, geranium, cardomon and other spice oils.

PRINCIPAL CONSTITUENTS Limonene (90 per cent), cadinene, paradisiol, neral, geraniol, citronellal, sinensal, as well as esters, coumarins and furocoumarins.

SAFETY DATA Non-toxic, non-irritant, non-sensitizing, non-phototoxic. It has a short shelf life – it oxidizes quickly.

AROMATHERAPY/HOME USE
SKIN CARE: Acne, congested and oily skin, promotes hair growth, tones the skin and tissues.
CIRCULATION, MUSCLES AND JOINTS: Cellulitis, exercise preparation, muscle fatigue, obesity, stiffness, water retention.
IMMUNE SYSTEM: Chills, colds, 'flu.
NERVOUS SYSTEM: Depression, headaches, nervous exhaustion, performance stress.

OTHER USES Employed as a fragrance component in soaps, detergents, cosmetics and perfumes. Extensively used in desserts, soft drinks and alcoholic beverages.

GUAIACWOOD
Bulnesia sarmienti

FAMILY Zygophyllaceae

SYNONYMS Champaca wood (oil), 'palo santo'.

GENERAL DESCRIPTION A small, wild tropical tree up to 4 metres high, with a decorative hard wood.

DISTRIBUTION Native to South America, especially Paraguay and Argentina. Some oil is distilled in Europe and the USA.

OTHER SPECIES Distinct from guaiac gum and guaiac resin, known as guaiacum, obtained from related trees *Guaiacum officinale* and *G. sanctum*. However, they are somewhat similar products and share common properties.

HERBAL/FOLK TRADITION The wood is much used for ornamental carving. It was formerly used for treating rheumatism and gout; guaiacum is still current in the British Herbal Pharmacopoeia as a specific for rheumatism and rheumatoid arthritis. Valnet includes guaiacum in his 'elixirs' for gout, venereal disease and in mouthwashes.

ACTIONS Anti-inflammatory, anti-oxidant, antirheumatic, antiseptic, diaphoretic, diuretic, laxative.

EXTRACTION Essential oil by steam distillation from the broken wood and sawdust.

CHARACTERISTICS A yellow, amber or greenish, soft or semi-solid mass with a pleasant, tearose type fragrance and sometimes an unpleasant smoky undertone. It blends well with geranium, neroli, oakmoss, rose, costus, sandalwood, amyris, spice and woody-floral bases.

PRINCIPAL CONSTITUENTS Guaiol (42–72 per cent), bulnesol, bulnesene, guaiene, patchoulene, guaioxide, among others.

SAFETY DATA Non-toxic, non-irritant, non-sensitizing.

AROMATHERAPY/HOME USE
CIRCULATION, MUSCLES AND JOINTS: Arthritis, gout, rheumatoid arthritis.

OTHER USES The fluid extract and tincture are used in pharmacology, mainly as a diagnostic reagent in blood tests. Used as a fixative and fragrance component in soaps, cosmetics and perfumes.

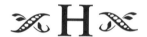

HELICHRYSUM
Helichrysum angustifolium

FAMILY Asteraceae (Compositae)

SYNOYNMS Immortelle, everlasting, St John's herb.

GENERAL DESCRIPTION A strongly aromatic herb, up to 0.6 metres high with a much-branched stem, woody at the base. The brightly coloured, daisy-like flowers become dry as the plant matures, yet retain their colour.

DISTRIBUTION Native to the Mediterranean region, especially the eastern part and North Africa. It is cultivated mainly in Italy, Yugoslavia, Spain and France.

OTHER SPECIES There are several other *Helichrysum* species such as *H. arenarium* found in florist shops and *H. stoechas* which is also used to produce an absolute. *H. orientale* is grown for its oil.

HERBAL/FOLK TRADITION In Europe it is used for respiratory complaints such as asthma, chronic bronchitis and whooping cough; also for headaches, migraine, liver ailments and skin conditions including burns, allergies and psoriasis. Usually taken in the form of a decoction or infusion.

ACTIONS Anti-allergenic, anti-inflammatory, antimicrobial, antitussive, antiseptic, astringent, cholagogue, cicatrisant, diuretic, expectorant, fungicidal, hepatic, nervine.

EXTRACTION 1. Essential oil by steam distillation from the fresh flowers and flowering tops. 2. An absolute (and concrete) are also produced by solvent extraction.

CHARACTERISTICS 1. A pale yellow to red oily liquid with a powerful, rich honeylike scent with a delicate tealike undertone. 2. A yellowy-brown viscous liquid with a rich, floral, tealike scent. It blends well with chamomile, boronia, labdanum, lavender, mimosa, oakmoss, geranium, clary sage, rose, Peru balsam, clove and citrus oils.

PRINCIPAL CONSTITUENTS Nerol and neryl acetate (30–50 per cent), geraniol, pinene, linalol, isovaleric aldehyde, sesquiterpenes, furfurol and eugenol, among others.

SAFETY DATA Non-toxic, non-irritant, non-sensitizing.

AROMATHERAPY/HOME USE
SKIN CARE: Abscess, acne, allergic conditions, boils, burns, cuts, dermatitis, eczema, inflammation, spots, wounds etc.
CIRCULATION, MUSCLES AND JOINTS: Muscular aches and pains, rheumatism, sprains, strained muscles.
RESPIRATORY SYSTEM: Asthma, bronchitis, chronic coughs, whooping cough.
DIGESTIVE SYSTEM: Liver congestion, spleen congestion.
IMMUNE SYSTEM: Bacterial infections, colds, 'flu, fever.
NERVOUS SYSTEM: Depression, debility, lethargy, nervous exhaustion, neuralgia, stress-related conditions.

OTHER USES Used as fixatives and fragrance components in soaps, cosmetics and perfumes. The absolute is used to flavour certain tobaccos; used for the isolation of natural anethole.

HOPS
Humulus lupulus

FAMILY Moraceae

SYNONYMS Common hop, European hop, lupulus.

GENERAL DESCRIPTION Perennial creeping, twining herb up to 8 metres high, which bears male and female flowers on separate plants. It has dark green, heart-shaped leaves and greeny-yellow flowers. A volatile oil, called lupulin, is formed in the glandular hairs of the cones or 'strobiles'.

DISTRIBUTION Native to Europe and North America; cultivated worldwide, especially in the USA (California and Washington), Yugoslavia and Germany. The oil is mainly produced in France, UK and Germany.

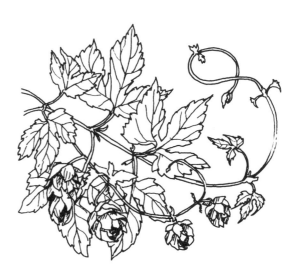

Hops

OTHER SPECIES Related to the common stinging nettle *(Urtica dioica)* and to the fig *(Ficus carica).*

HERBAL/FOLK TRADITION Best known as a nerve remedy, for insomnia, nervous tension, neuralgia, and also for sexual neurosis in both sexes. It supports the female oestrogens, and is useful for amenorrhoea (heavy periods). 'A mild sedative, well known in the form of the hop pillow where the heavy aromatic odour has been shown to relax by direct action at the olfactory centres ... it is the volatile aromatic component that appears to be the most active.'[42] It has also been used for heart disease, stomach and liver complaints, including bacterial dysentery.

In China it is used for pulmonary tuberculosis and cystitis. It is used to make beer. Current in the British Herbal Pharmacopoeia as a specific for restlessness with nervous headaches and/or indigestion.

ACTIONS Anodyne, an aphrodisiac, antimicrobial, antiseptic, antispasmodic, astringent, bactericidal, carminative, diuretic, emollient, oestrogenic properties, hypnotic, nervine, sedative, soporific.

EXTRACTION Essential oil by steam distillation from the dried cones or catkins, known as 'strobiles'. (An absolute is also produced by solvent extraction for perfumery use.)

CHARACTERISTICS A pale yellow to reddish-amber liquid with a rich, spicy-sweet odour. It blends well with pine, hyacinth, nutmeg, copaiba balsam, citrus and spice oils.

PRINCIPAL CONSTITUENTS Mainly humulene, myrcene, caryophyllene and farnesene, with over 100 other trace components.

SAFETY DATA Generally non-toxic (narcotic in excessive amounts) and non-irritant; may cause sensitization in some individuals. Should be avoided by those suffering from depression.

AROMATHERAPY/HOME USE
SKIN CARE: Dermatitis, rashes, rough skin, ulcers.

RESPIRATORY SYSTEM: Asthma, spasmodic cough.
DIGESTIVE SYSTEM: Indigestion, nervous dyspepsia.
GENITO-URINARY AND ENDOCRINE SYSTEMS: Amenorrhoea, menstrual cramp, supports female oestrogens, promotes feminine characteristics, reduces sexual overactivity.
NERVOUS SYSTEM: Headaches, insomnia, nervous tension, neuralgia, stress-related conditions.

OTHER USES Employed as a fragrance ingredient in perfumes, especially spicy or oriental types. Used in flavour work in tobacco, sauces and spice products, but mainly in alcoholic drinks, especially beer.

HORSERADISH
Armoracia rusticana

FAMILY Brassicaceae (Cruciferae)

SYNONYMS *Cochlearia armoracia, A. lapathifolia,* red cole, raifort.

GENERAL DESCRIPTION A perennial plant with large leaves up to 50 cms long, white flowers and a thick whitish tapering root, which is propagated easily.

DISTRIBUTION Its origins are uncertain, but probably native to eastern Europe. It is now common throughout Russia, Europe and Scandinavia.

OTHER SPECIES Possibly a cultivated form of *Cochlearia macrocarpa,* a native of Hungary.

HERBAL/FOLK TRADITION An extremely stimulating herb, once valued as a household remedy. Its action is similar to mustard seed and it was used for fever, digestive complaints, urinary infections and as a circulatory aid. Good for arthritis and rheumatism. It is still used as a condiment, especially on the Continent.

ACTIONS Antibiotic, antiseptic, diuretic, carminative, expectorant, laxative (mild), rubefacient, stimulant.

EXTRACTION Essential oil by water and steam distillation from the broken roots which have been soaked in water. (A resinoid or concrete is also produced by solvent extraction.)

CHARACTERISTICS A colourless or pale yellow mobile liquid with a sharp, potent odour and having a tear-producing effect.

PRINCIPAL CONSTITUENTS Allyl isothiocyanate (75 per cent), with phenylethyl isothiocyanate (which is only produced when the plant is bruised or crushed).

SAFETY DATA Oral toxin, dermal irritant, mucous membrane irritant. 'This is one of the most hazardous of all essential oils. It should not be used in therapy either externally or internally.'[43]

AROMATHERAPY/HOME USE None.

OTHER USES Mainly used in minute amounts in seasonings, ready-made salads, condiments and canned products.

HYACINTH
Hyacinthus orientalis

FAMILY Liliaceae

SYNONYMS *Scilla nutans*, bluebell.

GENERAL DESCRIPTION A much loved cultivated plant with fragrant, bell-shaped flowers of many colours, bright lance-shaped leaves and a round bulb.

DISTRIBUTION Native to Asia Minor, said to be of Syrian origin. Cultivated mainly in Holland and southern France.

OTHER SPECIES Closely related to garlic (*Allium sativum*), onion (*A. cepa*) and the wild bluebell (*H. non scriptus*). At one time bluebell essential oil was produced at Grasse in the south of France, which had a fresher and more flowery fragrance.

HERBAL/FOLK TRADITION The wild bluebell bulbs are poisonous; however, the white juice used to be employed as a substitute for starch or glue. 'The roots, dried and powdered, are balsamic, having some styptic properties that have not fully been investigated.'[44]

ACTIONS Antiseptic, balsamic, hypnotic, sedative, styptic.

EXTRACTION Concrete and absolute by solvent extraction from the flowers. (An essential oil is also obtained by steam distillation from the absolute.)

CHARACTERISTICS A reddish or greeny-brown viscous liquid with a sweet-green, floral fragrance and soft floral undertone. It blends well with narcissus, violet, ylang ylang, styrax, galbanum, jasmine, neroli and with oriental-type bases.

PRINCIPAL CONSTITUENTS Phenylethyl alcohol, benzaldehyde, cinnamaldehyde, benzyl alcohol, benzoic acid, benzyl acetate, benzyl benzoate, eugenol, methyl eugenol and hydroquinone, among others.

SAFETY DATA No safety data available at present. Most commercial hyacinth is nowadays adulterated or synthetic.

AROMATHERAPY/HOME USE
NERVOUS SYSTEM: The Greeks described the fragrance of hyacinth as being refreshing and invigorating to a tired mind. It may also be used for stress-related conditions, 'in self-hypnosis techniques ... and developing the creative right-hand side of the brain'.[45]

OTHER USES Used in high class perfumery, especially oriental/floral types.

HYSSOP
Hyssopus officinalis

FAMILY Lamiaceae (Labiatae)

SYNONYM Azob.

GENERAL DESCRIPTION An attractive perennial, almost evergreen subshrub up to 60 cms high with a woody stem, small, lance-shaped leaves and purplish-blue flowers.

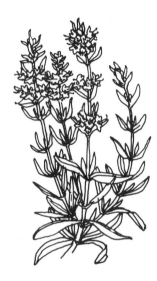

Hyssop

DISTRIBUTION Native to the Mediterranean region and temperate Asia; now grows wild throughout America, Russia and Europe. It is mainly cultivated in Hungary and France, and to a lesser degree in Albania and Yugoslavia.

OTHER SPECIES There are four main subspecies of hyssop, but *H. officinalis* is the main oil-producing variety. The species *H. officinalis var. decumbens* is less toxic than many other types, and well suited to aromatherapy use. To be distinguished from hedge hyssop *(Gratiola officinalis)* which is still used in herbal medicine but belongs to an entirely different family.

HERBAL/FOLK TRADITION Although hyssop is mentioned in the Bible, it probably

does not refer to this herb but to a form of wild marjoram or oregano, possibly *Oreganum syriacum*. Nevertheless *H. officinalis* has an ancient medical reputation and was used for purifying sacred places, and employed as a strewing herb. 'The healing virtues of the plant are due to a particular volatile oil.'[26]

It is used principally for respiratory and digestive complaints, and externally for rheumatism, bruises, sores, earache and toothache. It is also used to regulate the blood pressure, as a general nerve tonic, and for states of anxiety or hysteria. It is current in the British Herbal Pharmacopoeia as a specific for bronchitis and the common cold.

ACTIONS Astringent, antiseptic, antispasmodic, antiviral, bactericidal, carminative, cephalic, cicatrisant, digestive, diuretic, emmenagogue, expectorant, febrifuge, hypertensive, nervine, sedative, sudorific, tonic (heart and circulation), vermifuge, vulnerary.

EXTRACTION Essential oil by steam distillation from the leaves and flowering tops.

CHARACTERISTICS A colourless to pale yellowy-green liquid with a sweet, camphoraceous top note and warm spicy-herbaceous undertone. It blends well with lavender, rosemary, myrtle, bay leaf, sage, clary sage, geranium and citrus oils.

PRINCIPAL CONSTITUENTS Pinocamphone, isopinocamphone, estragole, borneol, geraniol, limonene, thujone, myrcene, caryophyllene, among others.

SAFETY DATA Non-irritant, non-sensitizing; the oil is moderately toxic due to the pinocamphone content. It should be used only in moderation and avoided in pregnancy and by epileptics.

AROMATHERAPY/HOME USE
SKIN CARE: Bruises, cuts, dermatitis, eczema, inflammation, wounds.
CIRCULATION, MUSCLES AND JOINTS: Low or high blood pressure, rheumatism.
RESPIRATORY SYSTEM: Asthma, bronchitis,

catarrh, cough, sore throat, tonsillitis, whooping cough.
DIGESTIVE SYSTEM: Colic, indigestion.
GENITO-URINARY SYSTEM: Amenorrhoea, leucorrhoea.
IMMUNE SYSTEM: Colds, 'flu.
NERVOUS SYSTEM: Anxiety, fatigue, nervous tension and stress-related conditions.

OTHER USES Employed as a fragrance component in soaps, cosmetics and perfumes, especially eau-de-cologne and oriental bases. Used as a flavour ingredient in many food products, mainly sauces and seasonings; also in alcoholic drinks, especially liqueurs such as chartreuse.

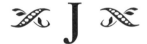

JABORANDI
Pilocarpus jaborandi

FAMILY Rutaceae

SYNONYMS *Pernambuco jaborandi, P. pennatifolius,* iaborandi, jamborandi, arrudo do mato, arruda brava, jamguaraddi, juarandi.

GENERAL DESCRIPTION A woody shrub up to 2 metres high with a smooth, greyish bark, large brownish-green leathery leaves containing big oil glands and reddish-purple flowers.

DISTRIBUTION Native to Brazil; other species are found in Paraguay, Cuba, the West Indies and Central America.

OTHER SPECIES There are many members of the *Rutaceae* and *Piperaceae* family known simply as jaborandi, such as *Piper jaborandi*. Others include maranham jaborandi *(P. microphyllus),* ceara jaborandi *(P. trachylophus)* and aracti jaborandi *(P. spicatus).*

There is consequently some confusion about the exact botanical source of the oil.

HERBAL/FOLK TRADITION Jaborandi induces salivation and most gland secretions; it was also used at one time to promote hair growth. 'Useful in psoriasis, prurigo, deafness ... chronic catarrh, tonsillitis and particularly dropsy.' [46].

ACTIONS Antiseptic, diaphoretic, emmenagogue, galactagogue, stimulant (nerve).

EXTRACTION Essential oil by steam distillation from the dried leaflets.

CHARACTERISTICS An orange or yellow liquid with a sweet-herbaceous fruity odour.

PRINCIPAL CONSTITUENTS Pilocarpine is the main active constituent; also isopilocarpine, pilocarpidine, methyl nonyl ketone, dipentene and other hydrocarbons.

SAFETY DATA Oral toxin, skin irritant, abortifacient.

AROMATHERAPY/HOME USE None.

OTHER USES Various hypodermic solutions are prepared from pilocarpine: the crude oil is rarely used. Little used in perfumery or flavour work due to toxicity.

JASMINE
Jasminum officinale

FAMILY Oleaceae

SYNONYMS Jasmin, jessamine, common jasmine, poet's jessamine.

GENERAL DESCRIPTION An evergreen shrub or vine up to 10 metres high with delicate, bright green leaves and star-shaped very fragrant white flowers.

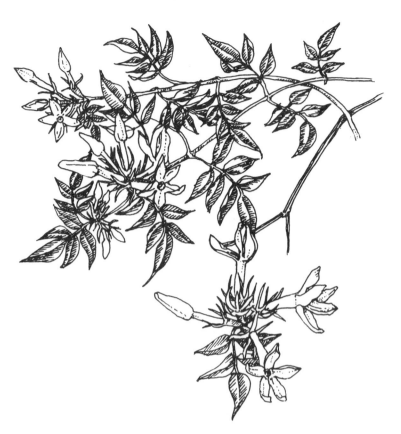

Jasmine

DISTRIBUTION Native to China, northern India and west Asia; cultivated in the Mediterranean region, China and India (depending on the exact species). The concrete is produced in Italy, France, Morocco, Egypt, China, Japan, Algeria and Turkey; the absolute is mainly produced in France.

OTHER SPECIES There are many species of jasmine used for medicine and perfumery work. Apart from the common jasmine, the most widespead varieties are the royal or Italian jasmine *(J. grandiflorum)* which is grown in the Mediterranean region, and its Eastern counterpart *J. officinale var. grandiflorum* or *J. auriculatum.* See the Botanical Classification section for a more comprehensive list.

HERBAL/FOLK TRADITION In China the flowers of *J. officinale var. grandiflorum* are used to treat hepatitis, liver cirrhosis and dysentery; the flowers of *J. sambac* are used for conjunctivitis, dysentery, skin ulcers and tumours. The root is used to treat headaches, insomnia, pain due to dislocated joints and rheumatism.

In the West, the common jasmine was said to 'warm the womb ... and facilitate the birth; it is useful for cough, difficulty of breathing, etc. It disperses crude humours, and is good for cold and catarrhous constitutions, but not for the hot.' It was also used for hard, contracted limbs and problems with the nervous and reproductive systems.

ACTIONS Analgesic (mild), antidepressant, anti-inflammatory, antiseptic, antispasmodic, aphrodisiac, carminative, cicatrisant, expectorant, galactagogue, parturient, sedative, tonic (uterine).

EXTRACTION A concrete is produced by solvent extraction; the absolute is obtained from the concrete by separation with alcohol. An essential oil is produced by steam distillation of the absolute.

CHARACTERISTICS The absolute is a dark orange-brown, viscous liquid with an intensely rich, warm, floral scent and a tealike undertone. It blends well with rose, sandalwood, clary sage, and all citrus oils. It has the ability to round off any rough notes and blend with virtually everything.

PRINCIPAL CONSTITUENTS There are over 100 constituents in the oil including benzyl acetate, linalol, phenylacetic acid, benzyl alcohol, farnesol, methyl anthranilate, cis-jasmone, methyl jasmonate, among others.

SAFETY DATA Non-toxic, non-irritant, generally non-sensitizing. (An allergic reaction has been known to occur in some individuals.)

AROMATHERAPY/HOME USE
SKIN CARE: Dry, greasy, irritated, sensitive skin.
CIRCULATION, MUSCLES AND JOINTS: Muscular spasm, sprains.
RESPIRATORY SYSTEM: Catarrh, coughs, hoarseness, laryngitis.
GENITO-URINARY SYSTEM: Dysmenorrhoea, frigidity, labour pains, uterine disorders.
NERVOUS SYSTEM: Depression, nervous exhaustion and stress-related conditions. 'It ... produces a feeling of optimism, confidence and euphoria. It is most useful in cases where there is apathy, indifference or listlessness.'[47]

OTHER USES Extensively used in soaps, toiletries, cosmetics and perfumes, especially high class floral and oriental fragrances. The oil and absolute are employed in a wide range of food products, alcoholic and soft drinks. The dried flowers of *J. sambac* are used in jasmine tea.

JUNIPER
Juniperus communis

FAMILY Cupressaceae

SYNONYM Common juniper.

GENERAL DESCRIPTION An evergreen shrub or tree up to 6 metres high, with bluish-green narrow stiff needles. It has small flowers and little round berries, which are green in the first year, turning black in the second and third.

DISTRIBUTION Native to the northern hemisphere: Scandinavia, Siberia, Canada, northern Europe and northern Asia. The oil is mainly produced in Italy, France, Yugoslavia, Austria, Czechoslovakia, Spain, Germany and Canada.

OTHER SPECIES In Yugoslavia an oil is produced from the fruit and twigs of *J. smerka*, less rich and sweet than that of common juniper. There are various other species of juniper such as *J. oxycedrus* which produces cade oil, *J. virginiana* which produces the so-called Virginian cedarwood oil, and *J. sabina* which produces savin oil. See also Botanical Classification section.

HERBAL/FOLK TRADITION The needles and berries have a long traditional history of use. It is used medicinally for urinary infections such as cystitis and urethritis; for respiratory problems such as bronchitis, colic and coughs; as well as gastro-intestinal infections and

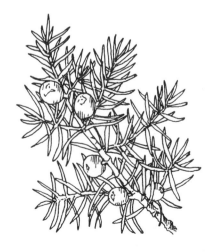
Juniper

worms. It helps expel the build-up of uric acid in the joints, and is employed in gout, rheumatism and arthritis. Current in the British Herbal Pharmacopoeia for rheumatic pain and cystitis.

ACTIONS Antirheumatic, antiseptic, antispasmodic, antitoxic, aphrodisiac, astringent, carminative, cicatrisant, depurative, diuretic, emmenagogue, nervine, parasiticide, rubefacient, sedative, stomachic, sudorific, tonic, vulnerary.

EXTRACTION Essential oil by steam distillation from   1. the berries (sometimes fermented first as a by-product of juniper-brandy manufacture – the oil is considered an inferior product), and   2. the needles and wood. A resinoid, concrete and absolute are also produced on a small scale.

CHARACTERISTICS 1. A water-white or pale yellow mobile liquid with a sweet, fresh, woody-balsamic odour. It blends well with vetiver, sandalwood, cedarwood, mastic, oakmoss, galbanum, elemi, cypress, clary sage, pine, lavender, lavandin, labdanum, fir needle, rosemary, benzoin, balsam tolu, geranium and citrus oils.   2. A water-white or pale yellow mobile liquid with a sweet-balsamic, fresh, turpentine-like odour.

PRINCIPAL CONSTITUENTS Mainly monoterpenes: pinene, myrcene, sabinene with limonene, cymene, terpinene, thujene and camphene, among others.

SAFETY DATA Non-sensitizing, may be slightly irritating, generally non-toxic. However, it stimulates the uterine muscle (an abortifacient) and must not be used during pregnancy. Neither should it be used by those with kidney disease due to its nephrotoxic effect. The wood oil is usually adulterated with turpentine oil. It is best to use only juniper berry oil, in moderation.

AROMATHERAPY/HOME USE
SKIN CARE: Acne, dermatitis, eczema, hair loss, haemorrhoids, oily complexions, as a skin

toner, wounds.
CIRCULATION, MUSCLES AND JOINTS: Accumulation of toxins, arteriosclerosis, cellulitis, gout, obesity, rheumatism.
IMMUNE SYSTEM: Colds, 'flu, infections.
GENITO-URINARY SYSTEM: Amenorrhoea, cystitis, dysmenorrhoea, leucorrhoea.
NERVOUS SYSTEM: Anxiety, nervous tension and stress-related conditions.

OTHER USES Berries and extracts are used in diuretic and laxative preparations; also veterinary preventatives of ticks and fleas. Employed as a fragrance component in soaps, detergents, cosmetics and perfumes, especially spicy fragrances and aftershaves. Extensively used in many food products but especially alcoholic and soft drinks : the berries are used to flavour gin.

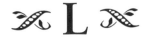

L

LABDANUM
Cistus ladaniferus

FAMILY Cistaceae

SYNONYMS Cistus (oil), gum cistus, ciste, cyste (absolute), labdanum gum, ambreine, European rock rose.

GENERAL DESCRIPTION A small sticky shrub up to 3 metres high with lance-shaped leaves which are white and furry on the underside, and fragrant white flowers. Labdanum gum, a dark brown solid mass, is a natural oleoresin which is obtained by boiling the plant material in water.

DISTRIBUTION Native to the Mediterranean mountainous regions and the Middle East. Now found throughout the Mediterranean region, especially southern France, Spain, Portugal, Greece, Morocco, Cyprus and Yugoslavia. The oil is mainly produced in Spain.

OTHER SPECIES Labdanum gum is also obtained from other *Cistus* species, notably *C. incanus*, and other subspecies: see Botanical Classification section.

HERBAL/FOLK TRADITION One of the early aromatic substances of the ancient world. The gum was used formerly for catarrh, diarrhoea, dysentery and to promote menstruation; externally it was used in plasters. The oil from the closely related plant frostwort *(Helianthemum canadense)*, also known as cistus, also has many medicinal qualities and is said to be useful for scrofulous skin conditions, ulcers and tumours, including cancer.

ACTIONS Antimicrobial, antiseptic, antitussive, astringent, balsamic, emmenagogue, expectorant, tonic.

EXTRACTION 1. A resinoid or resin concrete and absolute by solvent extraction from the crude gum. 2. An essential oil by steam distillation from the crude gum, the absolute, or from the leaves and twigs of the plant directly.

CHARACTERISTICS 1. Absolute – a semi-solid green or amber mass with a rich, sweet, herbaceous-balsamic odour. 2. Oil – a dark yellow or amber viscous liquid with a warm, sweet, dry-herbaceous musky scent. It blends well with oakmoss, clary sage, pine, juniper, calamus, opopanax, lavender, lavandin, bergamot, cypress, vetiver, sandalwood, patchouli, olibanum, chamomile maroc and oriental bases.

PRINCIPAL CONSTITUENTS It contains over 170 pinenes, including camphene, sabinene, myrcene, phellandrene, limonene, cymene, cineol, borneol, nerol, geraniol, fenchone, etc. Exact constituents vary according to source.

SAFETY DATA Generally non-toxic, non-irritant, non-sensitizing. Avoid during pregnancy.

AROMATHERAPY/HOME USE
SKIN CARE: Mature skin, wrinkles.
RESPIRATORY SYSTEM: Coughs, bronchitis, rhinitis, etc.
IMMUNE SYSTEM: Colds.

OTHER USES Used as a fixative and fragrance component in lotions, powders, soaps, detergents, colognes and perfumes, especially oriental perfumes and aftershaves. Employed in most major food categories, particularly meat products, as well as alcoholic and soft drinks.

LAVANDIN
Lavandula x intermedia

FAMILY Lamiaceae (Labiatae)

SYNONYMS *Lavandula hybrida, L. hortensis,* bastard lavender.

GENERAL DESCRIPTION A hybrid plant developed by crossing true lavender *(L. angustifolia)* with spike lavender or aspic *(L. latifolia)*. Due to its hybrid nature, lavandin has a variety of forms: in general, it is a larger plant than true lavender, with woody stems. Its flowers may be blue like true lavender, or greyish like aspic.

DISTRIBUTION A natural lavandin occurs in the mountainous regions of southern France where both parent plants grow wild, though at different altitudes. Still mainly cultivated in France, but also Spain, Hungary, Yugoslavia and Argentina.

OTHER SPECIES There are cultivars of lavender, such as 'Dwarf Blue', 'Hidcote Pink' and 'Bowles Early'; there are also many cultivars of lavandin such as 'Grey Hedge', 'Silver Grey' and 'Alba'. For further information see entries on true lavender and spike lavender; also the Botanical Classification section.

HERBAL/FOLK TRADITION Sixty years ago, when *A Modern Herbal* was written by Mrs

Grieve, lavandin was still unknown, so it does not have a long history of therapeutic use. Its properties seem to combine those of the true lavender and aspic.

ACTIONS See *true lavender*.

EXTRACTION Essential oil by steam distillation from the fresh flowering tops; it has a higher yield of oil than either true lavender or aspic. (A concrete and absolute are also produced by solvent extraction.)

CHARACTERISTICS A colourless or pale yellow liquid with a fresh camphoraceous topnote (which should not be too strong in a good quality oil), and a woody herbaceous undertone. It blends well with clove, bay leaf, cinnamon, citronella, cypress, pine, clary sage, geranium, thyme, patchouli, rosemary and citrus oils, especially bergamot and lime.

PRINCIPAL CONSTITUENTS Linalyl acetate (30–32 per cent), linalol, cineol, camphene, pinene and other trace constituents.

SAFETY DATA Non-toxic, non-irritant, non-sensitizing.

AROMATHERAPY/HOME USE Similar uses to true lavender, but it is more penetrating and rubefacient with a sharper scent – good for respiratory, circulatory or muscular conditions.

OTHER USES Extensively employed in soaps, detergents, room sprays, hair preparations and industrial perfumes. Used as a flavour ingredient in most major food categories, and also as a natural source of linalol and linalyl acetate.

LAVENDER, SPIKE
Lavandula latifolia

FAMILY Lamiaceae (Labiatae)

SYNONYMS *L. spica*, aspic, broad-leaved lavender, lesser lavender, spike.

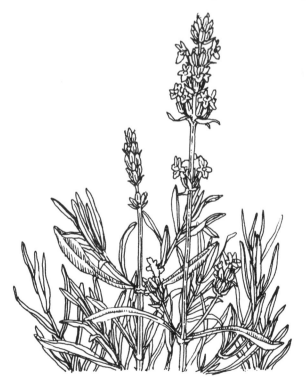

Spike Lavender

GENERAL DESCRIPTION An aromatic evergreen sub-shrub up to 1 metre high with lance-shaped leaves, broader and rougher than true lavender. The flower is more compressed and of a dull grey-blue colour.

DISTRIBUTION Native to the mountainous regions of France and Spain, also found in North Africa, Italy, Yugoslavia and the eastern Mediterranean countries. It is cultivated internationally; the oil is mainly produced in France and Spain.

OTHER SPECIES There are many different chemotypes of lavender in general, and this also applies to spike lavender. The French spike oil is reputed to be a more delicate, aromatic scent than the Spanish variety. For other varieties, see entries on lavandin, true lavender and the Botanical Classification section.

HERBAL/FOLK TRADITION Culpeper recommends spike lavender for a variety of ailments including 'pains of the head and brain which proceed from cold, apoplexy, falling sickness, the dropsy, or sluggish malady, cramps, convulsions, palsies, and often faintings.' He also warns that 'the oil of spike is of a fierce and piercing quality, and ought to be carefully used, a very few drops being sufficient for inward or outward maladies.'[48] The preparation 'oleum spicae' was made by mixing $1/_4$ spike oil with $3/_4$ turpentine, and used for paralysed limbs, old sprains and stiff joints (it was also said to encourage hair growth).
   Spike lavender is current in the British Herbal Pharmacopoeia, indicated for flatulent dyspepsia, colic, depressive headaches, and the oil (topically) for rheumatic pain.

ACTIONS See *true lavender*.

EXTRACTION Essential oil by water or steam distillation from the flowering tops.

CHARACTERISTICS A water-white or pale yellow liquid with a penetrating, fresh-herbaceous, camphoraceous odour. It blends well with rosemary, sage, lavandin, eucalyptus, rosewood, lavender, petitgrain, pine, cedarwood, oakmoss, patchouli and spice oils, particularly clove.

PRINCIPAL CONSTITUENTS Mainly cineol and camphor (40–60 per cent), with linalol and linalyl acetate, among others.

SAFETY DATA Non-toxic, non-irritant(except in concentration), non-sensitizing.

AROMATHERAPY/HOME USE See *true lavender.*

OTHER USES It is used in some pharmaceutical preparations and especially in veterinary practice as a prophylactic, in incipient paralysis, for rheumatism and arthritis and to get rid of lice. It is extensively employed as a fragrance component especially in soaps and industrial perfumes such as deodorants, disinfectants and cleaning agents, as well as insecticides and room sprays, etc. It is also used in the food industry and in the production of fine varnishes and lacquers.

LAVENDER, TRUE
Lavandula angustifolia

FAMILY Lamiaceae (Labiatae)

SYNONYMS *L. vera, L. officinalis*, garden lavender, common lavender

GENERAL DESCRIPTION An evergreen woody shrub, up to 1 metre tall, with pale green, narrow, linear leaves and flowers on blunt spikes of a beautiful violet-blue colour. The whole plant is highly aromatic.

DISTRIBUTION Indigenous to the Mediterranean region, now cultivated all over the world. The oil is produced mainly in France, also Spain, Italy, England, Australia, Tasmania, Yugoslavia, Turkey, Russia, Bulgaria, Greece, etc.

OTHER SPECIES There are many varieties of

lavender; *L. angustifolia* is divided into two subspecies – *L. delphinensis* and *L. fragrans*. French lavender *(L. stoechas)* is a smaller shrub with dark violet flowers; see also entries on spike lavender, lavandin and the Botanical Classification section. The so-called cotton lavender *(Santolina chamaecyparissus)* and the sea lavender *(Statice caroliniana)* belong to different botanical families.

HERBAL/FOLK TRADITION Lavender has a well-established tradition as a folk remedy, and its scent is still familiar to almost everyone. It was used to 'comfort the stomach' but above all as a cosmetic water, an insect repellent, to scent linen, and as a reviving yet soothing oil 'The essential oil, or a spirit of lavender made from it, proves admirably restorative and tonic against faintness, palpitations of a nervous sort, weak giddiness, spasms and colic ... A few drops of lavender in a hot footbath has a marked influence in relieving fatigue. Outwardly applied, it relieves toothache, neuralgia, sprains and rheumatism. In hysteria, palsy and similar disorders of debility and lack of nerve power, lavender will act as a powerful stimulant.'[49]

ACTIONS Analgesic, anticonvulsive, antidepressant, antimicrobial, antirheumatic, antiseptic, antispasmodic, antitoxic, carminative, cholagogue, choleretic, cicatrisant, cordial, cytophylactic, deodorant, diuretic, emmenagogue, hypotensive, insecticide, nervine, parasiticide, rubefacient, sedative, stimulant, sudorific, tonic, vermifuge, vulnerary.

EXTRACTION 1. Essential oil by steam distillation from the fresh flowering tops.
2. An absolute and concrete are also produced by solvent extraction in smaller quantities.

CHARACTERISTICS 1. The oil is a colourless to pale yellow liquid with a sweet, floral-herbaceous scent and balsamic-woody undertone; it has a more fragrant floral scent compared to spike lavender. It blends well with most oils, especially citrus and florals; also

cedarwood, clove, clary sage, pine, geranium, labdanum, oakmoss, vetiver, patchouli, etc.
2. The absolute is a dark green viscous liquid with a very sweet herbaceous, somewhat floral odour.

PR'NCIPAL CONSTITUENTS Over 100 constituents including linalyl acetate (up to 40 per cent), linalol, lavandulol, lavandulyl acetate, terpineol, cineol, limonene, ocimene, caryophyllene, among others. Constituents vary according to source: high altitudes generally produce more esters.

SAFETY DATA Non-toxic, non-irritant, non-sensitizing.

AROMATHERAPY/HOME USE Generally regarded as the most versatile essence therapeutically:
SKIN CARE: Abscesses, acne, allergies, athlete's foot, boils, bruises, burns, dandruff, dermatitis, earache, eczema, inflammations, insect bites and stings, insect repellent, lice, psoriasis, ringworm, scabies, sores, spots, all skin types, sunburn, wounds.
CIRCULATION, MUSCLES AND JOINTS: Lumbago, muscular aches and pains, rheumatism, sprains.
RESPIRATORY SYSTEM: Asthma, bronchitis, catarrh, halitosis, laryngitis, throat infections, whooping cough.
DIGESTIVE SYSTEM: Abdominal cramps, colic, dyspepsia, flatulence, nausea.
GENITO-URINARY SYSTEM: Cystitis, dysmenorrhoea, leucorrhoea.
IMMUNE SYSTEM: 'Flu.
NERVOUS SYSTEM: Depression, headache, hypertension, insomnia, migraine, nervous tension and stress-related conditions, PMT, sciatica, shock, vertigo.

OTHER USES Used in pharmaceutical antiseptic ointments and as a fragrance. Extensively employed in all types of soaps, lotions, detergents, cosmetics, perfumes, etc, especially toilet waters and colognes. Employed as a flavouring agent in most categories of food as well as alcoholic and soft drinks.

LEMON
Citrus limon

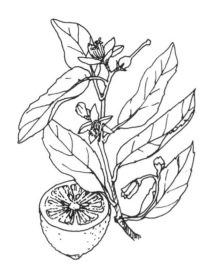

Lemon

FAMILY Rutaceae

SYNONYMS *C. limonum*, cedro oil.

GENERAL DESCRIPTION A small evergreen tree up to 6 metres high with serrated oval leaves, stiff thorns and very fragrant flowers. The fruit turns from green to yellow on ripening.

DISTRIBUTION Native to Asia, probably east India; it now grows wild in the Mediterranean region especially in Spain and Portugal. It is cultivated extensively worldwide in Italy, Sicily, Cyprus, Guinea, Israel, South and North America (California and Florida).

OTHER SPECIES There are about forty-seven varieties which are said to have been developed in cultivation, such as the Java lemon *(C. javanica)*. The lemon is also closely related to the lime, cedrat (or citron) and bergamot.

HERBAL/FOLK TRADITION The juice and peel are widely used as a domestic seasoning. It is very nutritious, being high in vitamins A, B and C. In Spain and other European countries, lemon is something of a 'cure-all', especially with regard to infectious illness. It was used for fever, such as malaria and typhoid, and employed specifically for scurvy on English ships at sea.

Taken internally, the juice is considered invaluable for acidic disorders, such as arthritis and rheumatism, and of great benefit in dysentery and liver congestion.

ACTIONS Anti-anaemic, antimicrobial, antirheumatic, antisclerotic, antiscorbutic, antiseptic, antispasmodic, antitoxic, astringent, bactericidal, carminative, cicatrisant, depurative, diaphoretic, diuretic, febrifuge, haemostatic, hypotensive, insecticidal, rubefacient, stimulates white corpuscles, tonic, vermifuge.

EXTRACTION Essential oil by cold expression from the outer part of the fresh peel. A terpeneless oil is also produced on a large scale (cedro oil).

CHARACTERISTICS A pale greeny-yellow liquid (turning brown with age), with a light, fresh, citrus scent. It blends well with lavender, neroli, ylang ylang, rose, sandalwood, olibanum, chamomile, benzoin, fennel, geranium, eucalyptus, juniper, oakmoss, lavandin, elemi, labdanum and other citrus oils.

PRINCIPAL CONSTITUENTS Limonene (approx. 70 per cent), terpinene, pinenes, sabinene, myrcene, citral, linalol, geraniol, octanol, nonanol, citronellal, bergamotene, among others.

SAFETY DATA Non-toxic; may cause dermal irritation or sensitization reactions in some individuals – apply in moderation. Phototoxic – do not use on skin exposed to direct sunlight.

AROMATHERAPY/HOME USE
SKIN CARE: Acne, anaemia, brittle nails, boils, chilblains, corns, cuts, greasy skin, herpes, insect bites, mouth ulcers, spots, varicose veins, warts.
CIRCULATION, MUSCLES AND JOINTS: Arthritis, cellulitis, high blood pressure, nosebleeds, obesity (congestion), poor circulation, rheumatism
RESPIRATORY SYSTEM: Asthma, throat infections, bronchitis, catarrh.
DIGESTIVE SYSTEM: Dyspepsia.
IMMUNE SYSTEM: Colds, 'flu, fever and infections.

OTHER USES   Used as a flavouring agent in pharmaceuticals. Extensively used as a fragrance component in soaps, detergents, cosmetics, toilet waters and perfumes. Extensively employed by the food industry in most types of product, including alcoholic and soft drinks.

LEMONGRASS
Cymbopogon citratus

FAMILY   Poaceae (Gramineae)

SYNONYMS   1. *Andropogon citratus*, *A. schoenathus*, West Indian lemongrass, Madagascar lemongrass, Guatemala lemongrass.   2. *Andropogon flexuosus*, *Cymbopogon flexuosus*, East Indian lemongrass, Cochin lemongrass, native lemongrass, British India lemongrass, 'vervaine Indienne' or France Indian verbena.

GENERAL DESCRIPTION   A fast-growing, tall, aromatic perennial grass up to 1.5 metres high, producing a network of roots and rootlets that rapidly exhaust the soil.

DISTRIBUTION   Native to Asia, there are two main types: 1. The West Indian lemongrass which is probably native to Sri Lanka, now cultivated mainly in the West Indies, Africa and tropical Asia. Main oil producers include Guatemala and India.   2. The East Indian lemongrass, which is native to east India (Travancore, etc.), now mainly cultivated in western India!

OTHER SPECIES   There are several varieties of lemongrass of which the East Indian and the West Indian types are the most common. Chemotypes within each variety are also quite pronounced.

HERBAL/FOLK TRADITION   Employed in traditional Indian medicine for infectious illness and fever; modern research carried out in India shows that it also acts as a sedative on the central nervous system. It is also used as an insecticide and for flavouring food. After the distillation process, the exhausted grass is used locally to feed cattle.

ACTIONS   Analgesic, antidepressant, antimicrobial, anti-oxidant, antipyretic, antiseptic, astringent, bactericidal, carminative, deodorant, febrifuge, fungicidal, galactagogue, insecticidal, nervine, sedative (nervous), tonic.

EXTRACTION   Essential oil by steam distillation from the fresh and partially dried leaves (grass), finely chopped.

CHARACTERISTICS   1. A yellow, amber or reddish-brown liquid with a fresh, grassy-citrus scent and an earthy undertone.   2. A yellow or amber liquid with a fresh, grassy-lemony scent, generally lighter than the West Indian type.

PRINCIPAL CONSTITUENTS   1. Citral (65–85 per cent), myrcene (12–25 per cent), dipentene, methylheptenone, linalol, geraniol, nerol, citronellol and farnesol, among others. 2. Citral (up to 85 per cent), geraniol, methyl eugenol, borneol, dipentene; constituents vary according to type.

SAFETY DATA   Non-toxic, possible dermal irritation and/or sensitization in some individuals – use with care.

AROMATHERAPY/HOME USE
SKIN CARE: Acne, athlete's foot, excessive perspiration, insect repellent (fleas, lice, ticks), open pores, pediculosis, scabies, tissue toner.
CIRCULATION, MUSCLES AND JOINTS: Muscular pain, poor circulation and muscle tone, slack tissue.
DIGESTIVE SYSTEM: Colitis, indigestion, gastro-enteritis.
IMMUNE SYSTEM: Fevers, infectious disease.
NERVOUS SYSTEM: Headaches, nervous exhaustion and stress-related conditions.

OTHER USES   Extensively used as a fragrance component in soaps, detergents, cosmetics and perfumes. Employed as a flavour ingredient in most major food categories including alcoholic and soft drinks. Also used for the isolation of citral and for the adulteration of more costly oils such as verbena or melissa.

LIME
Citrus aurantifolia

FAMILY Rutaceae

SYNONYMS *C. medica var. acida*, *C. latifolia*, Mexican lime, West Indian lime, sour lime.

GENERAL DESCRIPTION A small evergreen tree up to 4.5 metres high, with stiff sharp spines, smooth ovate leaves and small white flowers. The bitter fruit is a pale green colour, about half the size of a lemon.

DISTRIBUTION Probably native to south Asia; naturalized in many tropical and subtropical regions of the world. It is cultivated mainly in south Florida, the West Indies (Cuba), Central America (Mexico) and Italy.

OTHER SPECIES There are several species of lime such as the Italian lime *(C. limetta)* which is used to produce an oil called 'limette'; and the leech-lime *(C. hystrix)* which is occasionally used to produce an essential oil called combava.

HERBAL/FOLK TRADITION The fruit is often used indiscriminately in place of lemon with which it shares many qualities. It is used for similar purposes including fever, infections, sore throat, colds, etc. It used to be used as a remedy for dyspepsia with glycerin of pepsin.

ACTIONS Antirheumatic, antiscorbutic, antiseptic, antiviral, aperitif, bactericidal, febrifuge, restorative, tonic.

EXTRACTION Essential oil by 1. cold expression of the peel of the unripe fruit; the expressed oil is preferred in perfumery work, and 2. steam distillation of the whole ripe crushed fruit (a by-product of the juice industry).

CHARACTERISTICS 1. A pale yellow or olive-green liquid with a fresh, sweet, citrus-peel odour. 2. A water-white or pale yellow liquid with a fresh, sharp, fruity-citrus scent. It blends well with neroli, citronella, lavender, lavandin, rosemary, clary sage and other citrus oils.

PRINCIPAL CONSTITUENTS Limonene, pinenes, camphene, sabinene, citral, cymene, cineols and linalol, among others. The expressed 'peel' oil, but not the 'whole fruit' oil, also contains coumarins.

SAFETY DATA Non-toxic, non-irritant, non-sensitizing. However, the expressed 'peel' oil is phototoxic (but not the steam-distilled 'whole fruit' oil).

AROMATHERAPY/HOME USE See *lemon*.

OTHER USES Both oils, but mainly the expressed, are used as fragrance components in soaps, detergents, cosmetics and perfumes. Mainly the distilled oil, but also the terpeneless oil, is used by the food industry, especially in soft drinks – 'lemon and lime' flavour. The juice is used for the production of citric acid.

LINALOE
Bursera glabrifolia

FAMILY Burseraceae

SYNONYMS *B. delpechiana*, Mexican linaloe, 'copal limon'.

GENERAL DESCRIPTION A tall, bushy tropical shrub or tree, with a smooth bark and bearing fleshy fruit. The wood is only used for distillation purposes when the tree is twenty or thirty years old. The oil is partially a pathological product since its production is stimulated by lacerating the trunk – which apparently must be wounded on the night of the full moon for the tree to produce any oil!

DISTRIBUTION Native to Central and South America, especially Mexico. It is cultivated in the Far East particularly in India (Mysore). The wood oil is mainly produced in Mexico, the seed (and husk) oil in India.

OTHER SPECIES There are several species which are all known simply as linaloe: see Botanical Classification section. West Indian elemi *(B. simaruba)* is a close relative, as are myrrh and frankincense.

HERBAL/FOLK TRADITION The seed oil is known in India as 'Indian lavender oil' and used chiefly as a local perfume ingredient and in soaps by the cosmetics industry of Mysore state. It is not much found outside India. In Mexico the wood oil is used in a similar fashion to rosewood, which contains similar constituents.

ACTIONS Anticonvulsant, anti-inflammatory, antiseptic, bactericidal, deodorant, gentle tonic.

EXTRACTION Essential oil by steam distillation from the 1. Wood, and 2. Seed and husk. (An essential oil is also occasionally produced from the leaves and twigs.)

CHARACTERISTICS 1. A pale yellow liquid with a sweet-woody, floral scent, similar to rosewood. It blends well with rose, sandalwood, cedarwood, rosewood, frankincense, floral and woody fragrances. 2. A colourless liquid with a terpene-like odour, harsher than the wood oil.

PRINCIPAL CONSTITUENTS 1. Mainly linalol, some linalyl acetate. 2. Mainly linalyl acetate, some linalol.

SAFETY DATA Non-toxic, non-irritant, non-sensitizing.

AROMATHERAPY/HOME USE
SKIN CARE: Acne, cuts, dermatitis, wounds, etc., all skin types.
NERVOUS SYSTEM: Nervous tension and stress-related conditions.

OTHER USES The wood oil is used in soaps, toiletries and perfumes. It is also used for the production of natural linalol, although this is increasingly being replaced by synthetic linalol.

LINDEN
Tilia vulgaris

FAMILY Tiliaceae

SYNONYMS *T. europaea*, lime tree, common lime, lyne, tillet, tilea.

GENERAL DESCRIPTION A tall graceful tree up to 30 metres high with a smooth bark, spreading branches and bright green, heart-shaped leaves. It has yellowy-white flowers borne in clusters which have a very powerful scent.

DISTRIBUTION Native to Europe and the northern hemisphere. Common in England, France, Holland, etc.

OTHER SPECIES Several related types such as the broad-leaved lime *(T. platyphylla)* and the small-leaved lime *(T. cordata)*.

HERBAL/FOLK TRADITION Linden tea, known as 'tilleul', is drunk a great deal on the Continent, especially in France, as a general relaxant. The flowers are also used for indigestion, palpitations, nausea, hysteria and catarrhal symptoms following a cold. The honey from the flowers is highly regarded, and used in medicines and liqueurs. According to Culpeper the flowers are a 'good cephalic and

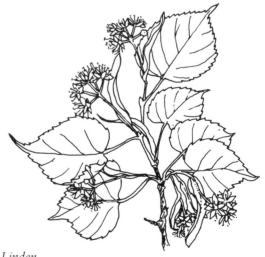

Linden

nervine, excellent for apoplexy, epilepsy, vertigo and palpitation of the heart.'[50] Lime flowers are current in the British Herbal Pharmacopoeia, indicated for migraine, hysteria, arteriosclerotic hypertension and feverish colds.

ACTIONS Astringent (mild), antispasmodic, bechic, carminative, cephalic, diaphoretic, diuretic, emollient, nervine, sedative, tonic.

EXTRACTION A concrete and absolute by solvent extraction from the dried flowers.

CHARACTERISTICS The concrete is a hard, brittle, dark green mass with a herbaceous, dry, haylike odour. The absolute is a yellow semi-solid mass with a green-herbaceous, dry, characteristic odour.

PRINCIPAL CONSTITUENTS Mainly farnesol – the concrete is very rich in waxes.

SAFETY DATA Most products are adulterated or synthetic. No safety data available at present.

AROMATHERAPY/HOME USE
DIGESTIVE SYSTEM: Cramps, indigestion, liver pains.
NERVOUS SYSTEM: Headaches, insomnia, migraine, nervous tension and stress-related conditions.

OTHER USES Occasionally used in high class perfumery.

LITSEA CUBEBA
Litsea cubeba

FAMILY Lauraceae

SYNONYMS *L. citrata*, 'may chang', exotic verbena, tropical verbena.

GENERAL DESCRIPTION A small tropical tree with fragrant, lemongrass-scented leaves and flowers. The small fruits are shaped like peppers, from which the name 'cubeba' derives.

DISTRIBUTION Native to east Asia, especially China; cultivated in Taiwan and Japan. China is the main producer of the oil, much of which is used by the Chinese themselves.

OTHER SPECIES Despite its folk names, this plant is not related to lemon verbena (*Aloysia triphylla*). It belongs to the same family as the laurel tree, rosewood and cinnamon.

HERBAL/FOLK TRADITION It is planted as a wind breaker in China.

ACTIONS Antiseptic, deodorant, digestive, disinfectant, insecticidal, stimulant, stomachic.

EXTRACTION Essential oil by steam distillation from the fruits.

CHARACTERISTICS A pale yellow mobile liquid with an intense, lemony, fresh-fruity odour (sweeter than lemongrass but less tenacious).

PRINCIPAL CONSTITUENTS Mainly citral (up to 85 per cent).

SAFETY DATA Non-toxic, non-irritant, possible sensitization in some individuals.

AROMATHERAPY/HOME USE
SKIN CARE: Acne, dermatitis, excessive perspiration, greasy skin, insect repellent, spots.
DIGESTIVE SYSTEM: Flatulence, indigestion.
IMMUNE SYSTEM: Epidemics, sanitation.

OTHER USES Extensively used as a fragrance component in air fresheners, soaps, deodorants, colognes, toiletries and perfumes. Employed in flavouring work, especially fruit products. It serves as a source of natural 'citral' all over the world.

LOVAGE
Levisticum officinale

FAMILY Apiaceae (Umbelliferae)

SYNONYMS *Angelica levisticum, Ligusticum*

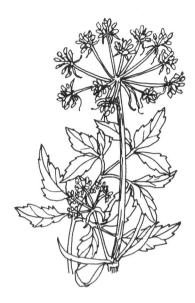

Lovage

levisticum, smellage, maggi herb, garden lovage, common lovage, old English lovage, Italian lovage, Cornish lovage.

GENERAL DESCRIPTION A large perennial herb up to 2 metres high with a stout hollow stem and dense ornamental foliage. It has a thick fleshy root and greenish-yellow flowers. The whole plant has a strong aromatic scent.

DISTRIBUTION Native to southern Europe and western Asia; naturalized in North America. It is cultivated in central and southern Europe, especially in France, Belgium, Czechoslovakia, Hungary, Yugoslavia and Germany.

OTHER SPECIES Several related plants are also used to produce essential oils, such as sea lovage *(Ligusticum scoticum)* and alpine lovage *(L. mutellina)*.

HERBAL/FOLK TRADITION A herb of ancient medical repute, used mainly for digestive complaints, oedema, skin problems, menstrual irregularities and fever. It was also believed to be good for the sight. The leaf stalks used to be blanched and used as a vegetable or in salads.   The root is current in the British Herbal Pharmacopoeia as a specific for flatulent dyspepsia and anorexia.

ACTIONS Antimicrobial, antiseptic, antispasmodic, diaphoretic, digestive, diuretic, carminative, depurative, emmenagogue, expectorant, febrifuge, stimulant (digestive), stomachic.

EXTRACTION Essential oil by steam distillation from   1. the fresh roots, and   2. the herb – fresh leaves and stalks.

CHARACTERISTICS 1. An amber or olive-brown liquid with a rich, spicy-warm, root-like odour.   2. A very pale yellow mobile liquid with a spicy, warm odour and sweet-floral undertone. It blends well with rose, galbanum, costus, opopanax, oakmoss, bay, lavandin and spice oils.

PRINCIPAL CONSTITUENTS Mainly phthalides (up to 70 per cent) such as butylidene, dihydrobutylidene, butylphthalides and ligostilides, with lesser amounts of terpenoids, volatile acids, coumarins and furocoumarins.

SAFETY DATA Non-toxic, non-irritant, possible sensitization/phototoxic effects. Use with care. Avoid during pregnancy.

AROMATHERAPY/HOME USE
CIRCULATION, MUSCLES AND JOINTS: Accumulation of toxins, congestion, gout, oedema, poor circulation, rheumatism, water retention.
DIGESTIVE SYSTEM: Anaemia, flatulence, indigestion, spasm.
GENITO-URINARY SYSTEM: Amenorrhoea, dysmenorrhoea, cystitis.

OTHER USES The root oil is used as a fragrance component in soaps, cosmetics and perfumes. The oils and extracts are used as savoury flavouring agents and in liqueurs and tobacco.

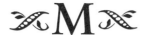

MANDARIN
Citrus reticulata

FAMILY Rutaceae

SYNONYMS *C. nobilis, C. madurensis, C. unshiu, C. deliciosa,* European mandarin, true mandarin, tangerine, satsuma.

GENERAL DESCRIPTION A small evergreen tree up to 6 metres high with glossy leaves, fragrant flowers and bearing fleshy fruit. The tangerine is larger than the mandarin and rounder, with a yellower skin, more like the original Chinese type.

DISTRIBUTION Native to southern China and the Far East. Brought to Europe in 1805 and to America forty years later, where it was renamed the tangerine. The mandarin is produced mainly in Italy, Spain, Algeria, Cyprus, Greece, the Middle East and Brazil; the tangerine in Texas, Florida, California and Guinea.

OTHER SPECIES There are many cultivars within this species: the terms tangerine *(C. reticulata)* and mandarin are used somewhat interchangeably, as is the word satsuma. They could be said to represent different chemotypes since the oils are quite different; see the Botanical Classification section.

HERBAL/FOLK TRADITION The name comes from the fruit which was a traditional gift to the Mandarins of China. In France it is regarded as a safe children's remedy for indigestion, hiccoughs, etc, and also for the elderly since it helps strengthen the digestive function and liver.

ACTIONS Antiseptic, antispasmodic, carminative, digestive, diuretic (mild), laxative (mild), sedative, stimulant (digestive and lymphatic), tonic.

EXTRACTION Essential oil by cold expression from the outer peel. A mandarin petitgrain oil is also produced in small quantities by steam distillation from the leaves and twigs.

CHARACTERISTICS Mandarin oil is a yellowy-orange mobile liquid with a blue-violet hint, having an intensely sweet, almost floral citrus scent. It blends well with other citrus oils, especially neroli, and spice oils such as nutmeg, cinnamon and clove. Tangerine oil is an orange mobile liquid with a fresh, sweet, orangelike aroma. It has less body than mandarin and is little used in perfumery work.

PRINCIPAL CONSTITUENTS Limonene, methyl methylanthranilate, geraniol, citral, citronellal, among others.

SAFETY DATA Non-toxic, non-irritant, non-sensitizing. Possibly phototoxic, although it has not been demonstrated decisively.

AROMATHERAPY/HOME USE
SKIN CARE: Acne, congested and oily skin, scars, spots, stretch marks, toner.
CIRCULATION, MUSCLES AND JOINTS: Fluid retention, obesity.
DIGESTIVE SYSTEM: Digestive problems, dyspepsia, hiccoughs, intestinal problems.
NERVOUS SYSTEM: Insomnia, nervous tension, restlessness. It is often used for children and pregnant women and is recommended in synergistic combinations with other citrus oils.

OTHER USES Mandarin oil is used in soaps, cosmetics and perfumes, especially colognes. It is employed as a flavouring agent especially in sweets, soft drinks and liqueurs.

MARIGOLD
Calendula officinalis

FAMILY Asteraceae (Compositae)

SYNONYMS Calendula, marygold, marybud, gold-bloom, pot marigold, hollygold, common marigold, poet's marigold.

GENERAL DESCRIPTION An annual herb up to 60 cms high with soft, oval, pale green leaves and bright orange daisylike flowers.

DISTRIBUTION Native to southern Europe and Egypt; naturalized throughout temperate regions of the world. Widely cultivated, especially in northern Europe for domestic and medicinal use. The absolute is only produced in France.

OTHER SPECIES There are several species of marigold, but the common marigold is the one generally used medicinally. It should not be confused with tagetes or taget from the Mexican marigold *(Tagetes minuta)* or the African marigold *(T. erecta)*, the oil of which is also often called 'calendula'.

HERBAL/FOLK TRADITION A herb of ancient medical repute, said to 'comfort the heart and spirits'.[51] It was also used for skin complaints, menstrual irregularities, varicose veins, haemorrhoids, conjunctivitis and poor eyesight. The flowers are current in the British Herbal Pharmacopoeia, specific for enlarged or inflamed lymph nodes, sebaceous cysts, duodenal ulcers and inflammatory skin lesions.
  The infused oil is useful for a wide range of skin problems including cracked and rough skin, nappy rash, grazes, cracked nipples, varicose veins and inflammations.

ACTIONS Antihaemorrhagic, anti-inflammatory, antiseptic, antispasmodic, astringent, diaphoretic, cholagogue, cicatrisant, emmenagogue, febrifuge, fungicidal, styptic, tonic, vulnerary.

EXTRACTION An absolute by solvent extraction from the flowers.

CHARACTERISTICS A dark greenish-brown viscous liquid with an intensely sharp, herbaceous odour. It blends well with oakmoss, hyacinth, floral and citrus oils.

PRINCIPAL CONSTITUENTS The absolute contains calendulin (a yellow resin), waxes and volatile oil.

SAFETY DATA Non-toxic, non-irritant, non-sensitizing. The real calendula absolute is only produced in small quantities, and is difficult to get hold of.

AROMATHERAPY/HOME USE
SKIN CARE: Burns, cuts, eczema, greasy skin, inflammations, insect bites, rashes, wounds. NB: 'The infused oil is very valuable in Aromatherapy for its powerful skin-healing properties.'[52]

OTHER USES Used in high class perfumery.

MARJORAM, SWEET
Origanum majorana

FAMILY Lamiaceae (Labiatae)

SYNONYMS *Marjorana hortensis*, knotted marjoram.

GENERAL DESCRIPTION A tender bushy perennial plant (cultivated as an annual in colder climates), up to 60 cms high with a hairy stem, dark green oval leaves and small greyish-white flowers in clusters or 'knots'. The whole plant is strongly aromatic.

DISTRIBUTION Native to the Mediterranean region, Egypt and North Africa. Major oil-producing countries include France, Tunisia, Morocco, Egypt, Bulgaria, Hungary and Germany.

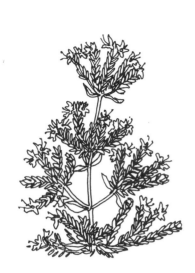

Sweet Marjoram

OTHER SPECIES There is a great deal of confusion regarding the various species of marjoram or oregano. The most common types are the pot or French marjoram *(Origanum onites* or *Marjorana onites)*, which is a hardier plant than the sweet marjoram and of a spreading nature; the Spanish marjoram or oregano *(Thymus mastichina)* and the wild or common marjoram or oregano *(Origanum vulgare)* which is used to produce the so-called 'oregano oil'. See entries on common oregano, Spanish oregano and also the Botanical Classification section.

HERBAL/FOLK TRADITION A traditional culinary herb and folk remedy. It was used by the ancient Greeks in their fragrances, cosmetics and medicines; the name oregano derives from a Greek word meaning 'joy of the mountains'. It is a versatile herb which has a soothing, fortifying and warming effect; it aids digestive and menstrual problems, as well as nervous and respiratory complaints.

It is 'comforting in cold diseases of the head, stomach, sinews and other parts, taken inwardly or outwardly applied ... helps diseases of the chest, obstructions of the liver and spleen.'[53] It is also very helpful for muscular and rheumatic pain, sprains, strains, stiff joints, bruises, etc.

ACTIONS Analgesic, anaphrodisiac, anti-oxidant, antiseptic, antispasmodic, antiviral, bactericidal, carminative, cephalic, cordial, diaphoretic, digestive, diuretic, emmenagogue, expectorant, fungicidal, hypotensive, laxative, nervine, sedative, stomachic, tonic, vasodilator, vulnerary.

EXTRACTION Essential oil by steam distillation of the dried flowering herb. An oleoresin is also produced in smaller quantities.

CHARACTERISTICS A pale yellow or amber-coloured mobile liquid with a warm, woody, spicy-camphoraceous odour. It blends well with lavender, rosemary, bergamot, chamomile, cypress, cedarwood, tea tree and eucalyptus.

PRINCIPAL CONSTITUENTS Terpinenes, terpineol, sabinenes, linalol, carvacrol, linalyl acetate, ocimene, cadinene, geranyl acetate, citral, eugenol, among others.

SAFETY DATA Non-toxic, non-irritant, non-sensitizing. Not to be used during pregnancy.

AROMATHERAPY/HOME USE
SKIN CARE: Chilblains, bruises, ticks.
CIRCULATION, MUSCLES AND JOINTS: Arthritis, lumbago, muscular aches and stiffness, rheumatism, sprains, strains.
RESPIRATORY SYSTEM: Asthma, bronchitis, coughs.
DIGESTIVE SYSTEM: Colic, constipation, dyspepsia, flatulence.
GENITO-URINARY SYSTEM: Amenorrhoea, dysmenorrhoea, leucorrhoea, PMT.
IMMUNE SYSTEM: Colds.
NERVOUS SYSTEM: Headache, hypertension, insomnia, migraine, nervous tension and stress-related conditions.

OTHER USES The oil and oleoresin are used as fragrance components in soaps, detergents, cosmetics and perfumes. Employed in most major food categories, especially meats, seasonings and sauces, as well as soft drinks and alcoholic beverages such as vermouths and bitters.

MASTIC
Pistacia lentiscus

FAMILY Anacardiaceae

SYNONYMS Mastick tree, mastick, mastix, mastich, lentisk.

GENERAL DESCRIPTION A small bushy tree or shrub up to 3 metres high, which produces a natural oleoresin from the trunk. Incisions are made in the bark in order to collect the liquid oleoresin, which then hardens into brittle pea-sized lumps.

DISTRIBUTION Native to the Mediterranean region (France, Spain, Portugal, Greece, Turkey) and also found in North Africa. Most mastic is produced on the Greek Island of Chios; some is also produced in Algeria, Morocco and the Canary Islands.

OTHER SPECIES It belongs to the same family as Peruvian pepper or Peruvian mastic *(Schinus molle)*. Mastic resembles the resin 'sanderach' but unlike the latter it can be chewed, rather than turning to powder.

HERBAL/FOLK TRADITION In the East it is used for the manufacture of sweets and cordials; it is still used medicinally for diarrhoea in children and is chewed to sweeten the breath. The oil was used in the West in a similar way to turpentine – 'It has many of the properties of coniferous turpentines and was formerly greatly used in medicine.'[54]

ACTIONS Antimicrobial, antiseptic, antispasmodic, astringent, diuretic, expectorant, stimulant.

EXTRACTION 1. A resinoid is produced by solvent extraction from the oleoresin, and 2. an essential oil is produced by steam distillation from the oleoresin or occasionally directly from the leaves and branches.

CHARACTERISTICS 1. A pale amber or greenish viscous mass with a faint balsamic turpentine-like odour. 2. A pale yellow mobile liquid with a fresh balsamic turpentine-like odour. It blends well with lavender, mimosa, citrus and floral oils.

PRINCIPAL CONSTITUENTS Mainly monoterpene hydrocarbons – mostly pinenes.

SAFETY DATA Non-toxic, non-irritant, possible sensitization in some individuals.

AROMATHERAPY/HOME USE See *turpentine*.

OTHER USES Used in dentistry and in the production of varnish. The resinoid and oil are employed in high class colognes and perfumes, and used as a flavouring agent, especially in liqueurs.

MELILOTUS
Melilotus officinalis

FAMILY Fabaceae (Leguminosae)

SYNONYMS Common melilot, yellow melilot, white melilot, corn melilot, melilot trefoil, sweet clover, plaster clover, sweet lucerne, wild laburnum, king's clover, melilotin (oleoresin).

GENERAL DESCRIPTION A bushy perennial herb up to 1 metre high with smooth erect stems, trifoliate oval leaves and small sweet-scented white or yellow flowers. The scent of the flowers becomes stronger on drying.

DISTRIBUTION Native to Europe and Asia Minor. Other similar species are found in Asia, the USA and Africa. The flowers are mainly cultivated in England, France, Germany and the USSR.

OTHER SPECIES There are several similar species such as *M. arvensis,* the oil of which is also used in perfumery and flavouring work.

HERBAL/FOLK TRADITION The leaves and shoots are used on the Continent for conditions which include sleeplessness, thrombosis, nervous tension, varicose veins, intestinal disorders, headache, earache and indigestion. In the form of an ointment or plaster, it is used externally for inflamed or swollen joints, abdominal and rheumatic pain, also bruises, cuts and skin eruptions.

ACTIONS Anti-inflammatory, antirheumatic, antispasmodic, astringent, emollient, expectorant, digestive, insecticidal (against moth), sedative.

EXTRACTION A concrete (usually called a resinoid or oleoresin) by solvent extraction from the dry flowers.

CHARACTERISTICS A viscous dark green liquid with a rich, sweet-herbaceous 'new-mown hay' scent.

PRINCIPAL CONSTITUENTS Mainly coumarins – melilotic acid and orthocoumaric acid.

SAFETY DATA In 1953 in some countries including the USA, coumarin was banned from use in flavourings due to toxicity levels. Some coumarins are also known to be phototoxic.

AROMATHERAPY/HOME USE None.

OTHER USES The oleoresin is used in high class perfumery work. Extensively used for flavouring tobacco in countries without the coumarin ban.

MIMOSA
Acacia dealbata

FAMILY Mimosaceae

SYNONYMS *A. decurrens var. dealbata,* Sydney black wattle.

GENERAL DESCRIPTION An attractive small tree up to 12 metres high, having a greyish-brown bark with irregular longitudinal ridges, delicate foliage and clusters of ball-shaped fragrant yellow flowers.

DISTRIBUTION Native to Australia; naturalized in North and Central Africa. It was brought to Europe as an ornamental plant in the early nineteenth century, but it now grows wild. The concrete (and absolute) is mainly produced in southern France, and also Italy.

OTHER SPECIES There are many varieties of *Acacia,* such as the East African type *(A. arabica)* which is very similar; the mimosa of the florist shop *(A. floribunda)*; and the Brazilian mimosa or sensitive plant *(Mimosa humilis)*, the homoeopathic tincture of which is used for swelling of the ankles. It is also closely related to cassie.

HERBAL/FOLK TRADITION The bark of mimosa which is known as 'wattle bark', has a leather-like odour and astringent taste. It contains up to 42 per cent tannins (also gallic acid) and is used extensively by the tanning industry. It is employed medicinally in similar ways to oak bark, as a specific for diarrhoea, and as an astringent gargle and ointment.
  The extract of black catechu *(A. catechu)* is current in the British Herbal Pharmacopoeia as a specific for chronic diarrhoea with colitis.

ACTIONS Antiseptic, astringent.

EXTRACTION A concrete and absolute by solvent extraction from the flowers and twig ends.

CHARACTERISTICS 1. Concrete – a hard wax-like yellow mass with a sweet-woody, deep floral fragrance. 2. Absolute – an amber-coloured viscous liquid with a slightly green, woody-floral scent. It blends well with lavandin, lavender, ylang ylang, violet, styrax, citronella, Peru balsam, cassie, floral and spice oils.

PRINCIPAL CONSTITUENTS Mainly hydrocarbons; palmic aldehyde, enanthic acid, anisic acid, acetic acid and phenols.

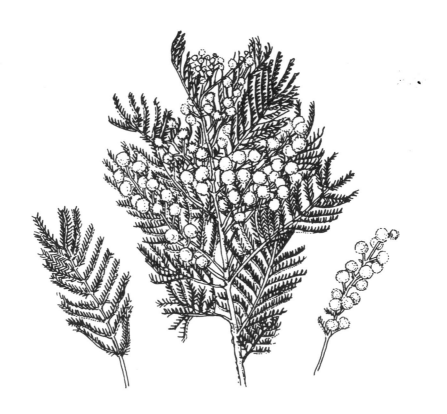

Mimosa

SAFETY DATA Non-toxic, non-irritant, non-sensitizing.

AROMATHERAPY/HOME USE
SKIN CARE: Oily, sensitive, general skin care.
NERVOUS SYSTEM: Anxiety, nervous tension, over-sensitivity, stress.

OTHER USES Employed largely in soaps, due to its good fixative properties. Also in high class perfumes, especially colognes, floral and oriental types.

MINT, CORNMINT
Mentha arvensis

FAMILY Lamiaceae (Labiatae)

SYNONYMS Field mint, Japanese mint.

GENERAL DESCRIPTION A rather fragile herb with leafy stems up to 60 cms high, lance-shaped leaves and lilac-coloured flowers borne in clustered whorls in the axils of the upper leaves.

DISTRIBUTION Native to Europe and parts of Asia (Japan and China); naturalized in North America. Major producers of the oil include China, Brazil, Argentina, India and Vietnam.

OTHER SPECIES There are many varieties and chemotypes of this herb, which is used for large scale oil production, such as the Chinese type *M. arvensis var. glabrata*, and the Japanese species *M. arvensis var. piperascens*.

HERBAL/FOLK TRADITION It is used therapeutically in many of the same ways as peppermint; the bruised leaves are applied to the forehead to relieve nervous headache. In the East it is used to treat rheumatic pain, neuralgia, toothache, laryngitis, indigestion, colds and bronchitis. In Chinese medicine, it is also employed for relieving earache, treating tumours and some skin conditions.

ACTIONS Anaesthetic, antimicrobial, antiseptic, antispasmodic, carminative, cytotoxic, digestive, expectorant, stimulant, stomachic.

EXTRACTION Essential oil by steam distillation from the flowering herb. The oil is usually dementholized since it contains so much menthol that it is otherwise solid at room temperature.

CHARACTERISTICS Dementholized oil – a colourless or pale yellow liquid with a strong, fresh, bitter-sweet minty odour, somewhat like peppermint.

PRINCIPAL CONSTITUENTS Menthol (70–95 per cent), menthone (10–20 per cent), pinene, menthyl acetate, isomenthone, thujone, phellandrene, piperitone and menthofuran, among others. Constituents vary according to source.

SAFETY DATA Non-toxic, non-irritant (except in concentration); may cause sensitization in some individuals. Menthol is a dermal irritant.

AROMATHERAPY/HOME USE None. Use peppermint in preference, since it is not fractionated like the commercial cornmint oil and has a more refined fragrance.

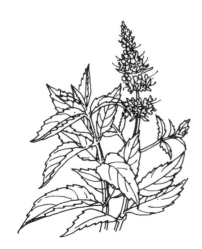

Peppermint

OTHER USES Used in some pharmaceutical preparations, such as cough lozenges, herb teas and syrups, mainly in the form of menthol. Extensively employed in soaps, toothpastes, detergents, cosmetics, perfumes and especially industrial fragrances. Used by the food industry especially for flavouring confectionery, liqueurs and chewing gum. However, it is mainly used for the isolation of natural menthol.

MINT, PEPPERMINT
Mentha piperita

FAMILY Lamiaceae (Labiatae)

SYNONYMS Brandy mint, balm mint.

GENERAL DESCRIPTION A perennial herb up to 1 metre high with underground runners by which it is easily propagated. The 'white' peppermint has green stems and leaves; the 'black' peppermint has dark green serrated leaves, purplish stems and reddish-violet flowers.

DISTRIBUTION Originally a cultivated hybrid between *M. viridis* and *M. aquatica*, known to have been propagated from before the seventeenth century in England. Naturalized throughout Europe and America, it is cultivated worldwide. The oil is produced mainly in France, England, America, Russia, Bulgaria, Italy, Hungary, Morocco and China.

OTHER SPECIES There are several different strains or chemotypes of peppermint. In addition there are numerous other species of mint, such as spearmint, apple mint, pennyroyal, water mint and pineapple mint – some of which are used to produce essential oils (see Botanical Classification section). Peppermints grown in northern regions, including the Mitcham peppermint, are considered of superior quality.

HERBAL/FOLK TRADITION Mints have been cultivated since ancient times in China and Japan. In Egypt evidence of a type of peppermint has been found in tombs dating from 1000BC. It has been used extensively in Eastern and Western medicine for a variety of complaints, including indigestion, nausea, sore throat, diarrhoea, headaches, toothaches and cramp.

It is current in the British Herbal Pharmacopoeia for intestinal colic, flatulence, common cold, vomiting in pregnancy and dysmenorrhoea.

ACTIONS Analgesic, anti-inflammatory, antimicrobial, antiphlogistic, antipruritic, antiseptic, antispasmodic, antiviral, astringent, carminative, cephalic, cholagogue, cordial, emmenagogue, expectorant, febrifuge, hepatic, nervine, stomachic, sudorific, vasoconstrictor, vermifuge.

EXTRACTION Essential oil by steam distillation from the flowering herb (approx. 3–4 per cent yield).

CHARACTERISTICS A pale yellow or greenish liquid with a highly penetrating, grassy-minty camphoraceous odour. It blends well with benzoin, rosemary, lavender, marjoram, lemon, eucalyptus and other mints.

PRINCIPAL CONSTITUENTS Menthol (29–48 per cent), menthone (20–31 per cent), menthyl acetate, menthofuran, limonene, pulegone, cineol, among others.

SAFETY DATA Non-toxic, non-irritant (except in concentration), possible sensitization due to menthol. Use in moderation.

AROMATHERAPY/HOME USE
SKIN CARE: Acne, dermatitis, ringworm, scabies, toothache.
CIRCULATION, MUSCLES AND JOINTS: Neuralgia, muscular pain, palpitations.
RESPIRATORY SYSTEM: Asthma, bronchitis, halitosis, sinusitis, spasmodic cough – 'When inhaled (in steam) it checks catarrh temporarily, and will provide relief from head colds and bronchitis: its antispasmodic action combines well with this to make it a most useful inhalation in asthma.'[55]
DIGESTIVE SYSTEM: Colic, cramp, dyspepsia, flatulence, nausea.

IMMUNE SYSTEM: Colds, 'flu, fevers.
NERVOUS SYSTEM: Fainting, headache, mental fatigue, migraine, nervous stress, vertigo.

OTHER USES Flavouring agent in pharmaceuticals, and ingredient in cough, cold and digestive remedies. Flavouring agent in many foods, especially chewing gum and sweets, alcoholic and soft drinks; also widely used to flavour tobacco. Fragrance component in soaps, toothpaste, detergents, cosmetics, colognes and perfumes.

MINT, SPEARMINT
Mentha spicata

FAMILY Lamiaceae (Labiatae)

SYNONYMS *M. viridis*, common spearmint, garden spearmint, spire mint, green mint, lamb mint, pea mint, fish mint.

GENERAL DESCRIPTION A hardy branched perennial herb with bright green, lance-shaped, sharply toothed leaves, quickly spreading underground runners and pink or lilac-coloured flowers in slender cylindrical spikes.

DISTRIBUTION Native to the Mediterranean region, now common throughout Europe, western Asia and the Middle East. It was introduced to the USA where it has become a very popular flavouring. The oil is produced in midwest USA, Hungary, Spain, Yugoslavia, the USSR and China.

OTHER SPECIES There are several different types of spearmint, especially in the USA, such as the curly mint *(M. spicata var. crispa)*. In Russia the oil from *M. verticellata* is also sold as spearmint oil.

HERBAL/FOLK TRADITION Valued all over the world as a culinary herb, as shown by its folk names. It was used by the ancient Greeks as a restorative and to scent their bathwater. The distilled water is used to relieve hiccough, colic, nausea, indigestion and flatulence. 'Applied to the forehead and temples, it eases the pains in the head, and is good to wash the heads of young children with, against all manner of breakings out, sores or scabs ... being smelled unto, it is comforting to the head.'[56]

ACTIONS Anaesthetic (local), antiseptic, antispasmodic, astringent, carminative, cephalic, cholagogue, decongestant, digestive, diuretic, expectorant, febrifuge, hepatic, nervine, stimulant, stomachic, tonic.

EXTRACTION Essential oil by steam distillation from the flowering tops.

CHARACTERISTICS A pale yellow or olive mobile liquid with a warm, spicy-herbaceous, minty odour. It blends well with lavender, lavandin, jasmine, eucalyptus, basil and rosemary and is often used in combination with peppermint.

PRINCIPAL CONSTITUENTS L-carvone (50–70 per cent), dihydrocarvone, phellandrene, limonene, menthone, menthol, pulegone, cineol, linalol, pinenes, among others.

SAFETY DATA Non-toxic, non-irritant, non-sensitizing.

AROMATHERAPY/HOME USE 'The properties of spearmint oil resemble those of peppermint but its effects are less powerful ... it is better adapted to children's maladies.'[57]
SKIN CARE: Acne, dermatitis, congested skin.
RESPIRATORY SYSTEM: Asthma, bronchitis, catarrhal conditions, sinusitis.
DIGESTIVE SYSTEM: Colic, dyspepsia, flatulence, hepatobiliary disorders, nausea, vomiting.
IMMUNE SYSTEM: Colds, fevers, 'flu.
NERVOUS SYSTEM: Fatigue, headache, migraine, nervous strain, neurasthenia, stress.

OTHER USES Used as a fragrance component, mainly in soaps and colognes. Primarily used as a flavour ingredient in a wide range of products, including toothpaste, chewing gum, sweets, alcoholic and soft drinks.

MUGWORT
Artemisia vulgaris

FAMILY Asteraceae (Compositae)

SYNONYMS Armoise, wild wormwood, felon herb, St John's plant.

GENERAL DESCRIPTION An erect, much-branched, perennial herb up to 1.5 metres high, with purplish stems, dark green divided leaves which are downy white beneath, and numerous small reddish-brown or yellow flowers.

DISTRIBUTION Believed to have originated in eastern Europe and western Asia; now found in temperate zones all over the world. The oil is produced in southern France, Morocco, Germany, Hungary, India, China and Japan.

OTHER SPECIES There are many different species in the *Artemisia* group (see Botanical Classification), which includes wormwood and tarragon. There are also several different types of mugwort such as the great mugwort (*A. arborescens*) and the Chinese mugwort (*A. moxa* and *A. sinensis*) which are both used to make 'moxa' in Japan, containing mainly borneol.

HERBAL/FOLK TRADITION In Europe, the herb has been associated with superstition and witchcraft, and was seen as a protective charm against evil and danger. It is said that St John the Baptist wore a girdle of the leaves in the wilderness. It was also seen as a woman's plant, used as a womb tonic, for painful or delayed menstruation and as a treatment for hysteria and epilepsy. It was also used to expel worms, control fever and as a digestive remedy.
　In the East the white fluffy underside of the leaves is used for moxibustion, a process often combined with acupuncture, in which the compressed dried herb is burned over a certain point in the body to stimulate it with heat. Moxa was also used in Europe to relieve gout and rheumatism.
　It is current in the British Herbal

Pharmacopoeia as a specific for amenorrhoea and dysmenorrhoea.

ACTIONS Anthelmintic, antispasmodic, carminative, choleretic, diaphoretic, diuretic, emmenagogue, nervine, orexigenic, stimulant, stomachic, tonic (uterine, womb), vermifuge.

EXTRACTION Essential oil by steam distillation from the leaves and flowering tops.

CHARACTERISTICS A colourless or pale yellow liquid with a powerful camphoraceous, bitter-sweet, herbaceous odour. It blends well with oakmoss, patchouli, rosemary, lavandin, pine, sage, clary sage and cedarwood.

PRINCIPAL CONSTITUENTS Thujone, cineol, pinenes and dihydromatricaria ester, among others.

SAFETY DATA Oral toxin, due to high thujone content. Abortifacient.

AROMATHERAPY/HOME USE None. 'It should not be used in therapy either internally or externally.'[58]

OTHER USES Used as a fragrance component in soaps, colognes and perfumes. Limited use in flavouring due to toxic levels of thujone.

MUSTARD
Brassica nigra

FAMILY Brassicaceae (Cruciferae)

SYNONYMS *Sinapsis nigra, B. sinapioides*, black mustard.

GENERAL DESCRIPTION An erect annual up to 3 metres high, with spear-shaped upper leaves, smooth flat pods containing about ten dark brown seeds, and bright yellow cabbagelike flowers.

DISTRIBUTION Common throughout south eastern Europe, southern Siberia, Asia Minor and North Africa; naturalized in North and South America. Cultivated for its seed and oil in England, Holland, Denmark, Germany and Italy.

OTHER SPECIES The Russian variety is known as brown mustard or 'sarepta' *(B. juncea)*; the white mustard *(B. alba)* does not contain any essential oil. Also closely related is rape *(B. napus)* and other local species which are used in India and China.

HERBAL/FOLK TRADITION The seeds are highly esteemed as a condiment and for their medicinal qualities. They have been used in the East and West to aid the digestion, warm the stomach and promote the appetite, and for cold, stiff or feverish conditions such as colds, chills, coughs, chilblains, rheumatism, arthritis, lumbago and general aches and pains.

ACTIONS Aperitif, antimicrobial, antiseptic, diuretic, emetic, febrifuge, rubefacient (produces blistering of the skin), stimulant.

EXTRACTION Essential oil by steam (or water) distillation from the black mustard seeds, which have been macerated in warm water.

CHARACTERISTICS A colourless or pale yellow liquid with a sharp, penetrating, acrid odour.

PRINCIPAL CONSTITUENTS Allyl isothiocyanate (99 per cent). NB: Black mustard seed or powder does not contain this constituent, which is only formed by contact with water during the production of the essential oil.

SAFETY DATA Oral toxin, dermal toxin, mucous membrane irritant. It is considered one of the most toxic of all essential oils.

AROMATHERAPY/HOME USE None. 'It should not be used in therapy either externally or internally.'[59]

OTHER USES Used in certain rubefacient or counter-irritant liniments. Used extensively by the food industry especially in pickles, seasonings and sauces. Little used as a fragrance component except in cat and dog repellents.

MYRRH
Commiphora myrrha

FAMILY Burseraceae

SYNONYMS *Balsamodendrom myrrha*, gum myrrh, common myrrh, hirabol myrrh, myrrha.

GENERAL DESCRIPTION The *Commiphora* species which yield myrrh are shrubs or small trees up to 10 metres high. They have sturdy knotted branches, trifoliate aromatic leaves and small white flowers. The trunk exudes a natural oleoresin, a pale yellow liquid which hardens into reddish-brown tears, known as myrrh. The native collectors make incisions in the bark of the tree to increase the yield.

DISTRIBUTION The *Commiphora* species are native to north east Africa and south west Asia, especially the Red Sea region (Somalia, Yemen and Ethiopia).

OTHER SPECIES There are several C. species which yield myrrh oleoresin: African or Somali myrrh *(C. molmol)* and Arabian or Yemen myrrh *(C. abyssinica)*. Bisabol myrrh or opopanax *(C. erthraea)* also belongs to the same family.

HERBAL/FOLK TRADITION Myrrh has been employed since the earliest times in Eastern and Western medicine; its use is mentioned some 3700 years ago. The ancient Egyptians used it for embalming purposes and in their perfumes and cosmetics. In China it is used for arthritis, menstrual problems, sores and haemorrhoids. In the West it is considered to have an 'opening, heating, drying nature' (Joseph Miller), good for asthma, coughs, common cold, catarrh, sore throat, weak gums and teeth, ulcers and sores. It has also been used to treat leprosy.

Current in the British Herbal Pharmacopoeia as a specific for mouth ulcers, gingivitis and pharyngitis.

ACTIONS Anticatarrhal, anti-inflammatory, antimicrobial, antiphlogistic, antiseptic, astringent, balsamic, carminative, cicatrisant, emmenagogue, expectorant, fungicidal, revitalizing, sedative, stimulant (digestive, pulmonary), stomachic, tonic, uterine, vulnerary.

EXTRACTION 1. Resinoid (and resin absolute) by solvent extraction of the crude myrrh. 2. Essential oil by steam distillation of the crude myrrh.

CHARACTERISTICS 1. The resinoid is a dark reddish-brown viscous mass, with a warm, rich, spicy-balsamic odour. It is not pourable at room temperature so a solvent, such as diethyl phthalate, is sometimes added. 2. The essential oil is a pale yellow to amber oily liquid with a warm, sweet-balsamic, slightly spicy-medicinal odour. It blends well with frankincense, sandalwood, benzoin, oakmoss, cypress, juniper, mandarin, geranium, patchouli, thyme, mints, lavender, pine and spices.

PRINCIPAL CONSTITUENTS The crude contains resins, gum and about 8 per cent essential oil composed mainly of heerabolene, limonene, dipentene, pinene, eugenol, cinnamaldehyde, cuminaldehyde, cadinene, among others.

SAFETY DATA Non-irritant, non-sensitizing, possibly toxic in high concentration. Not to be used during pregnancy.

AROMATHERAPY/HOME USE
SKIN CARE: Athlete's foot, chapped and cracked skin, eczema, mature complexions, ringworm, wounds, wrinkles.
CIRCULATION, MUSCLES AND JOINTS: Arthritis.
RESPIRATORY SYSTEM: Asthma, bronchitis, catarrh, coughs, gum infections, gingivitis, mouth ulcers, sore throat, voice loss.
DIGESTIVE SYSTEM: Diarrhoea, dyspepsia, flatulence, haemorrhoids, loss of appetite.
GENITO-URINARY SYSTEM: Amenorrhoea,

leucorrhoea, pruritis, thrush.
IMMUNE SYSTEM: Colds.

OTHER USES The oil, resinoid and tincture
are used in pharmaceutical products, including
mouthwashes, gargles and toothpaste; also used
in dentistry. The oil and resinoid are used as
fixatives and fragrance components in soaps,
detergents, cosmetics and perfumes, especially
oriental types and heavy florals. Used as flavour
ingredients in most major food categories,
alcoholic and soft drinks.

MYRTLE
Myrtus communis

FAMILY Myrtaceae

SYNONYM Corsican pepper.

GENERAL DESCRIPTION A large bush or
small tree with many tough but slender
branches, a brownish-red bark and small sharp-
pointed leaves. It has white flowers followed by
small black berries; both leaves and flowers are
very fragrant.

DISTRIBUTION Native to North Africa, it
now grows freely all over the Mediterranean
region; it is also cultivaedia as a garden shrub
throughout Europe. The oil is mainly produced
in Corsica, Spain, Tunisia, Morocco, Italy,
Yugoslavia and France.

OTHER SPECIES Part of the same large
aromatic family which includes eucalyptus and
tea tree; also bayberry or wax myrtle *(Myrica
cerifera)* and the Dutch myrtle or English bog
myrtle *(Myrica gale)* which are used in herbal
medicine (though their essential oils are said to
be poisonous). Not to be confused with iris,
sometimes called 'myrtle flower' or calamus,
which is also known as 'myrtle grass' or 'sweet
myrtle'.

HERBAL/FOLK TRADITION The leaves and
berries have been used for 'drying and binding,
good for diarrhoea and dysentery, spitting of
blood and catarrhous defluctions upon the
breast'.[60] Dioscorides prescribed it for lung and
bladder infections in the form of an extract
made by macerating the leaves in wine. The
leaves and flowers were a major ingredient of
'angel's water', a sixteenth-century skin care
lotion.

ACTIONS Anticatarrhal, antiseptic (urinary,
pulmonary), astringent, balsamic, bactericidal,
expectorant, regulator, slightly sedative.

EXTRACTION Essential oil by steam
distillation from the leaves and twigs
(sometimes the flowers).

CHARACTERISTICS A pale yellow or orange
liquid with a clear, fresh, camphoraceous,
sweet-herbaceous scent somewhat similar to
eucalyptus. It blends well with bergamot,
lavandin, lavender, rosemary, clary sage,
hyssop, bay leaf, lime, laurel, ginger, clove and
other spice oils.

PRINCIPAL CONSTITUENTS Cineol,
myrtenol, pinene, geraniol, linalol, camphene,
among others.

SAFETY DATA Non-toxic, non-irritant, non-
sensitizing.

AROMATHERAPY/HOME USE
SKIN CARE: Acne, haemorrhoids, oily skin, open
pores.
RESPIRATORY SYSTEM: Asthma, bronchitis,
catarrhal conditions, chronic coughs,
tuberculosis – 'Because of its relative mildness,
this is a very suitable oil to use for children's
coughs and chest complaints.'[61]
IMMUNE SYSTEM: Colds, 'flu, infectious disease.

OTHER USES Used mainly in eau-de-cologne
and toilet waters. Employed as a flavouring
ingredient in meat sauces and seasonings,
generally in combination with other herbs.

N

NARCISSUS
Narcissus poeticus

FAMILY Amaryllidaceae

SYNONYMS Pinkster lily, pheasant's eye, poet's narcissus.

GENERAL DESCRIPTION A familiar garden flower up to 50 cms high, with long sword-shaped leaves with very fragrant white flowers having a short yellow trumpet and crisped red edge.

DISTRIBUTION Native to the Middle East or the eastern Mediterranean region; naturalized in southern France. It is cultivated extensively for its flowers. Only Holland and the Grasse region of France produce the concrete and absolute.

OTHER SPECIES There are two main types produced in France: the cultivated or *des plaines* variety and the wild or *des montagnes* type. Narcissus is also closely related to the jonquil *(N. jonquilla)* and campernella *(N. odorus)*, which are also occasionally used to produce an absolute, as well as to the daffodil *(N. pseudo-narcissus)*.

HERBAL/FOLK TRADITION The name derives from the Greek *narkao* – to be numb – due to its narcotic properties. The Roman perfumers used 'narcissum', a solid unguent made from narcissus flowers, in the preparation of their elaborate fragrances. In France the flowers were used at one time for their antispasmodic properties, said to be useful in hysteria and epilepsy.
   In India the oil is applied to the body before prayer in temples, along with rose, sandalwood and jasmine. The Arabians recommend the oil as a cure for baldness, and as an aphrodisiac.

ACTIONS Antispasmodic, aphrodisiac, emetic, narcotic, sedative.

EXTRACTION A concrete and absolute by solvent extraction from the flowers.

CHARACTERISTICS The absolute is a dark orange, olive or green viscous liquid with a sweet, green-herbaceous odour and heavy floral undertone. It blends well with clove bud, jasmine, neroli, ylang ylang, rose, mimosa, sandalwood, oriental and floral fragrances.

PRINCIPAL CONSTITUENTS Quercetin, possibly narcissine (the alkaloid that causes nausea).

SAFETY DATA All members of the Amaryllidaceae family, especially the bulbs, have a profound effect on the nervous system, causing paralysis and even in some cases death. 'The bulbs of *N. poeticus* are more dangerous than those of the daffodil, being powerfully emetic and irritant. The scent of the flowers is deleterious, if they are present in any quantity in a closed room, producing in some persons headache and even vomiting.'[62]

AROMATHERAPY/HOME USE Perfume.

OTHER USES The absolute and concrete are used almost exclusively in high class perfumes of the narcotic/ floral type.

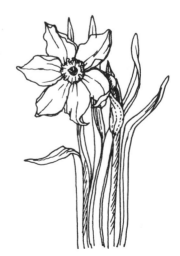

Narcissus

NIAOULI
Melaleuca viridiflora

FAMILY Myrtaceae

SYNONYMS *M. quinquenervia*, 'gomenol'.

GENERAL DESCRIPTION An evergreen tree with a flexible trunk and spongy bark, pointed linear leaves and bearing spikes of sessile yellowish flowers. The leaves have a strong aromatic scent when they are crushed.

DISTRIBUTION Native to Australia, New Caledonia, and the French Pacific Islands. The majority of the oil is produced in Australia and Tasmania.

OTHER SPECIES A typical member of the 'tea tree' group of oils; the oil is similar to cajuput. There is another physiological form of *M. viridiflora* called 'Variety A', which was originally developed to provide a natural source of nerolidol, the main constituent of its essential oil.

HERBAL/FOLK TRADITION It is used locally for a wide variety of ailments, such as aches and pains, respiratory conditions, cuts and infections; it is also used to purify the water. The name 'gomenol' derives from the fact that it used to be shipped from Gomen in the French East Indies.

ACTIONS Analgesic, anthelmintic, anticatarrhal, antirheumatic, antiseptic, antispasmodic, bactericidal, balsamic, cicatrisant, diaphoretic, expectorant, regulator, stimulant, vermifuge.

EXTRACTION Essential oil by steam distillation from the leaves and young twigs. (Usually rectified to remove irritant aldehydes.)

CHARACTERISTICS A colourless, pale yellow or greenish liquid with a sweet, fresh, camphoraceous odour.

PRINCIPAL CONSTITUENTS Cineol (50–65per cent), terpineol, pinene, limonene, citrene, terebenthene, valeric ester, acetic ester, butyric ester.

SAFETY DATA Non-toxic, non-irritant, non-sensitizing. Often subject to adulteration.

AROMATHERAPY/HOME USE
SKIN CARE: Acne, boils, burns, cuts, insect bites, oily skin, spots, ulcers, wounds.
CIRCULATION, MUSCLES AND JOINTS: Muscular aches and pains, poor circulation, rheumatism.
RESPIRATORY SYSTEM: Asthma, bronchitis, catarrhal conditions, coughs, sinusitis, sore throat, whooping cough.
GENITO-URINARY SYSTEM: Cystitis, urinary infection.
IMMUNE SYSTEM: Colds, fever, 'flu.

OTHER USES Used in pharmaceutical preparations such as gargles, cough drops, toothpastes, mouth sprays, etc.

NUTMEG
Myristica fragrans

FAMILY Myristicaceae

SYNONYMS *M. officinalis, M. aromata, Nux moschata,* myristica (oil), mace (husk), macis (oil).

GENERAL DESCRIPTION An evergreen tree up to 20 metres high with a greyish-brown smooth bark, dense foliage and small dull-yellow flowers. 'Mace' is the name given to the bright red netlike aril or husk surrounding the nutmeg shell and seed, which is contained within the fleshy fruit.

DISTRIBUTION Native to the Moluccas and nearby islands; cultivated in Indonesia, Sri Lanka and the West Indies, especially Grenada.

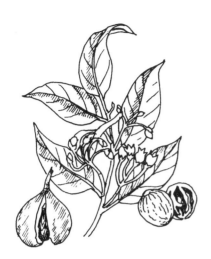

Nutmeg

EXTRACTION Essential oil by steam (or water) distillation from 1. the dried worm-eaten nutmeg seed (the worms eat away all the starch and fat content); 2. the dried orange-brown aril or husk – mace; and 3. an oleoresin is also produced in small quantities by solvent extraction from mace.

CHARACTERISTICS 1. A water-white or pale yellow mobile liquid with a sweet, warm-spicy odour and a terpeney top-note. 2. A water-white or pale yellow mobile liquid with a sweet, warm-spicy scent. 3. An orange-brown viscous liquid with a fresh, spicy-warm, balsamic fragrance. It has good masking power.

  They blend well with oakmoss, lavandin, bay leaf, Peru balsam, orange, geranium, clary sage, rosemary, lime, petitgrain, mandarin, coriander and other spice oils.

PRINCIPAL CONSTITUENTS Mainly monoterpene hydrocarbons (88 per cent approx.): camphene, pinene, dipentene, sabinene, cymene, with lesser amounts of geraniol, borneol, linalol, terpineol, myristicin (4–8 per cent), safrol and elemincin, among others. Mace oil contains similar constituents but contains more myristicin.

The oil is also distilled in the USA and Europe from the imported nutmegs.

OTHER SPECIES Indonesia and Sri Lanka produce the so-called 'East Indian' nutmeg which is considered superior, while Grenada produces the 'West Indian' nutmeg – see also Botanical Classification.

HERBAL/FOLK TRADITION Nutmeg and mace are widely used as domestic spices in the East and West. They have been used for centuries as a remedy mainly for digestive and kidney problems. In Malaysia they are used during pregnancy to strengthen and tone the uterine muscles. Grated nutmeg with lard is used for piles. A fixed oil of nutmeg is also used in soap and candle making.

  Nutmeg is current in the British Herbal Pharmacopoeia indicated for flatulent dyspepsia, nausea, diarrhoea, dysentery, and topically for rheumatism.

ACTIONS Analgesic, anti-emetic, anti-oxidant, antirheumatic, antiseptic, antispasmodic, aphrodisiac, carminative, digestive, emmenagogue, gastric secretory stimulant, larvicidal, orexigenic, prostaglandin inhibitor, stimulant, tonic.

SAFETY DATA Both nutmeg and mace are generally non-toxic, non-irritant and non-sensitizing. However, used in large doses they show signs of toxicity such as nausea, stupor and tachycardia, believed to be due to the myristicin content. 'Large quantities are hallucinogenic and excitant to the motor cortex.'[63] On this basis nutmeg (especially the West Indian type) is probably safer to use than mace. Use in moderation, and with care in pregnancy.

AROMATHERAPY/HOME USE
CIRCULATION, MUSCLES AND JOINTS: Arthritis, gout, muscular aches and pains, poor circulation, rheumatism.
DIGESTIVE SYSTEM: Flatulence, indigestion, nausea, sluggish digestion.
IMMUNE SYSTEM: Bacterial infection.
NERVOUS SYSTEM: Frigidity, impotence, neuralgia, nervous fatigue.

OTHER USES Used as a flavouring agent in pharmaceuticals, especially analgesic and tonic preparations. Nutmeg and mace oil are used in soaps, lotions, detergents, cosmetics and perfumes. Mace oleoresin is used in colognes and perfumes, especially men's fragrances. Both oils and oleoresin are used in most major food categories, including alcoholic and soft drinks.

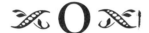

OAKMOSS
Evernia prunastri

FAMILY Usneaceae

SYNONYMS Mousse de chêne, treemoss.

GENERAL DESCRIPTION A light green lichen found growing primarily on oak trees, but sometimes other species.

DISTRIBUTION The oak *(Quercus robur)* is indigenous to Europe and North America; the lichen is collected all over central and southern Europe, especially France, Yugoslavia, Hungary, Greece, and also Morocco and Algeria. The aromatic materials are prepared mainly in France, but also in the USA, Bulgaria and Yugoslavia.

OTHER SPECIES There are many varieties of lichen used for their aromatic qualities, the most common being *E. furfuracea* and *Usnea barbata* which are frequently gathered from spruce and pine trees, and are known as fir moss or tree moss in Europe, but in the USA are also called oakmoss. However they are less refined than the 'true' oakmoss. Other species include *Sticta pulmonaceae* or *Lobaria pulmonaria, Usnea ceratina,* and some members of the *Ramalina, Alectoria* and *Parmelia* groups.

HERBAL/FOLK TRADITION *Sticta pulmonaceae,* a greeny-brown lichen also found growing on oak trees and frequently harvested along with *E. prunastri,* is also called oak lungs, lung moss, lungwort or 'lungs of oak' by the North American Indians who use it for respiratory complaints and for treating wounds. It is called lobaria in the British Herbal Pharmacopoeia and is used for asthma, bronchitis and coughs in children.
   Many types of lichen, especially the *Parmelia* group, are used as vegetable dyes.

ACTIONS Antiseptic, demulcent, expectorant, fixative.

EXTRACTION A range of products is produced: a concrete and an absolute by solvent extraction from the lichen which has often been soaked in lukewarm water prior to extraction; an absolute oil by vacuum distillation of the concrete; resins and resinoids by alcohol extraction of the raw material. Most important of these products is the absolute.

CHARACTERISTICS 1. The absolute is a dark green or brown, very viscous liquid with an extremely tenacious, earthy-mossy odour and a leatherlike undertone. 2. The absolute oil is a pale yellow or olive viscous liquid with a dry-earthy, barklike odour, quite true to nature. 3. The concrete, resin and resinoids are a very dark-coloured semi-solid or solid mass with a heavy, rich-earthy, extremely tenacious odour. They have a high fixative value and blend with virtually all other oils: they are extensively used in perfumery to lend body and rich natural undertones to all perfume types.

PRINCIPAL CONSTITUENTS Crystalline matter of so-called 'lichen acids' : mainly evernic acid, d-usnic acid, some atranorine and chloratronorine.

SAFETY DATA Extensively compounded or bouquetted' by cutting or adulteration with other lichen or synthetic perfume materials.

AROMATHERAPY/HOME USE As a fixative.

OTHER USES The concrete is used primarily in soaps; the absolute is the most versatile and is used in all perfume types (oriental, moss, fougère, new-mown hay, floral, colognes, aftershaves, etc.). The absolute oil is used in high class perfumes. The resins and resinoids, which have a poor solubility, are used in soaps, hair preparations, industrial perfumes and low cost products.

ONION
Allium cepa

FAMILY Liliaceae

SYNONYMS Common onion, Strasburg onion.

GENERAL DESCRIPTION A perennial or biennial herb up to 1.2 metres high with hollow leaves and flowering stem, and a globelike fleshy bulb.

DISTRIBUTION Native of western Asia and the Middle East, it has a long history of cultivation all over the world, mainly for culinary use. The essential oil is mainly produced in France, Germany and Egypt from the 'red' onion.

OTHER SPECIES There are numerous species of onion which have been developed, which include the Spanish or silver-skinned onion, the Tripoli and the red onion. See also Botanical Classification.

HERBAL/FOLK TRADITION Onion has an ancient reputation as a curative agent, highly extolled by the schools of Galen and Hippocrates. It is high in vitamins A, B and C and shares many of the properties of garlic, to which it is closely related. Raw onion helps to keep colds and infections at bay, promotes strong bones and a good blood supply to all the tissues. It acts as an effective blood cleanser

which, along with the sulphur it contains, helps to keep the skin clear and in good condition.

It has a sound reputation for correcting glandular imbalance and weight problems; it also improves lymphatic drainage which is often responsible for oedema and puffiness.

Onion has long been used as a home 'simple' for a wide range of conditions: 'As a poultice they are invaluable for the removal of hard tumours. In this form they afford relief in cases of suppressed gout or obstructed circulation ... Onions tend to soothe the nerves and induce sleep. They stimulate the action of the skin and remove obstructions of the viscera ... raw onions, bruised are good for burns and scalds in the absence of other remedies ... applied to the sting or bite of any poisonous insect often proves all that is desired.'[64]

ACTIONS Anthelmintic, antimicrobial, antirheumatic, antiseptic, antisclerotic, antispasmodic, antiviral, bactericidal, carminative, depurative, digestive, diuretic, expectorant, fungicidal, hypocholesterolaemic, hypoglycaemic, hypotensive, stomachic, tonic, vermifuge.

EXTRACTION Essential oil by steam distillation from the bulb. (An oleoresin is also produced in small quantities for flavouring use.)

CHARACTERISTICS A pale yellow or brownish-yellow mobile liquid with strong, unpleasant, sulphuraceous odour with a lachrymatory (tear-producing) effect.

PRINCIPAL CONSTITUENTS Mainly dipropyl disulphide, also methylpropyl disulphide, dipropyl trisulphide, methylpropyl trisulphide and allylpropyl disulphide, among others.

SAFETY DATA Specific safety data unavailable at present – probably similar to garlic, i.e. generally non-toxic, non-irritant, possible sensitization.

AROMATHERAPY/HOME USE None, due to its offensive smell.

OTHER USES Used in some pharmaceutical

preparations for colds, coughs, etc. The oil is extensively used in most major food categories, especially meats, savouries, salad dressings, as well as alcoholic and soft drinks. It is not used in perfumery work.

OPOPANAX
Commiphora erythraea

FAMILY Burseraceae

SYNONYMS *C. erythraea var. glabrascens,* bisabol myrrh, sweet myrrh.

GENERAL DESCRIPTION A tall tropical tree, similar to myrrh (to which it is closely related), which contains a natural oleogum resin in tubular vessels between the bark and wood of the trunk. The natives make incisions in the trunk of the tree to increase the yield. The crude gum dries to form dark reddish-brown tear-shaped lumps with a sweet-woody, rootlike odour.

DISTRIBUTION Native to East Africa (Somalia) and eastern Ethiopia (Harrar Province) where it grows wild. The essential oil production is generally carried out in the USA and Europe from the crude oleogum resin.

OTHER SPECIES The original or 'true' opopanax used in perfumery was derived from a large plant *Opopanax chironium* or *Pastinaca opopanax*, a plant similar to the parsnip of the Umbelliferae family and native to the Levant region, Sudan and Arabia. The oleogum resin was obtained by cutting into the stem at the base, which then produces reddish-yellow tears of a strong rootlike, parsnip or celery-type smell. This type of opopanax is now unavailable, and has been replaced by a similar type of oil known as 'bisabol myrrh'.
    Not to be confused with cassie *(Acacia farnesiana),* which is also known as 'opopanax'.

HERBAL/FOLK TRADITION Opopanax derived from *O. chironium* is described as having antispasmodic, expectorant, emmenagogue and antiseptic properties, which used to be employed in asthma, hysteria and visceral afflictions. In the Far East the bisabol myrrh is used extensively as an ingredient in incense.

ACTIONS Antiseptic, antispasmodic, balsamic, expectorant.

EXTRACTION 1. Essential oil by steam (or water) distillation from the crude oleogum resin. 2. A resinoid by solvent extraction from the crude oleogum resin.

CHARACTERISTICS 1. An orange, yellow or olive liquid with a sweet-balsamic, spicy, warm, animal-like odour (it does not contain a medicinal note like myrrh). It resinifies on exposure to air. 2. A solid dark mass with a warm, powdery, sweet-balsamic, rooty odour. It blends well with clary sage, coriander, labdanum, bergamot, myrrh, frankincense, vetiver, sandalwood, patchouli, mimosa, fir needle and neroli.

PRINCIPAL CONSTITUENTS The crude contains resins, gums (50–80 per cent) and essential oils (10–20 per cent), notably the sesquiterpene 'bisabolene' and sesquiterpene alcohols.

SAFETY DATA Frequently adulterated – it is more expensive than the 'hirabol myrrh'. The commercial resinoid is also usually mixed with a solvent such as myristate, because it is otherwise unpourable at room temperatures.

AROMATHERAPY/HOME USE Possibly similar uses to myrrh.

OTHER USES Used as a fixative and fragrance component in high class perfumery. Used in liqueurs to lend body and add winelike notes.

ORANGE, BITTER
Citrus aurantium var. amara

FAMILY Rutaceae

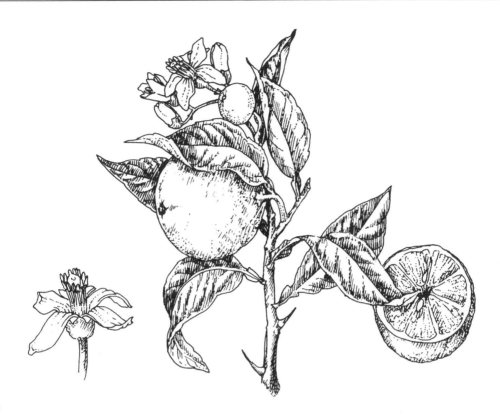

Orange

SYNONYMS *C. vulgaris, C. bigaradia*, Seville orange, sour orange bigarade (oil).

GENERAL DESCRIPTION An evergreen tree up to 10 metres high with dark green, glossy, oval leaves, paler beneath, with long but not very sharp spines. It has a smooth greyish trunk and branches, and very fragrant white flowers. The fruits are smaller and darker than the sweet orange. It is well known for its resistance to disease and is often used as root stock for other citrus trees, including the sweet orange.

DISTRIBUTION Native to the Far East, especially India and China, but has become well adapted to the Mediterranean climate. It also grows abundantly in the USA (California), Israel and South America. Main producers of the oil include Spain, Guinea, the West Indies, Italy, Brazil and the USA.

OTHER SPECIES There are numerous different species according to location – oils from Spain and Guinea are said to be of superior quality.

HERBAL/FOLK TRADITION 'Oranges and lemons strengthen the heart, are good for diminishing the coagubility of the blood, and are beneficial for palpitation, scurvy, jaundice, bleedings, heartburn, relaxed throat, etc. They are powerfully anti-scorbutic, either internally or externally applied.'[65] The dried bitter orange peel is used as a tonic and carminative in treating dyspepsia.

In Chinese medicine the dried bitter orange and occasionally its peel are used in treating prolapse of the uterus and of the anus, diarrhoea, and blood in the faeces. Ingestion of large amounts of orange peel in children, however, has been reported to cause toxic effects.

ACTIONS Anti-inflammatory, antiseptic, astringent, bactericidal, carminative, choleretic, fungicidal, sedative (mild), stomachic, tonic.

EXTRACTION An essential oil by cold expression (hand or machine pressing) from the outer peel of the almost ripe fruit. (A terpeneless oil is also produced.) The leaves are used for the production of petitgrain oil; the blossom for neroli oil.

CHARACTERISTICS A dark yellow or brownish-yellow mobile liquid with a fresh, dry, almost floral odour with a rich, sweet undertone.

PRINCIPAL CONSTITUENTS Over 90 per cent monoterpenes: mainly limonene, myrcene, camphene, pinene, ocimene, cymene, and small amounts of alcohols, aldehydes and ketones.

SAFETY DATA Phototoxic; otherwise generally non-toxic, non-irritant and non-sensitizing. Limonene has been reported to cause contact dermatitis in some individuals.

AROMATHERAPY/HOME USE See *sweet orange.*

OTHER USES Used in certain stomachic, laxative and carminative preparations. Employed as a fragrance component in soaps, detergents, cosmetics, colognes and perfumes. Extensively used as a flavouring material, especially in liqueurs and soft drinks. Also utilized as a starting material for the isolation of natural limonene.

ORANGE BLOSSOM
Citrus aurantium var. amara

FAMILY Rutaceae

SYNONYMS *C. vulgaris, C. bigaradia,* orange flower, neroli, neroli bigarade.

GENERAL DESCRIPTION An evergreen tree up to 10 metres high with glossy dark green leaves and fragrant white flowers. There are two flowering seasons when the blossom is picked, one in May and another in October (in mild weather). See also *bitter orange* .

DISTRIBUTION Native to the Far East, but well adapted to the Mediterranean climate. Major producers include Italy, Tunisia, Morocco, Egypt, America and especially France.

OTHER SPECIES The sweet orange (*C. aurantium var. dulcis)* is also used to make an absolute and oil called neroli Portugal or neroli petalae – however, it is less fragrant and considered of inferior quality.

HERBAL/FOLK TRADITION This oil was named after a princess of Nerola in Italy, who loved to wear it as a perfume. Orange flowers have many folk associations. They were used in bridal bouquets and wreaths, to calm any nervous apprehension before the couple retired to the marriage bed.
On the Continent an infusion of dried flowers is used as a mild stimulant of the nervous system, and as a blood cleanser. The distillation water, known as orange flower water, is a popular cosmetic and household article.

ACTIONS Antidepressant, antiseptic, antispasmodic, aphrodisiac, bactericidal, carminative, cicatrisant, cordial, deodorant, digestive, fungicidal, hypnotic (mild), stimulant (nervous), tonic (cardiac, circulatory).

EXTRACTION 1. A concrete and absolute are produced by solvent extraction from the freshly picked flowers. 2. An essential oil is produced by steam distillation from the freshly picked flowers. An orange flower water and an absolute are produced as a byproduct of the distillation process.

CHARACTERISTICS 1. The absolute is a dark brown or orange viscous liquid with a fresh, delicate yet rich, warm sweet-floral fragrance; very true to nature. It blends well with jasmine, benzoin, myrrh and all citrus oils. 2. The oil is a pale yellow mobile liquid (darkening with age) with a light, sweet-floral fragrance and terpeney topnote. Blends well with virtually all oils: chamomile, coriander, geranium, benzoin, clary sage, jasmine, lavender, rose, ylang ylang, lemon and other citrus oils.

PRINCIPAL CONSTITUENTS Linalol (34 per cent approx.), linalyl acetate (6–17 per cent), limonene (15 per cent approx.), pinene, nerolidol, geraniol, nerol, methyl anthranilate, indole, citral, jasmone, among others.

SAFETY DATA Non-toxic, non-irritant, non-sensitizing, non-phototoxic.

AROMATHERAPY/HOME USE

SKIN CARE: Scars, stretch marks, thread veins, mature and sensitive skin, tones the complexion, wrinkles.

CIRCULATION, MUSCLES AND JOINTS: Palpitations, poor circulation.

DIGESTIVE SYSTEM: Diarrhoea (chronic), colic, flatulence, spasm, nervous dyspepsia.

NERVOUS SYSTEM: Anxiety, depression, nervous tension, PMT, shock, stress-related conditions – 'I find that by far the most important uses of neroli are in helping with problems of emotional origin'.[66]

OTHER USES Neroli oil and orange flower water are used to flavour pharmaceuticals. The absolute is used extensively in high class perfumery work, especially oriental, floral and citrus blends; also as a fixative. The oil is used in eau-de-cologne and toilet waters (traditionally with lavender, lemon, rosemary and bergamot). Limited use as a flavour ingredient in foods, alcoholic and soft drinks.

ORANGE, SWEET
Citrus sinensis

FAMILY Rutaceae

SYNONYMS *C. aurantium var. dulcis, C. aurantium var. sinensis,* China orange, Portugal orange.

GENERAL DESCRIPTION An evergreen tree, smaller than the bitter variety, less hardy with fewer or no spines. The fruit has a sweet pulp and non-bitter membranes. Another distinguishing feature is the shape of the leaf stalk: the bitter orange is broader and in the shape of a heart.

DISTRIBUTION Native to China; extensively cultivated especially in America (California and Florida) and round the Mediterranean (France, Spain, Italy). The expressed oil is mainly produced in Israel, Cyprus, Brazil and North America; the distilled oil mainly comes from the Mediterranean and North America.

OTHER SPECIES There are numerous cultivated varieties of sweet orange, for example Jaffa, Navel and Valencia. There are also many other subspecies such as the Japanese orange *(C. aurantium var. natsudaidai)*. See also *bitter orange* .

HERBAL/FOLK TRADITION A very nutritious fruit, containing vitamins A, B and C. In Chinese medicine the dried sweet orange peel is used to treat coughs, colds, anorexia and malignant breast sores. Li Shih-chên says: 'The fruits of all the different species and varieties of citrus are considered by the Chinese to be cooling. If eaten in excess they are thought to increase the 'phlegm', and this is probably not advantageous to the health. The sweet varieties increase bronchial secretion, and the sour promote expectoration. They all quench thirst, and are stomachic and carminative.'[67]

ACTIONS Antidepressant, anti-inflammatory, antiseptic, bactericidal, carminative, choleretic, digestive, fungicidal, hypotensive, sedative (nervous), stimulant (digestive and lymphatic), stomachic, tonic.

EXTRACTION 1. Essential oil by cold expression (hand or machine) of the fresh ripe or almost ripe outer peel. 2. Essential oil by steam distillation of the fresh ripe or almost ripe outer peel. An oil of inferior quality is also produced by distillation from the essences recovered as a byproduct of orange juice manufacture. Distilled sweet orange oil oxidizes very quickly, and anti-oxidant agents are often added at the place of production. (An oil from the flowers is also produced occasionally called neroli Portugal or neroli petalae; an oil from the leaves is also produced in small quantities.)

CHARACTERISTICS 1. A yellowy-orange or dark orange mobile liquid with a sweet, fresh-fruity scent, richer than the distilled oil. It blends well with lavender, neroli, lemon, clary sage, myrrh and spice oils such as nutmeg, cinnamon and clove.
   2. A pale yellow or colourless mobile liquid with a sweet, light-fruity scent, but little tenacity.

PRINCIPAL CONSTITUENTS Over 90 per cent monoterpenes, mainly limonene. The cold expressed oil also contains bergapten, auraptenol and acids.

SAFETY DATA Generally non-toxic (although ingestion of large amounts of orange peel has been known to be fatal to children); non-irritant and non-sensitizing (although limonene has been found to cause dermatitis in a few individuals). Distilled orange oil is phototoxic: its use on the skin should be avoided if there is danger of exposure to direct sunlight. However, there is no evidence to show that expressed sweet orange oil is phototoxic although it too contains coumarins.

AROMATHERAPY/HOME USE
SKIN CARE: Dull and oily complexions, mouth ulcers.
CIRCULATION, MUSCLES AND JOINTS: Obesity, palpitations, water retention.
RESPIRATORY SYSTEM: Bronchitis, chills.
DIGESTIVE SYSTEM: Constipation, dyspepsia, spasm.
IMMUNE SYSTEM: Colds, 'flu.
NERVOUS SYSTEM: Nervous tension and stress-related conditions.

OTHER USES Sweet orange peel tincture is used to flavour pharmaceuticals. Extensively used as a fragrance component in soaps, detergents, cosmetics and perfumes, especially eau-de-colognes. Extensively used in all areas of the food and drinks industry (more so than the bitter orange oil). Used as the starting material for the isolation of natural limonene.

OREGANO, COMMON
Origanum vulgare

FAMILY Lamiaceae (Labiatae)

SYNONYMS European oregano, wild marjoram, common marjoram, grove marjoram, joy of the mountain, origanum (oil).

GENERAL DESCRIPTION A hardy, bushy, perennial herb up to 90 cms high with an erect hairy stem, dark green ovate leaves and pinky-purple flowers. A common garden plant with a strong aroma when the leaves are bruised.

DISTRIBUTION Native to Europe, now cultivated all over the world, including the USA, India and South America; the oil is mainly produced in the USSR, Bulgaria and Italy.

OTHER SPECIES There is much confusion concerning the exact botanical classification of the marjoram and oregano species. There are over thirty varieties some of which are used to produce essential oils, such as the winter or Greek marjoram *O. heracleoticum*, the African species *O. glandulosum*, the Moroccan species *O. virens*, as well as the Mexican oregano *Lippia graveolens* or *L. palmeri* and the Syrian oregano *(O. maru)*. However, most commercial 'oregano oil' is derived from the Spanish oregano *(Thymus capitatus)* and to a lesser degree from the common oregano or wild marjoram – see entries on Spanish oregano and sweet marjoram.

HERBAL/FOLK TRADITION This is the 'true' oregano of the herb garden, which also has a very ancient medical reputation. It has been used as a traditional remedy for digestive upsets, respiratory problems (asthma, bronchitis, coughs, etc), colds and 'flu as well as inflammations of the mouth and throat.
  In China it is also used to treat fever, vomiting, diarrhoea, jaundice and itchy skin conditions. The (diluted) oil has been used externally in herbal medicine for headaches, rheumatism, general aches and pains, and applied to stings and bites.

ACTIONS Analgesic, anthelmintic, antirheumatic, antiseptic, antispasmodic, antitoxic, antiviral, bactericidal, carminative, choleretic, cytophylactic, diaphoretic, diuretic, emmenagogue, expectorant, febrifuge, fungicidal, parasiticide, rubefacient, stimulant, tonic.

EXTRACTION Essential oil by steam distillation from the dried flowering herb.

CHARACTERISTICS A pale yellow liquid (browning with age), with a warm, spicy-herbaceous, camphoraceous odour. It blends well with lavandin, oakmoss, pine, spike lavender, citronella, rosemary, camphor and cedarwood.

PRINCIPAL CONSTITUENTS Carvacrol, thymol, cymene, caryophyllene, pinene, bisabolene, linalol, borneol, geranyl acetate, linalyl acetate, terpinene. NB: Constituents are highly variable according to source, but oils classified as 'oregano' or 'oreganum' have thymol and/or carvacrol as their major components.

SAFETY DATA Dermal toxin, skin irritant, mucous membrane irritant. Avoid during pregnancy.

AROMATHERAPY/HOME USE None. 'Should not be used on the skin at all.'[68]

OTHER USES Used as a fragrance component in soaps, colognes and perfumes, especially men's fragrances. Employed to some extent as a flavouring agent, mainly in meat products and pizzas.

OREGANO, SPANISH
Thymus capitatus

FAMILY Lamiaceae (Labiatae)

SYNONYMS *T. capitans, Coridothymus capitatus, Satureja capitata, Thymbra capitata*, oreganum (oil), Israeli oreganum (oil), Cretan thyme, corido thyme, conehead thyme, headed savory, thyme of the ancients.

GENERAL DESCRIPTION A perennial creeping herb with a woody stem, small dark green leaves and pink or white flowers borne in clusters.

DISTRIBUTION Native to the Middle East and Asia Minor; grows wild in Spain. The oil is produced mainly in Spain, Israel, Lebanon, Syria and Turkey.

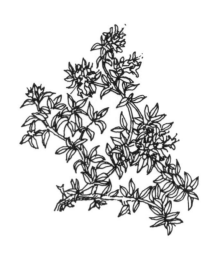

Common Oregano

OTHER SPECIES Although this herb is strictly a thyme, it serves as the source for most so-called 'oregano oil'. For other related species see entries on common thyme, common oregano and sweet marjoram; see also Botanical Classification section.

HERBAL/FOLK TRADITION According to Mrs Grieve the properties and oil of Spanish oregano (*Thymus capitatus*) are similar to the common thyme (*T. vulgaris*); it also shares many qualities with the common oregano or wild marjoram (*Origanum vulgare*).

ACTIONS See *common oregano*.

EXTRACTION Essential oil by steam distillation from the dried flowering tops.

CHARACTERISTICS A dark brownish-red or purple oil with a strong tarlike, herbaceous, refreshing odour.

PRINCIPAL CONSTITUENTS Carvacrol, thymol, cymene, caryophyllene, pinene, limonene, linalol, borneol, myrcene, thujone, terpinene.

SAFETY DATA Dermal toxin, skin irritant, mucous membrane irritant.

AROMATHERAPY/HOME USE None .
'Should not be used on the skin at all.'[68]

OTHER USES See *common oregano*.

ORRIS
Iris pallida

FAMILY Iridaceae

SYNONYMS Orris root, iris, flag iris, pale iris,
orris butter (oil).

GENERAL DESCRIPTION A decorative
perennial plant up to 1.5 metres high, with
sword-shaped leaves, a creeping fleshy rootstock
and delicate, highly scented, pale blue flowers.

DISTRIBUTION Native to the eastern
Mediterranean region; also found in northern
India and North Africa. Most commercial orris
is produced in Italy where it grows wild. The oil
is mainly produced in France and Morocco and
to lesser extent in Italy and the USA.

OTHER SPECIES There are many species of
iris; cultivation has also produced further types.
In Italy the pale iris (*I. pallida*) is collected
indiscriminately with the Florentine orris
(*I. florentina*) which has white flowers tinged
with pale blue, and the common or German iris
(*I. germanica*) which has deep purple flowers
with a yellow beard. Other species which have
been used medicinally include the American
blue flag (*I. versicolor*), and the yellow flag iris
(*I. pseudacorus*).

HERBAL/FOLK TRADITION In ancient
Greece and Rome orris root was used
extensively in perfumery, and its medicinal
qualities were held in high esteem by
Dioscorides. The juice of the root was used for
cosmetic purposes, and the root bruised in wine
was employed for dropsy, bronchitis, coughs,
hoarseness, chronic diarrhoea and congested
headaches. In Russia the root was used to make
a tonic drink with honey and ginger.

Iris is little used medicinally these days, but it
still appears in the British Herbal Pharmacopoeia
as being formerly used in upper respiratory
catarrh, coughs, and for diarrhoea in infants.

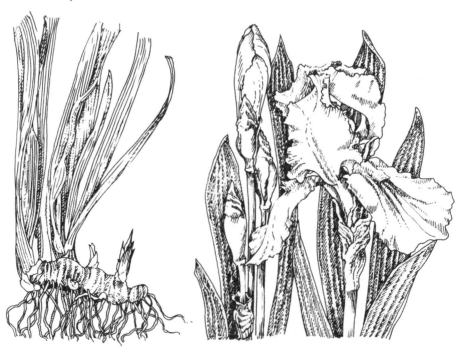

Orris

ACTIONS Dried Root – antidiarrhoeal, demulcent, expectorant. Fresh Root – diuretic, cathartic, emetic.

EXTRACTION 1. An essential oil (often called a 'concrete') by steam distillation from the rhizomes which have been peeled, washed, dried and pulverized. The rhizomes must be stored for a minimum of three years prior to extraction otherwise they have virtually no scent! 2. An absolute produced by alkali washing in ethyl ether solution to remove the myristic acid from the 'concrete' oil. 3. A resin or resinoid by alcohol extraction from the peeled rhizomes.

CHARACTERISTICS 1. The oil solidifies at room temperature to a cream-coloured mass with a woody, violetlike scent and a soft, floral-fruity undertone. 2. The absolute is a water-white or pale yellow oily liquid with a delicate, sweet, floral-woody odour. 3. The resin is a brown or dark orange viscous mass with a deep, woody-sweet, tobacco-like scent – very tenacious.
   Orris blends well with cedarwood, sandalwood, vetiver, cypress, mimosa, labdanum, bergamot, clary sage, rose, violet and other florals.

PRINCIPAL CONSTITUENTS Myristic acid, an odourless substance which makes the 'oil' solid (85–90 per cent), alpha-irone and oleic acid.

SAFETY DATA The fresh root causes nausea and vomiting in large doses. The oil and absolute are much adulterated or synthetic – 'true' orris absolute is three times the price of jasmine.

AROMATHERAPY/HOME USE None. However, the powdered orris, which is a common article, may be used as a dry shampoo, a body powder, a fixative for pot pourris, and to scent linen.

OTHER USES The powder is used to scent dentifrices, toothpowders, etc. The resin is used in soaps, colognes and perfumes; the absolute and 'concrete' oil are reserved for high class perfumery work. Occasionally used on the Continent for confectionery and fruit flavours.

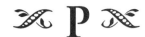

PALMAROSA
Cymbopogon martinii var. martinii

FAMILY Graminaceae

SYNONYMS *Andropogon martinii, A. martinii var. motia,* East Indian geranium, Turkish geranium, Indian rosha, motia.

GENERAL DESCRIPTION A wild-growing herbaceous plant with long slender stems and terminal flowering tops; the grassy leaves are very fragrant.

DISTRIBUTION Native to India and Pakistan; now grown in Africa, Indonesia, Brazil and the Comoro Islands.

OTHER SPECIES Of the same family as lemongrass and citronella; also closely related to gingergrass which is a different chemotype known as *C. martinii var. sofia.* Gingergrass is considered an inferior oil but in some parts of India the two types of grass are distilled together.

HERBAL/FOLK TRADITION ' The oil term "Indian" or "Turkish" geranium oil, which formerly was applied to palmarosa oil, dates back to the time when the oil was shipped from Bombay to ports of the Red Sea and transported partly by land, to Constantinople and Bulgaria, where the oil was often used for the adulteration of rose oil.'[70]

ACTIONS Antiseptic, bactericidal, cicatrisant, digestive, febrifuge, hydrating, stimulant (digestive, circulatory), tonic.

EXTRACTION Essential oil by steam or water distillation of the fresh or dried grass.

CHARACTERISTICS A pale yellow or olive

liquid with a sweet, floral, rosy, geranium-like scent. It blends well with cananga, geranium, oakmoss, rosewood, amyris, sandalwood, guaiacwood, cedarwood and floral oils.

PRINCIPAL CONSTITUENTS Mainly geraniol; also farnesol, geranyl acetate, methyl heptenone, citronellol, citral, dipentene and limonene, among others. Several chemotypes depending upon source – the cultivated varieties are considered of superior quality.

SAFETY DATA Non-toxic, non-irritant, non-sensitizing.

AROMATHERAPY/HOME USE
SKIN CARE: Acne, dermatitis and minor skin infections, scars, sores, wrinkles; valuable for all types of treatment for the face, hands, feet, neck and lips (moisturizes the skin, stimulates cellular regeneration, regulates sebum production).
DIGESTIVE SYSTEM: Anorexia, digestive atonia, intestinal infections – 'This is an essence which acts on the pathogenic intestinal flora, in particular on the colibacillus, the Eberth bacillus and the bacillus of dysentery ... this essence favours the transmutation of the pathogenic agent into normal cells of intestinal mucous membranes. Thus it arrests the degeneracy of the cells for the latter, swiftly impels groups of normal cells towards an inferior form in their hierarchy. The essence does not appear to contain any acid.'[71]
NERVOUS SYSTEM: Nervous exhaustion, stress-related conditions.

OTHER USES Used extensively as a fragrance component in cosmetics, perfumes and especially soaps due to excellent tenacity. Limited use as a flavouring agent, e.g. tobacco. Used for the isolation of natural geraniol.

PARSLEY
Petroselinum sativum

FAMILY Apiaceae (Umbelliferae)

SYNONYMS *P. hortense, Apium petroselinum, Carum petroselinum,* common parsley, garden parsley.

GENERAL DESCRIPTION A biennial or short-lived perennial herb up to 70 cms high with crinkly bright green foliage, small greenish-yellow flowers and producing small brown seeds.

DISTRIBUTION Native to the Mediterranean region, especially Greece. It is cultivated extensively, mainly in California, Germany, France, Belgium, Hungary and parts of Asia. The principal oil-producing countries are France, Germany, Holland and Hungary.

OTHER SPECIES There are over thirty-seven different varieties of parsley, such as the curly-leaved type *(P. crispum),* which is used in herbal medicine.

HERBAL/FOLK TRADITION It is used extensively as a culinary herb, both fresh and dried. It is a very nutritious plant, high in vitamins A and C; also used to freshen the breath. The herb and seed are used medicinally, princi-

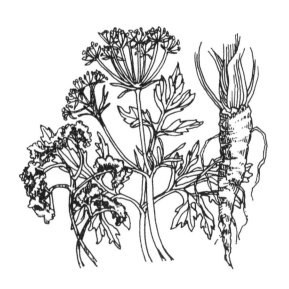

Parsley

pally for kidney and bladder problems, but it has also been employed for menstrual difficulties, digestive complaints and for arthritis, rheumatism, rickets and sciatica. It is said to stimulate hair growth, and help eliminate head lice.

The root is current in the British Herbal Pharmacopoeia as a specific for flatulent dyspepsia with intestinal colic.

ACTIONS Antimicrobial, antirheumatic, antiseptic, astringent, carminative, diuretic, depurative, emmenagogue, febrifuge, hypotensive, laxative, stimulant (mild), stomachic, tonic (uterine).

EXTRACTION Essential oil by steam distillation from 1. the seed, and 2. the herb. (An essential oil is occasionally extracted from the roots; an oleoresin is also produced by solvent extraction from the seeds.)

CHARACTERISTICS 1. A yellow, amber or brownish liquid with a warm woody-spicy herbaceous odour. 2. A pale yellow or greenish liquid with a heavy, warm, spicy-sweet odour, reminiscent of the herb. It blends well with rose, orange blossom, cananga, tea tree, oakmoss, clary sage and spice oils.

PRINCIPAL CONSTITUENTS 1. Mainly apiol, with myristicin, tetramethoxyallybenzene, pinene and volatile fatty acids. 2. Mainly myristicin (up to 85 per cent), with phellandrene, myrcene, apiol, terpinolene, menthatriene, pinene and carotel, among others.

SAFETY DATA Both oils are moderately toxic and irritant – myristicin has been shown to have toxic properties, and apiol has been shown to have irritant properties; otherwise non-sensitizing. Use in moderation. Avoid during pregnancy.

AROMATHERAPY/HOME USE
CIRCULATION, MUSCLES AND JOINTS: Accumulation of toxins, arthritis, broken blood vessels, cellulitis, rheumatism, sciatica.
DIGESTIVE SYSTEM: Colic, flatulence, indigestion, haemorrhoids.
GENITO-URINARY SYSTEM: Amenorrhoea,

dysmenorrhoea, to aid labour, cystitis, urinary infection.

OTHER USES Used in some carminative and digestive remedies, such as 'gripe waters'. The seed oil is used in soaps, detergents, colognes, cosmetics and perfumes, especially men's fragrances. The herb and seed oil as well as the oleoresin are used extensively in many types of food flavourings, especially meats, pickles and sauces, as well as alcoholic and soft drinks.

PATCHOULI
Pogostemon cablin

FAMILY Lamiaceae (Labiatae)

SYNONYMS *P. patchouly*, patchouly, puchaput.

GENERAL DESCRIPTION A perennial bushy herb up to 1 metre high with a sturdy, hairy stem, large, fragrant, furry leaves and white flowers tinged with purple.

DISTRIBUTION Native to tropical Asia, especially Indonesia and the Philippines. It is extensively cultivated for its oil in its native regions as well as India, China, Malaysia and South America. The oil is also distilled in Europe and America from the dried leaves.

OTHER SPECIES Closely related to the Java patchouli *(P. heyneanus)*, also known as false patchouli, which is also occasionally used to produce an essential oil.

HERBAL/FOLK TRADITION The oil is used in the East generally to scent linen and clothes, and is believed to help prevent the spread of disease (prophylactic). In China, Japan and Malaysia the herb is used to treat colds, headaches, nausea, vomiting, diarrhoea, abdominal pain and halitosis. In Japan and Malaysia it is used as an antidote to poisonous snakebites.

ACTIONS Antidepressant, anti-inflammatory, anti-emetic, antimicrobial, antiphlogistic, antiseptic, antitoxic, antiviral, aphrodisiac, astringent, bactericidal, carminative, cicatrisant, deodorant, digestive, diuretic, febrifuge, fungicidal, nervine, prophylactic, stimulant (nervous), stomachic, tonic.

EXTRACTION Essential oil by steam distillation of the dried leaves (usually subjected to fermentation previously). A resinoid is also produced, mainly as a fixative.

CHARACTERISTICS An amber or dark orange viscous liquid with a sweet, rich, herbaceous-earthy odour – it improves with age. It blends well with labdanum, vetiver, sandalwood, cedarwood, oakmoss, geranium, clove, lavender, rose, neroli, bergamot, cassia, myrrh, opopanax, clary sage and oriental-type bases.

PRINCIPAL CONSTITUENTS Patchouli alcohol (40 per cent approx.), pogostol, bulnesol, nor patchoulenol, bulnese, patchoulene, among others.

SAFETY DATA Non-toxic, non-irritant, non-sensitizing.

AROMATHERAPY/HOME USE
SKIN CARE: Acne, athlete's foot, cracked and chapped skin, dandruff, dermatitis, eczema (weeping), fungal infections, hair care, impetigo, insect repellent, sores, oily hair and skin, open pores, wounds, wrinkles.
NERVOUS SYSTEM: Frigidity, nervous exhaustion and stress-related complaints.

OTHER USES Extensively used in cosmetic preparations, and as a fixative in soaps and perfumes, especially oriental types. Extensively used in the food industry, in alcoholic and soft drinks. It makes a good masking agent for unpleasant tastes and smells.

PENNYROYAL
Mentha pulegium

FAMILY Lamiaceae (Labiatae)

SYNONYMS Pulegium, European pennyroyal, pudding grass.

GENERAL DESCRIPTION A perennial herb up to 50 cms tall with smooth roundish stalks, small, pale purple flowers and very aromatic, grey-green, oval leaves. Like other members of the mint family, it has a fibrous creeping root.

DISTRIBUTION Native to Europe and parts of Asia; it is cultivated mainly in southern Spain, Morocco, Tunisia, Portugal, Italy, Yugoslavia and Turkey.

OTHER SPECIES There are several different varieties of pennyroyal according to location: in Britain the 'erecta' and 'decumbens' types are most common. The North American pennyroyal *(Hedeoma pulegoides)*, which is also used to produce an essential oil, belongs to a slightly different species, though it shares similar properties with the European variety.

HERBAL/FOLK TRADITION A herbal remedy of ancient repute, used for a wide variety of ailments. It was believed to purify the blood and also be able to communicate its purifying qualities to water. 'Pennyroyal water' was distilled from the leaves and given as an antidote to spasmodic, nervous and hysterical affections. It was also used against cold and "affections of the joints".[72]
It is still current in the British Herbal Pharmacopoeia, indicated for flatulent dyspepsia, intestinal colic, the common cold, delayed menstruation, cutaneous eruptions and gout.

ACTIONS Antiseptic, antispasmodic, diaphoretic, carminative, digestive, emmenagogue, insect repellent, refrigerant, stimulant.

EXTRACTION Essential oil by steam distillation from the fresh or slightly dried herb.

CHARACTERISTICS A colourless or pale yellow liquid with a very fresh, minty-herbaceous odour. It blends well with geranium, rosemary, lavandin, sage and citronella.

PRINCIPAL CONSTITUENTS Mainly pulegone, with menthone, iso-menthone, octanol, piperitenone and trans-iso-pulegone. Constituents vary according to source – the Moroccan oil contains up to 96 per cent pulegone.

SAFETY DATA Oral toxin. Abortifacient (due to pulegone content). Ingestion of large doses has resulted in death.

AROMATHERAPY/HOME USE None. 'Should not be used in aromatherapy whether internally or externally.'[73]

OTHER USES Used as a fragrance material mainly in detergents or low-cost industrial perfumes. Mainly employed as a source of natural pulegone.

PEPPER, BLACK
Piper nigrum

FAMILY Piperaceae

SYNONYMS Piper, pepper.

GENERAL DESCRIPTION A perennial woody vine up to 5 metres high with heart-shaped leaves and small white flowers. The berries turn from red to black as they mature – black pepper is the dried fully grown unripe fruit.

DISTRIBUTION Native to south west India; cultivated extensively in tropical countries. Major producers are India, Indonesia, Malaysia, China and Madagascar. It is also distilled in Europe and America from the imported dried fruits.

OTHER SPECIES The so-called white pepper is the dried ripe fruit with the outer pericarp removed. Not to be confused with cayenne pepper or paprika from the capsicum species, which are used to make an oleoresin.

HERBAL/FOLK TRADITION Both black and white pepper have been used in the East for over

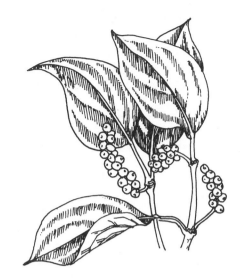

Black Pepper

4000 years for medicinal and culinary purposes. In Chinese medicine, white pepper is used to treat malaria, cholera, dysentery, diarrhoea, stomach ache and other digestive problems. In Greece it is used for intermittent fever and to fortify the stomach. 'The mendicant monks of India who cover daily considerable distances on foot, swallow 7–9 grains of pepper a day. This gives them remarkable endurance.'[74]

ACTIONS Analgesic, antimicrobial, antiseptic, antispasmodic, antitoxic, aperitif, aphrodisiac, bactericidal, carminative, diaphoretic, digestive, diuretic, febrifuge, laxative, rubefacient, stimulant (nervous, circulatory, digestive), stomachic, tonic.

EXTRACTION Essential oil by steam distillation from the black peppercorns, dried and crushed. ('Light' and 'heavy' oils are produced by the extraction of the low or high boiling fractions respectively.) An oleoresin is also produced by solvent extraction, mainly for flavour use.

CHARACTERISTICS A water-white to pale olive mobile liquid with a fresh, dry-woody, warm, spicy scent. It blends well with frankincense, sandalwood, lavender, rosemary, marjoram, spices and florals (in minute quantities).

PRINCIPAL CONSTITUENTS Mainly monoterpenes (70–80 per cent): thujene, pinene, camphene, sabinene, carene, myrcene, limonene, phellandrene, and sesquiterpenes (20–30 per cent) and oxygenated compounds.

SAFETY DATA Non-toxic, non-sensitizing, irritant in high concentration due to rubefacient properties. Use in moderation only.

AROMATHERAPY/HOME USE
SKIN CARE: Chilblains.
CIRCULATION, MUSCLES AND JOINTS: Anaemia, arthritis, muscular aches and pains, neuralgia, poor circulation, poor muscle tone (muscular atonia), rheumatic pain, sprains, stiffness.
RESPIRATORY SYSTEM: Catarrh, chills.
DIGESTIVE SYSTEM: Colic, constipation, diarrhoea, flatulence, heartburn, loss of appetite, nausea.
IMMUNE SYSTEM: Colds, 'flu, infections and viruses.

OTHER USES Used in certain tonic and rubefacient preparations. Used for unusual effects in perfumery work; for example, with rose or carnation in oriental or floral fragrances. The oil and oleoresin are used extensively in the food industry, as well as in alcoholic drinks.

PETITGRAIN
Citrus aurantium var. amara

FAMILY Rutaceae

SYNONYMS C. *bigaradia*, petitgrain bigarade (oil), petitgrain Paraguay (oil). See also *bitter orange*.

GENERAL DESCRIPTION The oil of petitgrain is produced from the leaves and twigs of the same tree that produces bitter orange oil and orange blossom oil: see *bitter orange* and *orange blossom*.

DISTRIBUTION Native to southern China and north east India. The best quality petitgrain oil comes from France but a good quality oil is also produced in North Africa, Paraguay and Haiti from semi-wild trees.

OTHER SPECIES A type of petitgrain is also produced in small quantities from the leaves, twigs and small unripe fruit of the lemon, sweet orange, mandarin and bergamot trees.

HERBAL/FOLK TRADITION At one time the oil used to be extracted from the green unripe oranges when they were still the size of a cherry – hence the name *petitgrains* or 'little grains'. One of the classic ingredients of eau-de-cologne.

ACTIONS Antiseptic, antispasmodic, deodorant, digestive, nervine, stimulant (digestive, nervous), stomachic, tonic.

EXTRACTION Essential oil by steam distillation from the leaves and twigs. An orange 'leaf and flower' water absolute is also produced, known as *petitgrain sur fleurs*.

CHARACTERISTICS A pale yellow to amber liquid with a fresh-floral citrus scent and a woody-herbaceous undertone. It blends well with rosemary, lavender, geranium, bergamot, bitter orange, orange blossom, labdanum, oakmoss, clary sage, jasmine, benzoin, palmarosa, clove and balsams.

PRINCIPAL CONSTITUENTS 40–80 per cent esters: mainly linalyl acetate and geranyl acetate, as well as linalol, nerol, terpineol, geraniol, nerolidol, farnesol, limonene, among others.

SAFETY DATA Non-toxic, non-irritant, non-sensitizing, non-phototoxic.

AROMATHERAPY/HOME USE
SKIN CARE: Acne, excessive perspiration, greasy skin and hair, toning.
DIGESTIVE SYSTEM: Dyspepsia, flatulence.
NERVOUS SYSTEM: Convalescence, insomnia, nervous exhaustion and stress-related conditions.

OTHER USES Extensively used as a fragrance component in soaps, detergents, cosmetics and perfumes, especially colognes (sometimes used to replace orange blossom). Employed as a flavour component in many foods, especially confectionery, as well as alcoholic and soft drinks.

PINE, DWARF
Pinus mugo var. pumilio

FAMILY Pinaceae

SYNONYMS *P. mugo, P. montana, P. pumilio,* mountain pine, Swiss mountain pine, pine needle (oil).

GENERAL DESCRIPTION A pyramidal shrub or small tree up to 12 metres high with a black bark, stiff and twisted needles borne in clusters, and brown cones, initially of a bluish hue.

DISTRIBUTION Native to the mountainous regions of central and southern Europe. The oil is mainly produced in Austria (Tirol), Yugoslavia, Denmark and Italy.

OTHER SPECIES There are very many species of pine used to produce essential oil from their needles and wood or employed in the production of turpentine. NB: The so-called huon pine *(Dacrydium franklinii)*, the essential oil of which is also a skin irritant, belongs to a different family, the Podcarpaceae. For further details see *Scotch pine* and the Botanical Classification section.

HERBAL/FOLK TRADITION A preparation made from the needles has been used internally for bladder, kidney and rheumatic complaints, as a liniment for rheumatism and muscular pain, and as an inhalant for bronchitis, catarrh, colds, etc.

ACTIONS Analgesic, antimicrobial, antiseptic, antitussive, antiviral, balsamic, diuretic, expectorant, rubefacient.

EXTRACTION Essential oil by steam distillation from the needles and twigs.

CHARACTERISTICS A water-white liquid with a very pleasant, balsamic-sweet, spicy-woody scent of good tenacity. This is the favoured pine fragrance for perfumery use due to its unique delicate odour, which blends well with cedarwood, lavandin, rosemary, sage, cananga, labdanum, juniper and other coniferous oils.

PRINCIPAL CONSTITUENTS Mainly monoterpene hydrocarbons; limonene, pinenes, phellandrene, dipentene, camphene, myrcene and bornyl acetate among others. The unusual scent is believed to be due to its aldehyde content.

SAFETY DATA Dermal irritant, common sensitizing agent; otherwise non-toxic. It is best avoided therapeutically due to irritant hazards.

AROMATHERAPY/HOME USE None.

OTHER USES Used as a fragrance and flavour component in pharmaceutical preparations for coughs and colds, nasal congestion and externally in analgesic ointments and liniments. Extensively employed in soaps, bath preparations, toiletries, cosmetics and perfumes, especially 'leather' and 'woody' type fragrances. It is also used in most major food categories, alcoholic and soft drinks.

PINE, LONGLEAF
Pinus palustris

FAMILY Pinaceae

SYNONYMS Longleaf yellow pine, southern yellow pine, pitch pine, pine (oil).

GENERAL DESCRIPTION A tall evergreen tree with long needles and a straight trunk, grown extensively for its timber. It exudes a natural oleoresin from the trunk, which provides the largest source for the production of turpentine in America – see also entry on turpentine.

DISTRIBUTION Native to south eastern USA, where the oil is largely produced.

OTHER SPECIES There are numerous other species of pine all over the world which are used to produce pine oil, as well as pine needle and turpentine oil – see Botanical Classification section.

HERBAL/FOLK TRADITION Pine sawdust has been used for centuries as a highly esteemed household remedy for a variety of ailments. 'It is a grand, gentle, although powerful external antiseptic remedy, applied as a poultice in rheumatism when localised, hard cancerous tumours, tuberculosis in the knee or ankle joints, disease of the bone, in short, all sluggish morbid deposits ... I have used it behind the head for failing sight, down the spine for general debility, on the loins for lumbago, etc. all with the best results.'[75]

ACTIONS Analgesic (mild), antirheumatic, antiseptic, bactericidal, expectorant, insecticidal, stimulant.

EXTRACTION The crude oil is obtained by steam distillation from the sawdust and wood chips from the heartwood and roots of the tree (wastage from the timber mills), and then submitted to fractional distillation under atmospheric pressure to produce pine essential oil.

CHARACTERISTICS A water-white or pale yellow liquid with a sweet-balsamic, pinewood scent. It blends well with rosemary, pine needle, cedarwood, citronella, rosewood, ho leaf and oakmoss.

PRINCIPAL CONSTITUENTS Terpineol, estragole, fenchone, fenchyl alcohol and borneol, among others.

SAFETY DATA Non-toxic; non-irritant (except in concentration); possible sensitization in some individuals.

AROMATHERAPY/HOME USE
CIRCULATION, MUSCLES AND JOINTS: Arthritis, debility, lumbago, muscular aches and pains, poor circulation, rheumatism, stiffness, etc. RESPIRATORY SYSTEM: Asthma, bronchitis, catarrh, sinusitis.

OTHER USES Used extensively in medicine, particularly in veterinary antiseptic sprays, disinfectants, detergents and insecticides (as a solvent carrier). Employed as a fragrance component in soaps, toiletries, bath products and perfumes. Also used in paint manufacture although it is increasingly being replaced by synthetic 'pine oil'.

PINE, SCOTCH
Pinus sylvestris

FAMILY Pinaceae

SYNONYMS Forest pine, Scots pine, Norway pine, pine needle (oil).

GENERAL DESCRIPTION A tall evergreen tree, up to 40 metres high with a flat crown. It has a reddish-brown, deeply fissured bark, long stiff needles which grow in pairs, and pointed brown cones.

DISTRIBUTION Native to Eurasia; cultivated in the eastern USA, Europe, Russia, the Baltic States and Scandinavia, especially Finland.

OTHER SPECIES Like the fir tree, there are numerous species of pine which yield an essential oil from their heartwood as well as from their twigs and needles and are also used to produce turpentine. The oil from the needles of the Scotch pine is one of the most useful and safest therapeutically. Other species which produce pine needle oil include the eastern white pine *(P. strobus)* from the eastern USA and Canada, the dwarf pine *(P. mugo var. pumilio)* grown in central and southern Europe, and the black pine *(P. nigra)* from Austria and Yugoslavia.

Many varieties, such as the longleaf pine *(Pinus palustris),* are used to produce turpentine. In addition, the oil commonly known as Siberian pine needle oil is actually from the Siberian fir *(Abies sibirica).* See also *dwarf pine* and the Botanical Classification section.

HERBAL/FOLK TRADITION The young macerated shoots are added to the bath for nervous exhaustion, circulatory disorders, slow, healing wounds, arthritis, rheumatism and skin disorders. It was used by the American Indians to prevent scurvy, and to stuff mattresses to repel lice and fleas.

As an inhalation it helps relieve bronchial catarrh, asthma, blocked sinuses, etc. The pine kernels are said to be excellent restoratives for consumptives, and after long illness.

ACTIONS Antimicrobial, antineuralgic, antirheumatic, antiscorbutic, antiseptic (pulmonary, urinary, hepatic), antiviral, bactericidal, balsamic, cholagogue, choleretic, deodorant, diuretic, expectorant, hypertensive, insecticidal, restorative, rubefacient, stimulant (adrenal cortex, circulatory, nervous), vermifuge.

EXTRACTION 1. Essential oil by dry distillation of the needles. 2. Gum turpentine is produced by steam distillation from the oleoresin: see entry on turpentine. (An inferior essential oil is also produced by dry distillation from the wood chippings, etc.)

CHARACTERISTICS 1. Pine needle oil is a colourless or pale yellow mobile liquid with a strong, dry-balsamic, turpentine-like aroma. It blends well with cedarwood, rosemary, tea tree, sage, lavender, juniper, lemon, niaouli, eucalyptus and marjoram. 2. See entry on turpentine.

PRINCIPAL CONSTITUENTS 50–90 per cent monoterpene hydrocarbons: pinenes, carene, dipentene, limonene, terpinenes, myrcene, ocimene, camphene, sabinene; also bornyl acetate, cineol, citral, chamazulene, among others.

SAFETY DATA Non-toxic, non-irritant (except in concentration), possible sensitization. Avoid in allergic skin conditions.

AROMATHERAPY/HOME USE
SKIN CARE: Cuts, lice, excessive perspiration, scabies, sores.

CIRCULATION, MUSCLES AND JOINTS: Arthritis, gout, muscular aches and pains, poor circulation, rheumatism.
RESPIRATORY SYSTEM: Asthma, bronchitis, catarrh, coughs, sinusitis, sore throat.
GENITO-URINARY SYSTEM: Cystitis, urinary infection.
IMMUNE SYSTEM: Colds, 'flu.
NERVOUS SYSTEM: Fatigue, nervous exhaustion and stress-related conditions, neuralgia.

OTHER USES Used as a fragrance component in soaps, detergents, cosmetics, toiletries (especially bath products) and, to a limited extent, perfumes. Employed as a flavour ingredient in major food products, alcoholic and soft drinks.

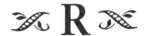

ROSE, CABBAGE
Rosa centifolia

FAMILY Rosaceae

SYNONYMS Rose maroc, French rose, Provence rose, hundred-leaved rose, Moroccan otto of rose (oil), French otto of rose (oil), rose de mai (absolute or concrete).

GENERAL DESCRIPTION The rose which is generally used for oil production is strictly a hybrid between *R. centifolia,* a pink rose, and *R. gallica,* a dark red rose. This variety, known as rose de mai, grows to a height of 2.5 metres and produces an abundance of flowers with large pink or rosy-purple petals. There are two subspecies – one is more spiny than the other.

DISTRIBUTION The birthplace of the cultivated rose is believed to be ancient Persia; now cultivated mainly in Morocco, Tunisia, Italy, France, Yugoslavia and China. The concrete,

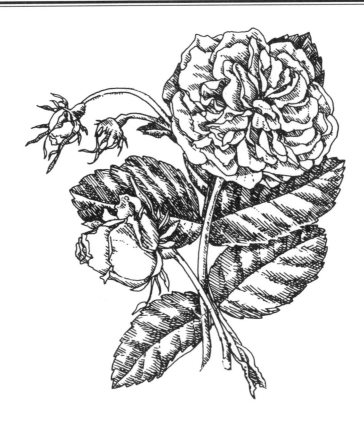

Cabbage Rose

absolute and oil are mainly produced in Morocco; the absolute in France, Italy and China.

OTHER SPECIES There are over 10,000 types of cultivated rose! There are several subspecies of *R. centifolia*, depending on the country of origin. Other therapeutic species are the red rose or apothecary rose *(R. gallica)* of traditional Western medicine, the oriental or tea rose *(R. indica)*, the Chinese or Japanese rose *(R. rugosa)* and the Turkish or Bulgarian rose *(R. damascena)* which is also extensively cultivated for its oil. Recently rosehip seed oil from *R. rubiginosa* has been found to be a very effective skin treatment; it promotes tissue regeneration and is good for scars, burns and wrinkles. See also entry on damask rose and the Botanical Classification section.

HERBAL/FOLK TRADITION The healing virtues of the rose have been known since antiquity and although roses are rarely used in herbal practice nowadays, up to the Middle Ages they played an essential part in the materia medica, and still fulfil an important role in Eastern medicine. They were used for a wide range of disorders, including digestive and menstrual problems, headaches and nervous tension, liver congestion, poor circulation, fever (plague), eye infections and skin complaints.

'The symbolism connected with the rose is perhaps one of the richest and most complex associated with any plant ... traditionally associated with Venus, the Goddess of love and beauty, and in our materialistic age the Goddess is certainly alive and well in the cosmetics industry for rose oil (mainly synthetic) is found as a component in 46% of men's perfumes and 98 % of women's fragrances.'[76]

The French or Moroccan rose possesses narcotic properties and has the reputation for being aphrodisiac (more so than the Bulgarian type), possibly due to the high percentage of phenyl ethanol in the former. For further distinctions between the different properties of rose types, see *damask rose*.

ACTIONS Antidepressant, antiphlogistic, antiseptic, antispasmodic, anti-tubercular agent, antiviral, aphrodisiac, astringent, bactericidal, choleretic, cicitrisant, depurative, emmenagogue, haemostatic, hepatic, laxative, regulator of appetite, sedative (nervous), stomachic, tonic (heart, liver, stomach, uterus).

EXTRACTION 1. Essential oil or otto by water or steam distillation from the fresh petals. (Rose water is produced as a byproduct of this process.) 2. Concrete and absolute by solvent extraction from the fresh petals. (A rose leaf absolute is also produced in small quantities in France.)

CHARACTERISTICS 1. The oil is a pale yellow liquid with a deep, sweet, rosy-floral, tenacious odour. 2. The absolute is a reddish-orange viscous liquid with a deep, rich, sweet, rosy-spicy, honeylike fragrance. It blends well with jasmine, cassie, mimosa, orange blossom, geranium, bergamot, lavender, clary sage, sandalwood, guaiacwood, patchouli, benzoin, chamomile, Peru balsam, clove and palmarosa.

PRINCIPAL CONSTITUENTS It has over 300 constituents, some in minute traces. Mainly citronellol (18–22 per cent), phenyl ethanol (63 per cent), geraniol and nerol (10–15 per cent), stearopten (8 per cent), farnesol (0.2–2 per cent), among others.

SAFETY DATA Non-toxic, non-irritant, non-sensitizing.

AROMATHERAPY/HOME USE
SKIN CARE: Broken capillaries, conjunctivitis (rose water), dry skin, eczema, herpes, mature and sensitive complexions, wrinkles.
CIRCULATION, MUSCLES AND JOINTS: Palpitations, poor circulation.
RESPIRATORY SYSTEM: Asthma, coughs, hay fever.
DIGESTIVE SYSTEM: Cholecystitis, liver congestion, nausea.
GENITO-URINARY SYSTEM: Irregular menstruation, leucorrhoea, menorrhagia, uterine disorders.
NERVOUS SYSTEM: Depression, impotence, insomnia, frigidity, headache, nervous tension and stress-related complaints – 'But the rose procures us one thing above all: a feeling of well being, even of happiness, and the individual under its influence will develop an amiable tolerance.'[77]

OTHER USES Rose water is used as a household cosmetic and culinary article (especially in Persian cookery). The concrete, absolute and oil are employed extensively in soaps, cosmetics, toiletries and perfumes of all types – floral, oriental, chyprès, etc. Some flavouring uses, especially fruit products and tobacco.

ROSE, DAMASK
Rosa damascena

FAMILY Rosaceae

SYNONYMS Summer damask rose, Bulgarian rose, Turkish rose (Anatolian rose oil), otto of rose (oil), attar of rose (oil).

GENERAL DESCRIPTION Small prickly shrub between 1 metre and 2 metres high, with pink, very fragrant blooms with thirty-six petals, and whitish hairy leaves. It requires a very specific soil and climate.

DISTRIBUTION Believed to be a native of the Orient, now cultivated mainly in Bulgaria, Turkey and France. Similar types are grown in China, India and Russia; however, India produces only rose water and *aytar* – a mixture of rose otto and sandalwood.

OTHER SPECIES There are many different subspecies: the Turkish variety is known simply as *R. damascena*. 'Trigintipetala' is the principal cultivar in commercial cultivation, known as the 'Kazanlik rose'. Bulgaria also grows the white rose *(R. damascena var. alba)* or the musk rose *(R. muscatta)* which is used as a windbreak around the damask rose plantations. See also *cabbage rose* and the Botanical Classification section.

HERBAL/FOLK TRADITION 'The damask rose, on account of its fragrance, belongs to the cephalics; but the next valuable virtue that it possesses consists in its cathartic quality ...oil of roses is used by itself to cool hot inflammations or swellings, and to bind and stay fluxes of humours to sores.'[78]

Rose hips are still current in the British Herbal Pharmacopoeia, mainly due to their high vitamin C content (also A and B). For further general properties, see entry for cabbage rose.

ACTIONS See *cabbage rose*.

EXTRACTION 1. Essential oil or otto by water or steam distillation from the fresh petals. 2. A concrete and absolute by solvent extraction from the fresh petals.

CHARACTERISTICS 1. A pale yellow or olive yellow liquid with a very rich, deep, sweet-floral, slightly spicy scent.   2. The absolute is a reddish-orange or olive viscous liquid with a rich, sweet, spicy-floral, tenacious odour. It blends well with most oils, and is useful for 'rounding off' blends. The Bulgarian type is considered superior in perfumery work, but in therapeutic practice it is more a matter of differing properties between the various types of rose.

PRINCIPAL CONSTITUENTS Mainly citronellol (34–55 per cent), geraniol and nerol (30–40 per cent), stearopten (16–22 per cent), phenyl ethanol (1.5–3 per cent) and farnesol (0.2–2 per cent), with many other trace contituents.

SAFETY DATA Non-toxic, non-irritant, non-sensitizing.

AROMATHERAPY/HOME USE See *cabbage rose*.

OTHER USES See *cabbage rose*.

ROSEMARY
Rosmarinus officinalis

FAMILY Lamiaceae (Labiatae)

SYNONYMS *R. coronarium*, compass plant, incensier.

GENERAL DESCRIPTION A shrubby evergreen bush up to 2 metres high with silvery-green, needle-shaped leaves and pale blue flowers. The whole plant is strongly aromatic.

DISTRIBUTION Native to the Mediterranean region, now cultivated worldwide in California, Russia, Middle East, England, France, Spain, Portugal, Yugoslavia, Morocco, China, etc. The main oil-producing countries are France, Spain and Tunisia.

OTHER SPECIES *R. officinalis* is the type used for oil production but it is generally not specified, although there are many different cultivars, for example pine-scented rosemary (*R. officinalis var. angustifolius*). See also Botanical Classification.

HERBAL/FOLK TRADITION One of the earliest plants to be used for food, medicine and magic, being regarded as sacred in many

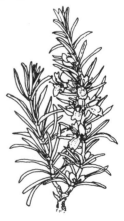

Rosemary

civilizations. Sprigs of rosemary were burnt at shrines in ancient Greece, fumigations were used in the Middle Ages to drive away evil spirits, and to protect against plague and infectious illness.

It has been used for a wide range of complaints including respiratory and circulatory disorders, liver congestion, digestive and nervous complaints, muscular and rheumatic pain, skin and hair problems.

It is current in the British Herbal Pharmacopoeia as a specific for 'depressive states with general debility and indications of cardiovascular weakness'. [79]

ACTIONS Analgesic, antimicrobial, antioxidant, antirheumatic, antiseptic, antispasmodic, aphrodisiac, astringent, carminative, cephalic, cholagogue, choleretic, cicatrisant, cordial, cytophylactic, diaphoretic, digestive, diuretic, emmenagogue, fungicidal, hepatic, hypertensive, nervine, parasiticide, restorative, rubefacient, stimulant (circulatory, adrenal cortex, hepatobiliary), stomachic, sudorific, tonic (nervous, general), vulnerary.

EXTRACTION Essential oil by steam distillation of the fresh flowering tops or (in Spain) the whole plant (poorer quality).

CHARACTERISTICS A colourless or pale yellow mobile liquid with a strong, fresh, minty-herbaceous scent and a woody-balsamic undertone. Poor quality oils have a strong camphoraceous note. It blends well with olibanum, lavender, lavandin, citronella, oregano, thyme, pine, basil, peppermint, labdanum, elemi, cedarwood, petitgrain, cinnamon and other spice oils.

PRINCIPAL CONSTITUENTS Mainly pinenes, camphene, limonene, cineol, borneol with camphor, linalol, terpineol, octanone, bornyl acetate, among others.

SAFETY DATA Non-toxic, non-irritant (in dilution only), non-sensitizing. Avoid during pregnancy. Not to be used by epileptics.

AROMATHERAPY/HOME USE
SKIN CARE: Acne, dandruff, dermatitis, eczema, greasy hair, insect repellent, promotes hair growth, regulates seborrhoea, scabies, stimulates scalp, lice, varicose veins.
CIRCULATION, MUSCLES AND JOINTS: Arteriosclerosis, fluid retention, gout, muscular pain, palpitations, poor circulation, rheumatism.
RESPIRATORY SYSTEM: Asthma, bronchitis, whooping cough.
DIGESTIVE SYSTEM: Colitis, dyspepsia, flatulence, hepatic disorders, hypercholesterolaemia, jaundice.
GENITO-URINARY: Dysmenorrhoea, leucorrhoea.
IMMUNE SYSTEM: Colds, 'flu, infections.
NERVOUS SYSTEM: Debility, headaches, hypotension, neuralgia, mental fatigue, nervous exhaustion and stress-related disorders.

OTHER USES Extensively used in soaps, detergents, cosmetics, household sprays and perfumes, especially colognes. Also used as a masking agent. Extensively employed in most major food categories, especially meat products, as well as alcoholic and soft drinks. Serves as a source of natural anti-oxidants.

ROSEWOOD
Aniba rosaeodora

FAMILY Lauraceae

SYNONYMS *A. rosaeodora var. amazonica*, bois de rose, Brazilian rosewood.

GENERAL DESCRIPTION Medium-sized, tropical, evergreen tree with a reddish bark and heartwood, bearing yellow flowers. Used extensively for timber. NB: This is one of the trees that is being extensively felled in the clearing of the South American rainforests; the continual production of rosewood oil is consequently enviromentally damaging.

DISTRIBUTION Native to the Amazon region; Brazil and Peru are the main producers.

OTHER SPECIES There are several species of timber all known as rosewood; however, the essential oil is only distilled from the above species. French Guiana used to produce the cayenne rosewood *(Ocotea caudata)*, which is superior in quality to the Peruvian or Brazilian type.

HERBAL/FOLK TRADITION Used for building, carving and French cabinet making. Nowadays, most rosewood goes to Japan for the production of chopsticks.

ACTIONS Mildly analgesic, anticonvulsant, antidepressant, anti-microbial, antiseptic, aphrodisiac, bactericidal, cellular stimulant, cephalic, deodorant, stimulant (immune system), tissue regenerator, tonic.

EXTRACTION Essential oil by steam distillation of the wood chippings.

CHARACTERISTICS Colourless to pale yellow liquid with a very sweet, woody-floral fragrance with a spicy hint. Blends well with most oils, especially citrus, woods and florals. It helps give body and rounds off sharp edges.

PRINCIPAL CONSTITUENTS Linalol (90–97 per cent) in cayenne rosewood; in the Brazilian oil slightly less (80–90 per cent). Also cineol, terpineol, geraniol, citronellal, limonene, pinene, among others.

SAFETY DATA Non-toxic, non-irritant, non-sensitizing.

AROMATHERAPY/HOME USE
SKIN CARE: Acne, dermatitis, scars, wounds, wrinkles and general skin care: sensitive, dry, dull, combination oily/dry, etc. 'Although it does not have any dramatic curative power ... I find it very useful especially for skin care. It is very mild and safe to use.'[80]
IMMUNE SYSTEM: Colds, coughs, fever, infections, stimulates the immune system.
NERVOUS SYSTEM: Frigidity, headaches, nausea, nervous tension and stress-related conditions.

OTHER USES Once extensively used as a source of natural linalol, now increasingly replaced by the synthetic form. Acetylated rosewood oil is used extensively in perfumery work – soaps, toiletries, cosmetics and perfumes. The oil is employed in most major food categories, alcoholic and soft drinks.

RUE
Ruta graveolens

FAMILY Rutaceae

SYNONYMS Garden rue, herb-of-grace, herbygrass.

GENERAL DESCRIPTION An ornamental, shrubby herb with tough, woody branches, small, smooth, bluish-green leaves and greeny-yellow flowers. The whole plant has a strong, aromatic, bitter or acrid scent.

DISTRIBUTION Native to the Mediterranean region; found growing wild extensively in Spain, Morocco, Corsica, Sardinia and Algeria. It is cultivated mainly in France and Spain for its oil; also in Italy and Yugoslavia.

OTHER SPECIES There are several different types of rue, such as the summer rue *(R. montana)*, winter rue *(R. chalepensis)* and Sardinian rue *(R. angustifolia)*, which are also used to produce essential oils.

HERBAL/FOLK TRADITION A favoured remedy of the ancients, especially as an antidote to poison. It was seen as a magic herb by many cultures and as a protection against evil. It was also used for nervous afflictions. 'It helps disorders in the head, nerves and womb, convulsions and hysteric fits, the colic, weakness of the stomach and bowels; it resists poison and cures venomous bites.'[81]

ACTIONS Antitoxic, antitussive, antiseptic, antispasmodic, diuretic, emmenagogue, insecticidal, nervine, rubefacient, stimulant, tonic, vermifuge.

EXTRACTION Essential oil by steam distillation from the fresh herb.

CHARACTERISTICS A yellow or orange viscous mass which generally solidifies at room temperature, with a sharp, herbaceous-fruity acrid odour. The winter rue oil does not solidify at room temperature.

PRINCIPAL CONSTITUENTS Mainly methyl nonyl ketone (90 per cent in summer rue oil).

SAFETY DATA Oral toxin (due to main constituent). Skin and mucous membrane irritant. Abortifacient. 'Rue oil should never be used in perfumery or flavour work.'[82]

AROMATHERAPY/HOME USE None. 'Should not be used at all in aromatherapy.'[83]

OTHER USES Employed as a source of methyl nonyl ketone.

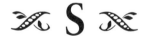

SAGE, CLARY
Salvia sclarea

FAMILY Lamiaceae (Labiatae)

SYNONYMS Clary, clary wort, muscatel sage, clear eye, see bright, common clary, clarry, eye bright.

GENERAL DESCRIPTION Stout biennial or perennial herb up to 1 metre high with large, hairy leaves, green with a hint of purple, and small blue flowers.

DISTRIBUTION Native to southern Europe; cultivated worldwide especially in the Mediterranean region, Russia, the USA,

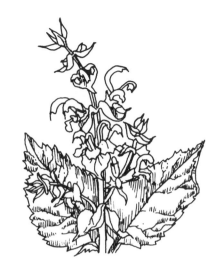

Clary Sage

England, Morocco and central Europe. The French, Moroccan and English clary are considered of superior quality for perfumery work.

OTHER SPECIES Closely related to the garden sage *(S. officinalis)* and the Spanish sage *(S. lavendulaefolia)*, which are both used to produce essential oils. Other types of sage include meadow clary *(S. pratensis)* and vervain sage *(S. verbenaca)*. Clary sage should not be confused with the common wayside herb eyebright *(Euphrasia)*.

HERBAL/FOLK TRADITION This herb, highly esteemed in the Middle Ages, has now largely fallen out of use. It was used for digestive disorders, kidney disease, uterine and menstrual complaints, for cleansing ulcers and as a general nerve tonic. The mucilage from the seeds was used for treating tumours and for removing dust particles from the eyes.

Like garden sage, it cools inflammation and is especially useful for throat and respiratory infections.

ACTIONS Anticonvulsive, antidepressant, antiphlogistic, antiseptic, antispasmodic, aphrodisiac, astringent, bactericidal, carminative, cicatrisant, deodorant, digestive, emmenagogue, hypotensive, nervine, regulator (of seborrhoea), sedative, stomachic, tonic, uterine.

EXTRACTION Essential oil by steam distillation from the flowering tops and leaves. (A concrete and absolute are also produced by solvent extraction in small quantities.)

CHARACTERISTICS A colourless or pale yellowy-green liquid with a sweet, nutty-herbaceous scent. It blends well with juniper, lavender, coriander, cardomon, geranium, sandalwood, cedarwood, pine, labdanum, jasmine, frankincense, bergamot and other citrus oils.

PRINCIPAL CONSTITUENTS Linalyl acetate (up to 75 per cent), linalol, pinene, myrcene and phellandrene, among others. Constituents vary according to geographical origin – there are several different chemotypes.

SAFETY DATA Non-toxic, non-irritant, non-sensitizing. Avoid during pregnancy. Do not use clary sage oil while drinking alcohol since it can induce a narcotic effect and exaggerate drunkenness. Clary sage is generally used in preference to the garden sage in aromatherapy due to its lower toxicity level.

AROMATHERAPY/HOME USE
SKIN CARE: Acne, boils, dandruff, hair loss, inflamed conditions, oily skin and hair, ophthalmia, ulcers, wrinkles.
CIRCULATION, MUSCLES AND JOINTS: High blood pressure, muscular aches and pains.
RESPIRATORY SYSTEM: Asthma, throat infections, whooping cough.
DIGESTIVE SYSTEM: Colic, cramp, dyspepsia, flatulence.
GENITO-URINARY SYSTEM: Amenorrhoea, labour pain, dysmenorrhoea, leucorrhoea.
NERVOUS SYSTEM: Depression, frigidity, impotence, migraine, nervous tension and stress-related disorders.

OTHER USES The oil and absolute are used as fragrance components and fixatives in soaps, detergents, cosmetics and perfumes. The oil is used extensively by the food and drink industry, especially in the production of wines with a muscatel flavour.

SAGE, COMMON
Salvia officinalis

FAMILY Lamiaceae (Labiatae)

SYNONYMS Garden sage, true sage, Dalmatian sage.

GENERAL DESCRIPTION An evergreen, shrubby, perennial herb up to 80 cms high with a woody base, soft, silver, oval leaves and a mass of deep blue or violet flowers.

DISTRIBUTION Native to the Mediterranean region; cultivated worldwide especially in Albania, Yugoslavia, Greece, Italy, Turkey, France, China and the USA.

OTHER SPECIES There are several different species and cultivars which have been developed, such as the Mexican sage (*S. azurea grandiflora*) and the red sage (*S. colorata*) both of which are used medicinally. Essential oils are also produced from other species including the Spanish sage (*S. lavendulaefolia*) and clary sage (*S. sclarea*) – see separate entries and Botanical Classification section.

HERBAL/FOLK TRADITION A herb of ancient repute, valued as a culinary and medicinal plant – called *herba sacra* or 'sacred herb' by the Romans. It has been used for a variety of disorders including respiratory infections, menstrual difficulties and digestive complaints. It was also believed to strengthen the senses and the memory.
  It is still current in the British Herbal Pharmacopoeia as a specific for inflammations of the mouth, tongue and throat.

ACTIONS Anti-inflammatory, antimicrobial, anti-oxidant, antiseptic, antispasmodic, astringent, digestive, diuretic, emmenagogue, febrifuge, hypertensive, insecticidal, laxative, stomachic, tonic.

EXTRACTION Essential oil by steam distillation from the dried leaves. (A so-called 'oleoresin' is also produced from the exhausted plant material.)

CHARACTERISTICS A pale yellow mobile liquid with a fresh, warm-spicy, herbaceous, somewhat camphoraceous odour. It blends well with lavandin, rosemary, rosewood, lavender, hyssop, lemon and other citrus oils. The common sage oil is preferred in perfumery work to the Spanish sage oil which, although safer, has a less refined fragrance.

PRINCIPAL CONSTITUENTS Thujone (about 42 per cent), cineol, borneol, caryophyllene and other terpenes.

SAFETY DATA Oral toxin (due to thujone). Abortifacient; avoid in pregnancy. Avoid in epilepsy. Use with care or avoid in therapeutic work altogether – Spanish sage or clary sage are good alternatives.

AROMATHERAPY/HOME USE None.

OTHER USES Used in some pharmaceutical preparations such as mouthwashes, gargles, toothpastes, etc. Employed as a fragrance component in soaps, shampoos, detergents, anti-perspirants, colognes and perfumes, especially men's fragrances. The oil and oleoresin are extensively used for flavouring foods (mainly meat products), soft drinks and alcoholic beverages, especially vermouth. It also serves as a source of natural anti-oxidants.

SAGE, SPANISH
Salvia lavendulaefolia

FAMILY Lamiaceae (Labiatae)

SYNONYMS Lavender-leaved sage.

GENERAL DESCRIPTION An evergreen shrub, similar to the garden sage but with narrower leaves and small purple flowers. The whole plant is aromatic with a scent reminiscent of spike lavender.

DISTRIBUTION Native to the mountains in Spain, it also grows in south west France and Yugoslavia. The oil is mainly produced in Spain.

OTHER SPECIES A very similar oil is distilled in Turkey from a Greek variety, *S. triloba,* which is used for pharmaceutical purposes. See also entries on clary sage and common sage for other types of sage.

HERBAL/FOLK TRADITION In Spain it is regarded as something of a 'cure-all'. Believed to promote longevity and protect against all types of infection (such as plague). Used to treat rheumatism, digestive complaints, menstrual problems, infertility and nervous weakness.

ACTIONS Antidepressant, anti-inflammatory, antimicrobial, antiseptic, antispasmodic, astringent, carminative, deodorant, depurative, digestive, emmenagogue, expectorant, febrifuge, hypotensive, nervine, regulator (of seborrhoea), stimulant (hepatobiliary, adrenocortical glands, circulation), stomachic, tonic (nerve and general).

EXTRACTION Essential oil by steam distillation from the leaves.

CHARACTERISTICS A pale yellow mobile liquid with a fresh-herbaceous, camphoraceous, slightly pinelike odour. It blends well with rosemary, lavandin, lavender, pine, citronella, eucalyptus, juniper, clary sage and cedarwood.

PRINCIPAL CONSTITUENTS Camphor (up to 34 per cent), cineol (up to 35 per cent), limonene (up to 41 per cent), camphene (up to 20 per cent), pinene (up to 20 per cent) and other minor constituents.

SAFETY DATA Relatively non-toxic, non-irritant, non-sensitizing. Avoid during pregnancy; use in moderation.

AROMATHERAPY/HOME USE

SKIN CARE: Acne, cuts, dandruff, dermatitis, eczema, excessive sweating, hair loss, gingivitis, gum infections, sores.

CIRCULATION, MUSCLES AND JOINTS: Arthritis, debility, fluid retention, muscular aches and pains, poor circulation, rheumatism.

RESPIRATORY SYSTEM: Asthma, coughs, laryngitis.

DIGESTIVE SYSTEM: Jaundice, liver congestion.

GENITO-URINARY SYSTEM: Amenorrhoea, dysmenorrhoea, sterility.

IMMUNE SYSTEM: Colds, fevers, 'flu.

NERVOUS SYSTEM: Headaches, nervous exhaustion and stress-related conditions.

OTHER USES Extensively used as a fragrance component in soaps, cosmetics, toiletries and perfumes, especially 'industrial' type fragrances. Extensively employed in foods (especially meat products), as well as alcoholic and soft drinks.

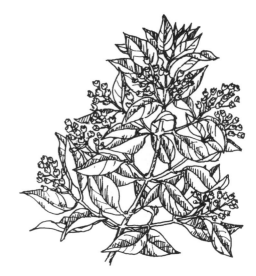

Sandalwood

SANDALWOOD

Santalum album

FAMILY Santalaceae

SYNONYMS White sandalwood, yellow sandalwood, East Indian sandalwood, sandalwood Mysore, sanders-wood, santal (oil), white saunders (oil), yellow saunders (oil).

GENERAL DESCRIPTION A small, evergreen, parasitic tree up to 9 metres high with brown-grey trunk and many smooth, slender branches. It has leathery leaves and small pinky-purple flowers. The tree must be over thirty years old before it is ready for the production of sandalwood oil.

DISTRIBUTION Native to tropical Asia, especially India, Sri Lanka, Malaysia, Indonesia and Taiwan. India is the main essential oil producer; the region of Mysore exports the highest quality oil, although some oil is distilled in Europe and the USA.

OTHER SPECIES The Australian sandalwood (*S. spicatum* or *Eucarya spicata*) produces a very similar oil, but with a dry-bitter top note. The so-called West Indian sandalwood or amyris (*Amyris balsamifera*) is a poor substitute and bears no botanical relation to the East Indian sandalwood.

HERBAL/FOLK TRADITION One of the oldest known perfume materials, with at least 4000 years of uninterrupted use. It is used as a traditional incense, as a cosmetic, perfume and embalming material all over the East. It is also a popular building material, especially for temples.

In Chinese medicine it is used to treat stomach ache, vomiting, gonorrhoea, choleraic difficulties and skin complaints. In the Ayurvedic tradition it is used mainly for urinary and respiratory infections, for acute and chronic diarrhoea.

In India it is often combined with rose in the famous scent *aytar*.

ACTIONS Antidepressant, antiphlogistic, antiseptic (urinary and pulmonary), antispasmodic, aphrodisiac, astringent, bactericidal, carminative, cicatrisant, diuretic, expectorant, fungicidal, insecticidal, sedative, tonic.

EXTRACTION Essential oil by water or steam distillation from the roots and heartwood, powdered and dried.

CHARACTERISTICS A pale yellow, greenish or brownish viscous liquid with a deep, soft, sweet-woody balsamic scent of excellent tenacity. It blends well with rose, violet, tuberose, clove, lavender, black pepper, bergamot, rosewood, geranium, labdanum, oakmoss, benzoin, vetiver, patchouli, mimosa, cassie, costus, myrrh and jasmine.

PRINCIPAL CONSTITUENTS About 90 per cent santalols, 6 per cent sesquiterpene hydrocarbons: santene, teresantol, borneol, santalone, tri-cyclo-ekasantalal, among others.

SAFETY DATA Non-toxic, non-irritant, non-sensitizing.

AROMATHERAPY/HOME USE
SKIN CARE: Acne, dry, cracked and chapped skin, aftershave (barber's rash), greasy skin, moisturizer.
RESPIRATORY SYSTEM: Bronchitis, catarrh, coughs (dry, persistent), laryngitis, sore throat.
DIGESTIVE SYSTEM: Diarrhoea, nausea.
GENITO-URINARY SYSTEM: Cystitis.
NERVOUS SYSTEM: Depression, insomnia, nervous tension and stress-related complaints.

OTHER USES Used to be used as a pharmaceutical disinfectant, now largely abandoned. Extensively employed as a fragrance component and fixative in soaps, detergents, cosmetics and perfumes – especially oriental, woody, aftershaves, chyprès, etc. Extensively used in the production of incense. Employed as a flavour ingredient in most major food categories, including soft and alcoholic drinks.

SANTOLINA
Santolina chamaecyparissus

FAMILY Asteraceae (Compositae)

SYNONYMS *Lavandula taemina,* cotton lavender

GENERAL DESCRIPTION An evergreen, woody shrub with whitish-grey foliage and small, bright yellow, ball-shaped flowers borne on long single stalks. The whole plant has a strong rather rank odour, a bit like chamomile.

DISTRIBUTION Native to Italy, now common throughout the Mediterranean region. Much grown as a popular border herb.

OTHER SPECIES There are several varieties such as *S. fragrantissima.* It is not related to true lavender *(Lavandula angustifolia)* despite the common name.

HERBAL/FOLK TRADITION It was used as an antidote to all sorts of poison, and to expel worms; also 'good against obstruction of the liver, the jaundice and to promote the menses'.[84] It was used to keep away moths from linen, to repel mosquitos, and as a remedy for insect bites, warts, scabs and veruccae. The Arabs are said to have used the juice for bathing the eyes.

ACTIONS Antispasmodic, antitoxic, anthelmintic, insecticidal, stimulant, vermifuge.

EXTRACTION Essential oil by steam distillation from the seeds.

CHARACTERISTICS A pale yellow liquid with a strong, acrid, herbaceous odour.

PRINCIPAL CONSTITUENTS Only one principal constituent: santolinenone.

SAFETY DATA Oral toxin. 'There is no safety data available ... likely to be dangerously toxic.'[85]

AROMATHERAPY/HOME USE None.

OTHER USES Little used in flavour or perfumery work due to toxicity.

SASSAFRAS
Sassafras albidum

FAMILY Lauraceae

SYNONYMS *S. officinale, Laurus sassafras, S. variifolium,* common sassafras, North American sassafras, sassafrax.

GENERAL DESCRIPTION A deciduous tree up to 40 metres high with many slender branches, a soft and spongy orange-brown bark and small yellowy-green flowers. The bark and wood are aromatic.

DISTRIBUTION Native to eastern parts of the USA; the oil is mainly produced from Florida to Canada and in Mexico.

OTHER SPECIES There are several other species, notably the Brazilian sassafras *(Ocotea pretiosa)* which is also used to produce an essential oil (also highly toxic). See also Botanical Classification section.

HERBAL/FOLK TRADITION It has been used for treating high blood pressure, rheumatism, arthritis, gout, menstrual and kidney problems, and for skin complaints. 'Sassafras pith – used as a demulcent, especially for inflammation of the eyes, and as a soothing drink in catarrhal affection.'[86] The wood and bark yield a bright yellow dye.

ACTIONS Antiviral, diaphoretic, diuretic, carminative, pediculicide (destroys lice), stimulant.

EXTRACTION Essential oil by steam distillation from the dried root bark chips.

CHARACTERISTICS A yellowy-brown, oily liquid with a fresh, sweet-spicy, woody-camphoraceous odour. (A safrol-free sassafras oil is produced by alcohol extraction.)

PRINCIPAL CONSTITUENTS Safrole (80–90 per cent), pinenes, phellandrenes, asarone, camphor, thujone, myristicin and menthone, among others.

SAFETY DATA Highly toxic – ingestion of even small amounts has been known to cause death. Carcinogen. Irritant. Abortifacient.

AROMATHERAPY/HOME USE None. 'Should not be used in therapy, whether internally or externally.'[87]

OTHER USES Sassafras oil and crude are banned from food use; safrol-free extract is used to a limited extent in flavouring work. Safrol is used as a starting material for the fragrance item 'heliotropin'.

SAVINE
Juniperus sabina

FAMILY Cupressaceae

SYNONYMS *Sabina cacumina,* savin (oil).

GENERAL DESCRIPTION A compact evergreen shrub about 1 metre high (though much taller in the Mediterranean countries), which tends to spread horizontally. It has a pale green bark becoming rough with age, small, dark green leaves and purplish-black berries containing three seeds.

DISTRIBUTION Native to North America, middle and southern Europe. The oil is produced mainly in Austria (the Tirol), a little in France and Yugoslavia.

OTHER SPECIES Closely related to the common juniper *(J. communis)* and other members of the family – see *juniper.*

HERBAL/FOLK TRADITION It was used at one time as an ointment or dressing for blisters, in order to promote discharge, and for syphilitic warts and other skin problems. It is rarely administered nowadays because of its possible toxic effects.

ACTIONS Powerful emmenagogue, rubefacient, stimulant.

EXTRACTION Essential oil by steam distillation from the twigs and leaves.

CHARACTERISTICS A pale yellow or olive oily liquid with a disagreeable, bitter, turpentine-like odour.

PRINCIPAL CONSTITUENTS Sabinol, sabinyl acetate, terpinene, pinene, sabinene, decyl aldehyde, citronellol, geraniol, cadinene and dihydrocuminyl alcohol.

SAFETY DATA Oral toxin. Dermal irritant. Abortifacient. 'The oil is banned from sale to the public in many countries due to its toxic effects (nerve poison and blood circulation stimulant).'[88]

AROMATHERAPY/HOME USE None. 'Should not be used in therapy, whether internally or externally.'[89]

OTHER USES Occasional perfumery use. Little employed nowadays.

SAVORY, SUMMER
Satureja hortensis

FAMILY Lamiaceae (Labiatae)

SYNONYMS *Satureia hortensis, Calamintha hortensis,* garden savory.

GENERAL DESCRIPTION An annual herb up to 45 cms high with slender, erect, slightly hairy stems, linear leaves and small, pale lilac flowers.

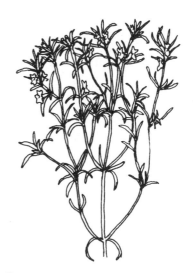

Summer Savory

DISTRIBUTION Native to Europe, naturalized in North America. Extensively cultivated, especially in Spain, France, Yugoslavia and the USA for its essential oil.

OTHER SPECIES Closely related to the thyme family, with which it shares many characteristics. There are several different types 'of savory' which include *S. thymbra,* found in Spain, which contains mainly thymol, and the winter savory (*S. montana*) – see separate entry.

HERBAL/FOLK TRADITION A popular culinary herb, with a peppery flavour. It has been used therapeutically mainly as a tea for various ailments including digestive complaints (cramp, nausea, indigestion, intestinal parasites), menstrual disorders and respiratory conditions (asthma, catarrh, sore throat). Applied externally, the fresh leaves bring instant relief from insect bites, bee and wasp stings.
'This kind is both hotter and drier than the winter kind ... it expels tough phlegm from the chest and lungs, quickens the dull spirits in the lethargy.'[90]

ACTIONS Anticatarrhal, antiputrescent, antispasmodic, aphrodisiac, astringent, bactericidal, carminative, cicatrisant, emmenagogue, expectorant, fungicidal, stimulant, vermifuge.

EXTRACTION Essential oil by steam distillation from the whole dried herb. (An oleoresin is also produced by solvent extraction.)

CHARACTERISTICS A colourless or pale yellow oil with a fresh, herbaceous, spicy odour. It blends well with lavender, lavandin, pine needle, oakmoss, rosemary and citrus oils.

PRINCIPAL CONSTITUENTS Carvacrol, pinene, cymene, camphene, limonene, phellandrene and borneol, among others.

SAFETY DATA Dermal toxin, dermal irritant, mucous membrane irritant. Avoid during pregnancy.

AROMATHERAPY/HOME USE None. 'Should not be used on the skin at all.'[91]

OTHER USES Occasionally used in perfumery work for its fresh herbaceous notes. The oil and oleoresin are used in most major food categories, especially meat products and canned food.

SAVORY, WINTER
Satureja montana

FAMILY Lamiaceae (Labiatae)

SYNONYMS *S. obovata, Calamintha montana*.

GENERAL DESCRIPTION A bushy perennial subshrub up to 40 cms high with woody stems at the base, linear leaves and pale purple flowers.

DISTRIBUTION Native to the Mediterranean region, now found all over Europe, Turkey and the USSR. The oil is mainly produced in Spain, Morocco and Yugoslavia.

OTHER SPECIES The creeping variety of the winter savory {*S. montana subspicata*) is also a well-known garden herb. See also *summer savory (S. hortensis)* and Botanical Classification section.

HERBAL/FOLK TRADITION It has been used as a culinary herb since antiquity, much in the same way as summer savory. It was used as a digestive remedy especially good for colic, and in Germany it is used particularly for diarrhoea.

When compared against many varieties of thyme, rosemary and lavender, recent research has shown 'the net superiority of the anti-microbial properties of essence of savory'.[92]

ACTIONS See *summer savory*.

EXTRACTION Essential oil by steam distillation from the whole herb. (An oleoresin is also produced by solvent extraction.)

CHARACTERISTICS A colourless or pale yellow liquid with a sharp, medicinal, herbaceous odour.

PRINCIPAL CONSTITUENTS Mainly carvacrol, cymene and thymol, with lesser amounts of pinenes, limonene, cineol, borneol and terpineol.

SAFETY DATA See *summer savory*.

AROMATHERAPY/HOME USE None. 'Should not be used on the skin at all.'[93]

OTHER USES Occasionally used in perfumery work. The oil and oleoresin are employed to some extent in flavouring, mainly meats and seasonings.

SCHINUS MOLLE
Schinus molle

FAMILY Anacardiaceae

SYNONYMS Peruvian pepper, Peruvian mastic, Californian pepper tree.

GENERAL DESCRIPTION A tropical evergreen tree up to 20 metres high with graceful, drooping branches, feathery foliage and fragrant yellow flowers. The berries or fruit have an aromatic, peppery flavour.

DISTRIBUTION Native to South America; found growing wild in Mexico, Peru, Guatemala and other tropical regions, including California. It has been introduced into North and South Africa and the Mediterranean region. The fruits are collected for essential oil production in Spain, Guatemala and Mexico.

OTHER SPECIES Closely related to the mastic tree *(Pistacia lentiscus)* – see entry on mastic.

HERBAL/FOLK TRADITION In Greece and other Mediterranean countries an intoxicating beverage is made from the fruits of the tree. The fruit is also used as a substitute for black pepper in the growing areas. During World War II, the oil of black pepper was unavailable and was consequently replaced by schinus molle.

ACTIONS Antiseptic, antiviral, bactericidal, carminative, stimulant, stomachic.

EXTRACTION Essential oil by steam distillation from the fruit or berries. (An oil from the leaves is also produced in small quantities.)

CHARACTERISTICS A pale green or olive, oily liquid with a warm, woody-peppery scent with a smoky undertone. It blends well with oakmoss, clove, nutmeg, cinnamon, black pepper and eucalyptus.

PRINCIPAL CONSTITUENTS Mainly phellandrene, also caryophyllene, pinene and carvacrol.

SAFETY DATA Non-toxic, non-irritant, non-sensitizing.

AROMATHERAPY/HOME USE See *black pepper.*

OTHER USES Used as a substitute for black pepper in perfumery and flavouring work.

SNAKEROOT
Asarum canadense

FAMILY Aristolochiaceae

SYNONYMS Wild ginger, Indian ginger.

GENERAL DESCRIPTION An inconspicuous but fragrant little plant not more than 35 cms high with a hairy stem, two glossy, kidney-shaped leaves and a creeping rootstock. The solitary bell-shaped flower is brownish purple, and creamy white inside.

DISTRIBUTION Native to North America, especially North Carolina, Kansas and Canada. The oil is produced in the USA mainly from wild-growing plants.

OTHER SPECIES It should not be confused with 'serpentaria oil' from the Virginian snakeroot *(Aristolochia serpentaria)* which belongs to the same botanical family but contains asarone and is considered toxic.

HERBAL/FOLK TRADITION This plant has been employed for centuries in folk medicine but is now little prescribed. It used to be used for chronic chest complaints, dropsy, rheumatism and painful bowel and stomach spasms. It was also considered a 'valuable stimulant in cases of amenorrhoea and colds' and for 'promoting a copious perspiration'.[94]
The name (of the Virginian variety at least) derives from its use in aiding the body to combat nettle rash, poison ivy and some snake bites.

ACTIONS Anti-inflammatory, antispasmodic, carminative, diuretic, diaphoretic, emmenagogue, expectorant, febrifuge, stimulant, stomachic.

EXTRACTION Essential oil by steam

distillation from the dried rhizomes and crushed roots.

CHARACTERISTICS A brownish-yellow or amber liquid with a warm, woody-spicy, rich, gingerlike odour. It blends well with bergamot, costus, oakmoss, patchouli, pine needle, clary sage, mimosa, cassie and other florals.

PRINCIPAL CONSTITUENTS Pinene, linalol, borneol, terpineol, geraniol, eugenol and methyl eugenol, among others.

SAFETY DATA Non-toxic, non-irritant, non-sensitizing. Avoid during pregnancy.

AROMATHERAPY/HOME USE May possibly be used for its antispasmodic qualities, for example for period pains or indigestion.

OTHER USES Occasionally used in perfumery work. Mainly used as a flavouring agent with other spicy materials, especially in confectionery.

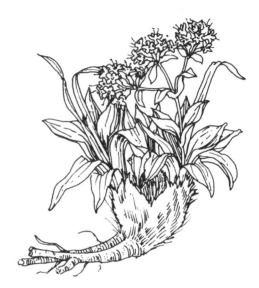

Spikenard

SPIKENARD
Nardostachys jatamansi

FAMILY Valerianaceae

SYNONYMS Nard, 'false' Indian valerian root (oil).

GENERAL DESCRIPTION A tender aromatic herb with a pungent rhizome root.

DISTRIBUTION Native to the mountainous regions of northern India; also China and Japan (see Other Species). The oil is mainly distilled in Europe or the USA.

OTHER SPECIES Closely related to the common valerian *(Valeriana officinalis)* and the Indian valerian *(V. wallichii)* with which it shares many qualities. There are also several other similar species, notably the Chinese spikenard *(N. chinensis)* which is also used to

produce an essential oil. Not to be confused with aspic or spike lavender *(Lavandula latifolia)*, nor with essential oils from the musk root *(Ferula sumbul)* which is collected from the same area. The roots of several other plants are also commonly sold as 'Indian valerian root'.

HERBAL/FOLK TRADITION Spikenard is one of the early aromatics used by the ancient Egyptians and is mentioned in the Song of Solomon in the Bible. It is also the herb which Mary used to anoint Jesus before the Last Supper; 'Then took Mary a pound of ointment of spikenard, very costly, and anointed the feet of Jesus, and wiped his feet with her hair; and the house was filled with the odour of the ointment.'[95]

The oil was also used by the Roman perfumers, or *unguentarii*, in the preparation of *nardinum*, one of their most celebrated scented oils, and by the Mughal empress Nur Jehan in her rejuvenating cosmetic preparations.

It was also a herb known to Dioscorides as 'warming and drying', good for nausea, flatulent indigestion, menstrual problems, inflammations and conjunctivitis.

ACTIONS Anti-inflammatory, antipyretic, bactericidal, deodorant, fungicidal, laxative, sedative, tonic.

EXTRACTION Essential oil by steam distillation from the dried and crushed rhizome and roots.

CHARACTERISTICS A pale yellow or amber-coloured liquid with a heavy, sweet-woody, spicy-animal odour, somewhat similar to valerian oil. It blends well with labdanum, lavender, oakmoss, patchouli, pine needle, vetiver and spice oils.

PRINCIPAL CONSTITUENTS Bornyl acetate, isobornyl valerianate, borneol, patchouli alcohol, terpinyl valerianate, terpineol, eugenol and pinenes, among others.

SAFETY DATA Probably similar to valerian, i.e. non-toxic, non-irritant, non-sensitizing.

AROMATHERAPY/HOME USE
SKIN CARE: Allergies, inflammation, mature skin (rejuvenating), rashes, etc.
NERVOUS SYSTEM: Insomnia, nervous indigestion, migraine, stress and tension.

OTHER USES Little used these days, usually as a substitute for valerian oil.

SPRUCE, HEMLOCK
Tsuga canadensis

FAMILY Pinaceae

SYNONYMS *Pinus canadensis, Abies canadensis,* spruce, eastern hemlock, common hemlock, hemlock (oil), spruce (oil), fir needle (oil).

GENERAL DESCRIPTION A large evergreen tree up to 50 metres tall, with slender horizontal branches, finely toothed leaves and smallish brown cones, which yields a natural exudation from its bark.

DISTRIBUTION Native to the west coast of the USA. The oil is produced in Vermont, New York, New Hampshire, Virginia and Wisconsin.

OTHER SPECIES Numerous cultivars of this species exist; often the oil is produced from a mixture of different types. Similar oils, also called simply 'spruce oil' are produced from the black spruce (*Picea nigra* or *mariana)*, the Norway spruce *(P. abies)* and the white or Canadian spruce *(P. glauca).* The essential oil from the western hemlock *(Tsuga heterophylla),* contains quite different constituents. It is also closely related to the Douglas fir (*Pseudotsuga taxifolia),* which is also used to produce an essential oil and a balsam.

HERBAL/FOLK TRADITION The bark of the hemlock spruce (which contains tannins and resin as well as volatile oil) is current in the British Herbal Pharmacopoeia indicated for diarrhoea, cystitis, mucous colitis, leucorrhoea, uterine prolapse, pharyngitis, stomatitis, and gingivitis. An extract of the bark is also used in the tanning industry.

ACTIONS Antimicrobial, antiseptic, antitussive, astringent, diaphoretic, diuretic, expectorant, nervine, rubefacient, tonic.

EXTRACTION Essential oil by steam distillation from the needles and twigs.

CHARACTERISTICS A colourless or pale yellow liquid with a pleasing, fresh-balsamic, sweet-fruity odour. It blends well with pine, oakmoss, cedarwood, galbanum, benzoin, lavender, lavandin and rosemary.

PRINCIPAL CONSTITUENTS Mainly pinenes, limonene, bornyl acetate, tricyclene, phellandrene, myrcene, thujone, dipentene and cadinene, among others. Constituents vary according to source and exact botanical species (sometimes mixed).

SAFETY DATA Non-toxic, non-irritant, non-sensitizing.

AROMATHERAPY/HOME USE
CIRCULATION, MUSCLES AND JOINTS: Muscular aches and pains, poor circulation, rheumatism.
RESPIRATORY SYSTEM: Asthma, bronchitis, coughs, respiratory weakness.

IMMUNE SYSTEM: Colds, 'flu, infections.
NERVOUS SYSTEM: Anxiety, stress-related
conditions – 'opening and elevating though
grounding ... excellent for yoga and
meditation.'[96]

OTHER USES Used in veterinary liniments.
Extensively used for room spray perfumes,
household detergents, soaps, bath preparations
and toiletries, especially in the USA.

STYRAX, LEVANT
Liquidambar orientalis

FAMILY Hamamelidaceae

SYNONYMS *Balsam styracis*, oriental
sweetgum, Turkish sweetgum, asiatic styrax,
styrax, storax, liquid storax.

GENERAL DESCRIPTION A deciduous tree
up to 15 metres high with a purplish-grey bark,
leaves arranged into five three-lobed sections,
and white flowers. The styrax is a pathological
secretion produced by pounding the bark,
which induces the sapwood to produce a liquid
from beneath the bark. It hardens to form a
semi-solid greenish-brown mass with a sweet
balsamic odour.

DISTRIBUTION Native to Asia Minor. It
forms forests around Bodrum, Milas, Mugla
and Marmaris in Turkey.

OTHER SPECIES Very similar to the American
styrax *(L. styraciflua)* or red gum, which
produces a natural exudation slightly darker
and harder than the Levant type. There are also
many other types of styrax; *Styrax officinale*
produced the styrax of ancient civilizations.
NB: *Styrax benzoin* is the botanical name for
benzoin, with which it shares similar qualities.

HERBAL/FOLK TRADITION In China it is
used for coughs, colds, epilepsy and skin
problems, including cuts, wounds and scabies.
In the West it has been recommended as a
remedy for catarrh, diphtheria, gonorrhoea,
leucorrhoea, ringworm, etc. A syrup made
from the bark of the American styrax is used
for diarrhoea and dysentery in the western
USA.

ACTIONS Anti-inflammatory, antimicrobial,
antiseptic, antitussive, bactericidal, balsamic,
expectorant, nervine, stimulant.

EXTRACTION Essential oil by steam
distillation from the crude. (A resinoid and
absolute are also produced by solvent
extraction).

CHARACTERISTICS A water-white or pale
yellow liquid with a sweet-balsamic, rich,
tenacious odour. It blends well with ylang ylang,
jasmine, mimosa, rose, lavender, carnation,
violet, cassie and spice oils.

PRINCIPAL CONSTITUENTS Mainly styrene
with vanillin, phenylpropyl alcohol, cinnamic
alcohol, benzyl alcohol and ethyl alcohol,
among others.

SAFETY DATA Non-toxic, non-irritant,
possible sensitization in some individuals.
Frequently adulterated.

AROMATHERAPY/HOME USE
SKIN CARE: Cuts, ringworm, scabies, wounds.
RESPIRATORY SYSTEM: Bronchitis, catarrh,
coughs.
NERVOUS SYSTEM: Anxiety, stress-related
conditions.

OTHER USES Used in compound benzoin
tincture, mainly for respiratory conditions. The
oil and resinoid are used as fixatives and
fragrance components mainly in soaps, floral
and oriental perfumes. The resinoid and
absolute are used in most major food categories,
including alcoholic and soft drinks.

❦ T ❦

TAGETES
Tagetes minuta

FAMILY Asteraceae (Compositae)

SYNONYMS *T. glandulifera,* tagette, taget, marigold, Mexican marigold, wrongly called 'calendula' (oil).

GENERAL DESCRIPTION A strongly scented annual herb about 30 cms high with bright orange, daisylike flowers and soft green oval leaves.

DISTRIBUTION Native to South America and Mexico. Now grows wild in Africa, Europe, Asia and North America. The oil is mainly produced in South Africa, France, Argentina and Egypt, the absolute in Nigeria and France.

OTHER SPECIES There are several other types of tagetes which share similar characteristics and are used to produce essential oils, notably the French marigold *(T. patula)* and the African or Aztec marigold *(T. erecta)* – see also Botanical Classification section.
   NB: Not to be confused with the 'true' marigold *(Calendula officinalis)* which has very different properties and constituents, and is used extensively in herbal medicine (and occasionally to make an absolute). See entry on marigold.

HERBAL/FOLK TRADITION In India the locally grown flowering tops of the French marigold are distilled into a receiver which contains a solvent, often sandalwood oil, to produce 'attar genda' – a popular Indian perfume material. In China the flowers of the African marigold are used for whooping cough, colds, colic, mumps, sore eyes and mastitis – usually as a decoction.

ACTIONS Anthelmintic, antispasmodic, bactericidal, carminative, diaphoretic, emmenagogue, fungicidal, stomachic.

EXTRACTION 1. An essential oil by steam distillation from the fresh flowering herb. 2. An absolute (and concrete) by solvent extraction from the fresh flowering herb.

CHARACTERISTICS 1. A dark orange or yellow mobile liquid which slowly solidifies on exposure to air and light, with a bitter-green, herby odour. 2. An orange, olive or brown semi-liquid mass with an intense, sweet, green-fruity odour. It blends well with clary sage, lavender, jasmine, bergamot and other citrus oils in very small percentages.

PRINCIPAL CONSTITUENTS Mainly tagetones, with ocimene, myrcene, linalol, limonene, pinenes, carvone, citral, camphene, valeric acid and salicylaldehyde, among others.

SAFETY DATA 'It is quite possible that "tagetone" (the main constituent) is harmful to the human organism.'[97] Some reported cases of dermatitis with the tagetes species. Use with care, in moderation.

AROMATHERAPY/HOME USE
SKIN CARE: Bunions, calluses, corns, fungal infections.

OTHER USES Used in some pharmaceutical products. The absolute and oil are employed to a limited extent in herbaceous and floral perfumes. Used for flavouring tobacco and in most major food categories, including alcoholic and soft drinks.

TANSY
Tanacetum vulgare

FAMILY Asteraceae (Compositae)

SYNONYMS *Chrysanthemum vulgare,*

C. tanacetum, buttons, bitter buttons, bachelor's buttons, scented fern, cheese.

GENERAL DESCRIPTION A hardy perennial wayside herb, up to 1 metre high with a smooth stem, dark ferny leaves and small, round, brilliant yellow flowers borne in clusters. The whole plant is strongly scented.

DISTRIBUTION Native to central Europe; naturalized in North America and now found in most temperate regions of the world. The essential oil is mainly produced in France, Germany, Hungary, Poland and the USA.

OTHER SPECIES Closely related to the medicinal herb feverfew *(Tanacetum parthenium)*, the marigolds and daisy family.

HERBAL/FOLK TRADITION Traditionally used to flavour eggs and omelettes. It has a long history of medicinal use, especially among gypsies, and is regarded as something of a 'cure all'. It was used to expel worms, to treat colds and fever, prevent possible miscarriage and ease dyspepsia and cramping pains. Externally, the distilled water was used to keep the complexion pale, and the bruised leaves employed as a remedy for scabies, bruises, sprains and rheumatism. It was also used generally for nervous disorders and to keep flies and vermin away.

The flowers are still current in the British Herbal Pharmacopoeia as a specific (used externally) for worms in children.

ACTIONS Anthelmintic, anti-inflammatory, antispasmodic, carminative, diaphoretic, digestive, emmenagogue, febrifuge, nervine, stimulant, tonic, vermifuge.

EXTRACTION Essential oil by steam distillation from the whole herb (aerial parts).

CHARACTERISTICS A yellow, olive or orange liquid (darkening with age) with a warm, sharp-spicy herbaceous odour.

PRINCIPAL CONSTITUENTS Thujone (66–81 per cent), camphor, borneol, among others.

SAFETY DATA Oral toxin – poisonous due to high thujone content. Abortifacient.

AROMATHERAPY/HOME USE None. 'Should not be used in aromatherapy whether internally or externally.'[98]

OTHER USES Occasionally used in herbaceous-type perfumes. The oil used to be used in alcoholic drinks – it is no longer used for flavouring.

TARRAGON
Artemisia dracunculus

FAMILY Asteraceae (Compositae)

SYNONYMS Estragon (oil), little dragon, Russian tarragon.

GENERAL DESCRIPTION A perennial herb with smooth narrow leaves; an erect stem up to 1.2 metres tall, and small yellowy-green, inconspicuous flowers.

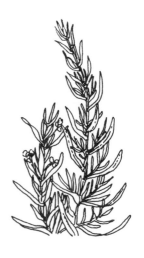

Tarragon

DISTRIBUTION Native to Europe, southern Russia and western Asia. Now cultivated worldwide, especially in Europe and the USA. The oil is mainly produced in France, Holland, Hungary and the USA.

OTHER SPECIES The so-called French tarragon or 'sativa', which is cultivated as a garden herb, is a smaller plant with a sharper flavour than the Russian type and is a sterile derivative of the wild species.

HERBAL/FOLK TRADITION The leaf is commonly used as domestic herb, especially with chicken or fish, and to make tarragon vinegar. The name is thought to derive from an ancient use as an antidote to the bites of venomous creatures and 'madde dogges'. It was favoured by the maharajahs of India who took it as a tisane, and in Persia it was used to induce appetite.

'The leaves, which are chiefly used, are heating and drying, and good for those that have the flux, or any prenatural discharge.'[99] The leaf was also formerly used for digestive and menstrual irregularities, while the root was employed as a remedy for toothache.

ACTIONS Anthelmintic, antiseptic, antispasmodic, aperitif, carminative, digestive, diuretic, emmenagogue, hypnotic, stimulant, stomachic, vermifuge.

EXTRACTION Essential oil by steam distillation from the leaves.

CHARACTERISTICS A colourless or pale yellow mobile liquid (turning yellow with age), with a sweet-anisic, spicy-green scent. It blends well with labdanum, galbanum, lavender, oakmoss, vanilla, pine and basil.

PRINCIPAL CONSTITUENTS Estragole (up to 70 per cent), capillene, ocimene, nerol, phellandrene, thujone and cineol, among others.

SAFETY DATA Moderately toxic due to 'estragole' (methyl chavicol) : use in moderation only. Possibly carcinogenic. Otherwise non-irritant, non-sensitizing. Avoid during pregnancy.

AROMATHERAPY/HOME USE
DIGESTIVE SYSTEM: Anorexia, dyspepsia, flatulence, hiccoughs, intestinal spasm, nervous indigestion, sluggish digestion.
GENITO-URINARY SYSTEM: Amenorrhoea, dysmenorrhoea, PMT.

OTHER USES Used as a fragrance component in soaps, detergents, cosmetics and perfumes. Employed as a flavour ingredient in most major food categories, especially condiments and relishes, as well as alcoholic and soft drinks.

TEA TREE
Melaleuca alternifolia

FAMILY Myrtaceae

SYNONYMS Narrow-leaved paperbark tea tree, ti-tree, ti-trol, melasol.

GENERAL DESCRIPTION A small tree or shrub (smallest of the tea tree family), with needlelike leaves similar to cypress, with heads of sessile yellow or purplish flowers.

DISTRIBUTION Native to Australia. Other varieties have been cultivated elsewhere, but *M. alternifolia* is not produced outside Australia, mainly in New South Wales.

OTHER SPECIES Tea tree is a general name for members of the *Melaleuca* family which exists in many physiological forms including cajeput *(M. cajeputi)* and niaouli *(M. viridiflora)*, and many others such as *M. bracteata* and *M. linariifolia* – see Botanical Classification section.

HERBAL/FOLK TRADITION The name derives from its local usage as a type of herbal tea, prepared from the leaves. Our present knowledge of the properties and uses of tea tree is based on a very long history of use by the aboriginal people of Australia. It has been

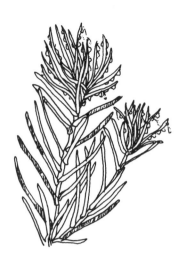

Tea Tree

extensively researched recently by scientific methods with the following results:

'1. This oil is unusual in that it is active against all three varieties of infectious organisms: bacteria, fungi and viruses. 2. It is a very powerful immuno-stimulant, so when the body is threatened by any of these organisms ti-tree increases its ability to respond.'[100]

ACTIONS Anti-infectious, anti-inflammatory, antiseptic, antiviral, bactericidal, balsamic, cicatrisant, diaphoretic, expectorant, fungicidal, immuno-stimulant, parasiticide, vulnerary.

EXTRACTION Essential oil by steam or water distillation from the leaves and twigs.

CHARACTERISTICS A pale yellowy-green or water-white mobile liquid with a warm, fresh, spicy-camphoraceous odour. It blends well with lavandin, lavender, clary sage, rosemary, oakmoss, pine, cananga, geranium, marjoram, and spice oils, especially clove and nutmeg.

PRINCIPAL CONSTITUENTS Terpinene-4-ol (up to 30 per cent), cineol, pinene, terpinenes, cymene, sesquiterpenes, sesquiterpene alcohols, among others.

SAFETY DATA Non-toxic, non-irritant, possible sensitization in some individuals.

AROMATHERAPY/HOME USE
SKIN CARE: Abscess, acne, athlete's foot, blisters, burns, cold sores, dandruff, herpes, insect bites, oily skin, rashes (nappy rash), spots, veruccae, warts, wounds (infected).
RESPIRATORY SYSTEM: Asthma, bronchitis, catarrh, coughs, sinusitis, tuberculosis, whooping cough.
GENITO-URINARY SYSTEM: Thrush, vaginitis, cystitis, pruritis.
IMMUNE SYSTEM: Colds, fever, 'flu, infectious illnesses such as chickenpox.

OTHER USES Employed in soaps, toothpastes, deodorants, disinfectants, gargles, germicides and, increasingly, in aftershaves and spicy colognes.

THUJA
Thuja occidentalis

FAMILY Cupressaceae

SYNONYMS Swamp cedar, white cedar, northern white cedar, eastern white cedar, tree of life, American arborvitae, cedarleaf (oil).

GENERAL DESCRIPTION A graceful pyramid-shaped coniferous tree up to 20 metres high with scale-like leaves and broadly-winged seeds, sometimes planted as hedging. The tree must be at least fifteen years old before it is ready to be used for essential oil production.

DISTRIBUTION Native to north eastern North America; cultivated in France. The oil is produced mainly in Canada and the USA, similar oils are also produced in the East – see below.

OTHER SPECIES There are many forms and cultivated varieties of this tree: the western red cedar or Washington cedar *(T. plicata)*; the Chinese or Japanese cedar *(T. orientalis* or *Biota orientalis)*; the North African variety

(T. articulata) which yields a resin known as 'sanderac'.

The hiba tree *(Thujopsis dolobrata)* is used to produce hiba wood oil and hiba leaf oil in Japan. Hiba wood oil, according to available data, is non-toxic, non-irritant and non-sensitizing (unlike the other thuja oils), and has excellent resistance to fungi and bacteria due to the ketonic substances found in the oil. It is used extensively in Japan as an industrial perfume.

HERBAL/FOLK TRADITION Used as an incense by ancient civilizations for ritual purposes. A decoction of leaves has been used for coughs, fever, intestinal parasites, cystitis and venereal diseases. The ointment has been used for rheumatism, gout, warts, veruccae, psoriasis and other ailments.

The twigs are current in the British Herbal Pharmacopoeia, used specifically for bronchitis with cardiac weakness, and warts.

ACTIONS Antirheumatic, astringent, diuretic, emmenagogue, expectorant, insect repellent, rubefacient, stimulant (nerve, uterus and heart muscles), tonic, vermifuge.

EXTRACTION Essential oil by steam distillation from the fresh leaves, twigs and bark.

CHARACTERISTICS A colourless to pale yellowy-green liquid with a sharp, fresh, camphoraceous odour.

PRINCIPAL CONSTITUENTS Thujone (approx. 60 per cent), fenchone, camphor, sabinene and pinene, among others.

SAFETY DATA Oral toxin – poisonous due to high thujone content. Abortifacient.

AROMATHERAPY/HOME USE None. 'Should not be used in aromatherapy either internally or externally.'[101]

OTHER USES Used in pharmaceutical products such as disinfectants and sprays; also as a counter-irritant in analgesic ointments and liniments. A fragrance component in some toiletries and perfumes. Employed as a flavour ingredient in most major food categories (provided that the finished food is recognized thujone-free).

THYME, COMMON
Thymus vulgaris

FAMILY Lamiaceae (Labiatae)

SYNONYMS *T. aestivus, T. ilerdensis, T. webbianus, T. valentianus,* French thyme, garden thyme, red thyme (oil), white thyme (oil).

GENERAL DESCRIPTION A perennial evergreen subshrub up to 45 cms high with a woody root and much-branched upright stem. It has small, grey-green, oval, aromatic leaves and pale purple or white flowers.

DISTRIBUTION Native to Spain and the Mediterranean region; now found throughout Asia Minor, Algeria, Turkey, Tunisia, Israel, the USA, Russia, China and central Europe. The oil is mainly produced in Spain but also in France, Israel, Greece, Morocco, Algeria, Germany and the USA.

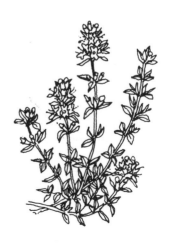

Thyme

OTHER SPECIES There are numerous varieties of thyme – the common thyme is believed to have derived from the wild thyme or mother-of-thyme *(T. serpyllum)*, which is also used to produce an essential oil called serpolet, similar in effect to the common thyme oil.

Another species used for the production of the so-called red thyme oil is particularly the Spanish sauce thyme *(T. zygis),* a highly penetrating oil good for cellulitis, sports injuries, etc. (although, like the common thyme, it is a skin irritant). Other species used for essential oil production include lemon thyme *(T. citriodorus)*, a fresh scented oil good for asthma and other respiratory conditions, safe for children. See also Botanical Classification section.

HERBAL/FOLK TRADITION One of the earliest medicinal plants employed throughout the Mediterranean region, well known to both Hippocrates and Dioscorides. It was used by the ancient Egyptians in the embalming process, and by the ancient Greeks to fumigate against infectious illness; the name derives from the Greek *thymos* meaning 'to perfume'. It is also a long-established culinary herb, especially used for the preservation of meat.

It has a wide range of uses, though in Western herbal medicine its main areas of application are respiratory problems, digestive complaints and the prevention and treatment of infection. In the British Herbal Pharmacopoeia it is indicated for dyspepsia, chronic gastritis, bronchitis, pertussis, asthma, children's diarrhoea, laryngitis, tonsillitis and enuresis in children.

ACTIONS Anthelmintic, antimicrobial, anti-oxidant, antiputrescent, antirheumatic, antiseptic (intestinal, pulmonary, genito-urinary), antispasmodic, antitussive, antitoxic, aperitif, astringent, aphrodisiac, bactericidal, balsamic, carminative, cicatrisant, diuretic, emmenagogue, expectorant, fungicidal, hypertensive, nervine, revulsive, rubefacient, parasiticide, stimulant (immune system, circulation), sudorific, tonic, vermifuge.

EXTRACTION Essential oil by water or steam distillation from the fresh or partially dried leaves and flowering tops. 1. 'Red thyme oil' is the crude distillate. 2. 'White thyme oil' is produced by further redistillation or rectification. (An absolute is also produced in France by solvent extraction for perfumery use.)

CHARACTERISTICS 1. A red, brown or orange liquid with a warm, spicy-herbaceous, powerful odour. 2. A clear, pale yellow liquid with a sweet, green-fresh, milder scent. It blends well with bergamot, lemon, rosemary, melissa, lavender, lavandin, marjoram, Peru balsam, pine, etc.

PRINCIPAL CONSTITUENTS Thymol and carvacrol (up to 60 per cent), cymene, terpinene, camphene, borneol, linalol; depending on the source it can also contain geraniol, citral and thuyanol, etc.

There are many chemotypes of thyme oil: notably the 'thymol' and 'carvacrol' types (warming and active); the 'thuyanol' type (penetrating and antiviral); and the milder 'linalol' or 'citral' types (sweet-scented, non-irritant).

SAFETY DATA Red thyme oil, serpolet (from wild thyme), 'thymol' and 'carvacrol' type oils all contain quite large amounts of toxic phenols (carvacrol and thymol). They can irritate mucous membranes, cause dermal irritation and may cause sensitization in some individuals. Use in moderation, in low dilution only. They are best avoided during pregnancy.

White thyme is not a 'complete' oil and is often adulterated. Lemon thyme and 'linalol' types are in general less toxic, non-irritant, with less possibility of sensitization – safe for use on the skin and with children.

AROMATHERAPY/HOME USE
SKIN CARE: Abscess, acne, bruises, burns, cuts, dermatitis, eczema, insect bites, lice, gum infections, oily skin, scabies.
CIRCULATION, MUSCLES AND JOINTS: Arthritis, cellulitis, gout, muscular aches and pains, obesity, oedema, poor circulation, rheumatism, sprains, sports injuries.
RESPIRATORY SYSTEM: Asthma, bronchitis, catarrh, coughs, laryngitis, sinusitis, sore throat, tonsillitis.

DIGESTIVE SYSTEM: Diarrhoea, dyspepsia, flatulence.

GENITO-URINARY SYSTEM: Cystitis, urethritis.

IMMUNE SYSTEM: Chills, colds, 'flu, infectious diseases.

NERVOUS SYSTEM: Headaches, insomnia, nervous debility and stress-related complaints – 'helps to revive and strengthen both body and mind'.[44]

OTHER USES The oil is used in mouthwashes, gargles, toothpastes and cough lozenges. 'Thymol' is isolated for pharmaceutical use in surgical dressings, disinfectants etc. Used as a fragrance component in soaps, toiletries, aftershaves, perfumes, colognes, etc. Extensively employed by the food and drink industry, especially in meat products.

TONKA
Dipteryx odorata

FAMILY Leguminosae

SYNONYMS *Coumarouna odorata,* tonquin bean, Dutch tonka bean.

GENERAL DESCRIPTION A very large tropical tree with big elliptical leaves and violet flowers, bearing fruit which contain a single black seed or 'tonka bean', about the size of a butter bean. The beans, known as 'rumara' by the natives, are collected and dried, then soaked in alcohol or rum for twelve to fifteen hours to make them swell. When they are removed from the bath they become dried and shrunken, covered in a whitish powder of crystallized coumarin.

The 'curing' of the beans is partly a conventional 'sales promotion' technique rather than an indication of quality, since the frosted appearance has come to be expected of the product.

DISTRIBUTION Native to South America, especially Venezuela, Guyana and Brazil; cultivated in Nigeria and elsewhere in West Africa. Most beans come from South America

after 'curing', to be processed in Europe and the USA.

OTHER SPECIES There are many species of *Dipteryx* which produce beans suitable for extraction.

HERBAL/FOLK TRADITION In Holland the fatty substance from the beans is sold as 'tarquin butter', which used to be used as an insecticide against moth in linen cupboards. 'The fluid extract has been used with advantage in whooping cough, but it paralyses the heart if used in large doses.'[103]

ACTIONS Insecticidal, narcotic, tonic (cardiac).

EXTRACTION A concrete and absolute by solvent extraction from the 'cured' beans.

CHARACTERISTICS The absolute is a semi-solid yellow or amber mass with a very rich, warm and sweet herbaceous-nutty odour. It blends well with lavender, lavandin, clary sage, styrax, bergamot, oakmoss, helichrysum and citronella.

PRINCIPAL CONSTITUENTS Mainly coumarin (20–40 per cent) in the absolute.

SAFETY DATA Oral and dermal toxin, due to high coumarin content.

AROMATHERAPY/HOME USE None.

OTHER USES Used to a limited extent as a pharmaceutical masking agent. The absolute is employed as a fixative and fragrance component in oriental, new-mown hay and chyprès type perfumes. It is no longer used as a flavouring (due to the coumarin ban in many countries), though it is still used to flavour tobacco.

TUBEROSE
Polianthes tuberosa

FAMILY Agavaceae

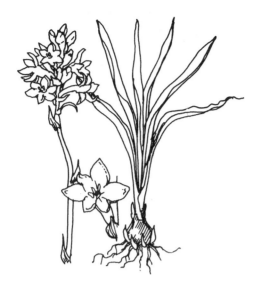

Tuberose

SYNONYMS Tuberosa, tubereuse

GENERAL DESCRIPTION A tender, tall, slim perennial up to 50 cms high, with long slender leaves, a tuberous root and large, very fragrant, white lilylike flowers.

DISTRIBUTION Native of Central America, where it is found growing wild. Cultivated for its oil in southern France, Morocco, China, Taiwan and Egypt.

OTHER SPECIES Related to the narcissus and jonquil. The Chinese species of tuberose is somewhat different from the French and Moroccan type, although both are single-flowered varieties.

HERBAL/FOLK TRADITION The double-flowered variety is grown for ornamental purposes and for use by the cut flower trade. 'Pure absolute extraction of tuberose is perhaps the most expensive natural flower oil at the disposal of the modern perfumer.'[104]

ACTIONS Narcotic.

EXTRACTION A concrete and absolute by solvent extraction from the fresh flowers, picked before the petals open. (An essential oil is also obtained by distillation of the concrete.)

CHARACTERISTICS The absolute is a dark orange or brown soft paste, with a heavy, sweet-floral, sometimes slightly spicy, tenacious fragrance. It blends well with gardenia, violet, opopanax, rose, jasmine, carnation, orris, Peru balsam, neroli and ylang ylang.

PRINCIPAL CONSTITUENTS Methyl benzoate, methyl anthranilate, benzyl alcohol, butyric acid, eugenol, nerol, farnesol, geraniol, among others.

SAFETY DATA No safety data available – often adulterated.

AROMATHERAPY/HOME USE Perfume.

OTHER USES Used in high class perfumes, especially of an oriental, floral or fantasy type. Occasionally used for flavouring confectionery and some beverages.

TURMERIC
Curcuma longa

FAMILY Zingiberaceae

SYNONYMS *C. domestica, Amomoum curcuma*, curcuma, Indian saffron, Indian yellow root, curmuma (oil).

GENERAL DESCRIPTION A perennial tropical herb up to 1 metre high, with a thick rhizome root, deep orange inside, lanceolate root leaves tapering at each end, and dull yellow flowers.

DISTRIBUTION Native to southern Asia; extensively cultivated in India, China, Indonesia, Jamaica and Haiti. The oil is mainly distilled in India, China and Japan. Some roots are imported to Europe and the USA for distillation.

OTHER SPECIES Closely related to the common ginger *(Zingiber officinale)*. Not to be confused with the Indian turmeric or American yellow root *(Hydrastis canadensis)*.

HERBAL/FOLK TRADITION A common household spice, especially for curry powder. It is high in minerals and vitamins, especially vitamin C. It is also used extensively as a local home medicine.

In Chinese herbalism it is used for bruises, sores, ringworm, toothache, chest pains, colic and menstrual problems, usually in combination with remedies. It was once used as a cure for jaundice.

ACTIONS Analgesic, anti-arthritic, anti-inflammatory, anti-oxidant, bactericidal, cholagogue, digestive, diuretic, hypotensive, insecticidal, laxative, rubefacient, stimulant.

EXTRACTION Essential oil by steam distillation from the 'cured' rhizome – boiled, cleaned and sun-dried. (An oleoresin, absolute and concrete are also produced by solvent extraction.)

CHARACTERISTICS A yellowy-orange liquid with a faint blue fluorescence and a fresh spicy-woody odour. It blends well with cananga, labdanum, elecampane, ginger, orris, cassie, clary sage and mimosa.

PRINCIPAL CONSTITUENTS Mainly tumerone (60 per cent), with ar-tumerone, atlantones, zingiberene, cineol, borneol, sabinene and phellandrene, among others.

SAFETY DATA The ketone 'tumerone' is moderately toxic and irritant in high concentration. Possible sensitization problems. 'The essential oil of turmeric must be used in moderation and with care for a fairly limited period.'[105]

AROMATHERAPY/HOME USE
CIRCULATION, MUSCLES AND JOINTS: Arthritis, muscular aches and pains, rheumatism.
DIGESTIVE SYSTEM: Anorexia, sluggish digestion, liver congestion.

OTHER USES Employed in perfumery work, for oriental and fantasy-type fragrances. The oleoresin is used as a flavour ingredient in some foods, mainly curries, meat products and condiments.

TURPENTINE
Pinus palustris and other *Pinus* species

FAMILY Pinaceae

SYNONYMS Terebinth, therebentine, gum thus, gum turpentine, turpentine balsam, spirit of turpentine (oil).

GENERAL DESCRIPTION 'Gum turpentine' is a term loosely applied to the natural oleoresin formed as a physiological product in the trunks of various *Pinus, Picea* and *Abies* species. Turpentine refers both to the crude oleoresin (a mixture of oil and resin) and to the distilled and rectified essential oils.

DISTRIBUTION All over the world. The largest producer is the USA, also Mexico, France, Portugal, Spain, Greece, Scandinavia, New Zealand, Tasmania, India, China, the USSR, etc.

OTHER SPECIES Apart from the longleaf pine *(Pinus palustris),* which is the leading source of American gum turpentine, other sources in the USA include the slash pine *(P. elliottii)* and the Mexican white pine *(P. ayacahuite).* In India the chir pine *(P. roxburghii);* in Tasmania the lodgepole pine *(P. contorta var. latifolia);* in China the masson or Southern red pine *(P. massoniana);* in Europe and Scandinavia the Scotch pine *(P. sylvestris)* and the sea pine *(P. pinaster),* as well as many others. See Botanical Classification section.

HERBAL/FOLK TRADITION Known to Galen and Hippocrates for its many applications, especially with regard to pulmonary and genito-urinary infections, digestive complaints and externally as a treatment for rheumatic or neuralgic pain and skin conditions. In China the oleoresin has been used (both internally and externally) for centuries for excess phlegm, bronchitis, rheumatism, stiff joints, toothache, boils, sores, ringworm and dermatitis.

The turpentine essence or spirit of turpentine is said to be four times more active than the crude turpentine.

ACTIONS Analgesic, antimicrobial, antirheumatic, antiseptic, antispasmodic, balsamic, diuretic, cicatrisant, counter-irritant, expectorant, haemostatic, parasiticide, rubefacient, stimulant, tonic, vermifuge.

EXTRACTION Essential oil by steam (or water) distillation from the crude oleoresin, then rectified. 'It has to be purified because it is viscous, coloured and acidic.'[106]

CHARACTERISTICS A colourless, water-white mobile liquid with a fresh, warm-balsamic, familiar odour.

PRINCIPAL CONSTITUENTS Mainly alphapinene (approx. 50 per cent), betapinene (25–35 per cent) and carene (20–60 per cent) in the American oils. In European oils the alphapinene can constitute up to 95 per cent – constituents vary according to source.

SAFETY DATA Environmental hazard – marine pollutant. Relatively non-toxic and non-irritant; possible sensitization in some individuals. Avoid therapeutic use or employ in moderation only.

AROMATHERAPY/HOME USE
Use with care for:
SKIN CARE: Boils, cuts, fleas, insect repellent, lice, ringworm, scabies, wounds.
CIRCULATION, MUSCLES AND JOINTS: Arthritis, gout, muscular aches and pains, rheumatism, sciatica.
RESPIRATORY SYSTEM: Bronchitis, catarrh, whooping cough.
GENITO-URINARY SYSTEM: Cystitis, leucorrhoea, urethritis.
IMMUNE SYSTEM: Colds.
NERVOUS SYSTEM: Neuralgia.

OTHER USES Used in many ointments and lotions for aches and pains; and in cough and cold remedies. Neither oil nor oleoresin is used in perfumery work, although resin derivatives are used as fixative agents and in pine and industrial perfumes. Mainly known as a paint and stain remover, solvent and insecticide. Also used as a starting material for the production of terpineol, etc.

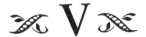

VALERIAN
Valeriana fauriei

FAMILY Valerianaceae

SYNONYMS *V. officinalis*, *V. officinalis var. angustifolium*, *V. officinalis var. latifolia*, European valerian, common valerian, Belgian valerian, fragrant valerian, garden valerian.

GENERAL DESCRIPTION A perennial herb up to 1.5 metres high with a hollow, erect stem, deeply dissected dark leaves and many purplish-white flowers. It has short, thick, greyish roots, largely showing above ground, which have a strong odour.

DISTRIBUTION Native to Europe and parts of Asia; naturalized in North America. It is mainly cultivated in Belgium for its oil, also in France, Holland, England, Scandinavia, Yugoslavia, Hungary, China and the USSR.

OTHER SPECIES There are over 150 species of valerian found in different parts of the world. The Eastern varieties are slightly different from the Western types: the oil from the Japanese plant called 'kesso root'(*V. officinalis*) is more woody; the oil from the Indian valerian (*V. wallichii*) is more musky. Also closely related to spikenard (*Nardostachys jatamansi*) – see entry.

HERBAL/FOLK TRADITION This herb has been highly esteemed since medieval times, and used to be called 'all heal'. It has been used in the West for a variety of complaints, especially where there is nervous tension or restlessness, such as insomnia, migraine, dysmenorrhoea, intestinal colic, rheumatism, and as a pain reliever.

On the Continent the oil has been used for cholera, epilepsy and for skin complaints. In China it is used for backache, colds, menstrual problems, bruises and sores.

The root is current in the British Herbal Pharmacopoeia as a specific for 'conditions presenting nervous excitability'.[107]

ACTIONS Anodyne (mild), antidandruff, diuretic, antispasmodic, bactericidal, carminative, depressant of the central nervous system, hypnotic, hypotensive, regulator, sedative, stomachic.

EXTRACTION 1. Essential oil by steam distillation from the rhizomes. 2. An absolute (and concrete) by solvent extraction of the rhizomes.

CHARACTERISTICS 1. An olive to brown liquid (darkening with age) with a warm-woody, balsamic, musky odour; a green topnote in fresh oils. 2. An olive-brown viscous liquid with a balsamic-green, woody, bitter-sweet strong odour. It blends well with patchouli, costus, oakmoss, pine, lavender, cedarwood, mandarin, petitgrain and rosemary.

PRINCIPAL CONSTITUENTS Mainly bornyl acetate and isovalerate, with caryophyllene, pinenes, valeranone, ionone, eugenyl isovalerate, borneol, patchouli alcohol and valerianol, among others.

SAFETY DATA Non-toxic, non-irritant, possible sensitization. Use in moderation.

AROMATHERAPY/HOME USE
NERVOUS SYSTEM: Insomnia, nervous indigestion, migraine, restlessness and tension states.

OTHER USES Used in pharmaceutical preparations as a relaxant and in herbal teas. The oil and absolute are used as fragrance components in soaps and in 'moss' and 'forest' fragrances. Used to flavour tobacco, root beer, liqueurs and apple flavourings.

VANILLA
Vanilla planifolia

FAMILY Orchidaceae

SYNONYMS *V. fragrans*, common vanilla, Mexican vanilla, Bourbon vanilla, Reunion vanilla.

GENERAL DESCRIPTION A perennial herbaceous climbing vine up to 25 metres high, with green stems and large white flowers which have a deep narrow trumpet. The green capsules or fruits are ready to pick after eight or nine months on the plant, and then have to be 'cured'. The immature vanilla 'pod' or 'bean' which is from 14 cms to 22 cms long, has to be fermented and dried to turn it into the fragrant brown vanilla pods of commerce – a process which can take up to six months to complete. During the drying process vanillin can accumulate as white crystals on the surface of the bean.

DISTRIBUTION Native to Central America and Mexico; cultivated mainly in Madagascar and Mexico; also Tahiti, the Comoro Islands, East Africa and Indonesia, although the pods are often processed in Europe or the USA.

OTHER SPECIES There are several different species of vanilla, such as the Tahiti vanilla (*V. tahitensis*) which is a smaller bean, and the 'vanillons' type (*V. pompona*) which produces an inferior quality oil.

HERBAL/FOLK TRADITION When vanilla is grown in cultivation the deep trumpet-shaped flowers have to be hand-pollinated; except in Mexico where the native humming birds do most of the work!

ACTIONS Balsamic.

EXTRACTION A resinoid (often called an oleoresin) by solvent extraction from the 'cured' vanilla beans. (An absolute is occasionally produced by further extraction from the resinoid.)

CHARACTERISTICS A viscous dark brown liquid with a rich, sweet, balsamic, vanilla-like odour. It blends well with sandalwood, vetiver, opopanax, benzoin, balsams and spice oils.

PRINCIPAL CONSTITUENTS Vanillin (1.3–2.9 per cent) with over 150 other constituents, many of them traces: hydroxybenzaldehyde, acetic acid, isobutyric acid, caproic acid, eugenol and furfural, among others.

SAFETY DATA Non-toxic, common sensitizing agent. Widely adulterated.

AROMATHERAPY/HOME USE None.

OTHER USES Used in pharmaceutical products as a flavouring agent. Used as a fragrance ingredient in perfumes, especially oriental types. Widely used to flavour tobacco and as a food flavouring, mainly in ice cream, yoghurt and chocolate.

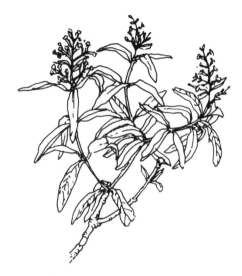

Lemon Verbena

VERBENA, LEMON
Aloysia triphylla

FAMILY Verbenaceae

SYNONYMS *A. citriodora, Verbena triphylla, Lippia citriodora, L. triphylla,* verbena, herb Louisa.

GENERAL DESCRIPTION A handsome deciduous perennial shrub up to 5 metres high with a woody stem, very fragrant, delicate, pale green, lanceolate leaves arranged in threes, and small, pale purple flowers. Often grown as an ornamental bush in gardens.

DISTRIBUTION Native of Chile and Aregentina; cultivated (and found semi-wild) in the Mediterranean region – France, Tunisia, Algeria – as well as Kenya and China. The oil is mainly produced in southern France and North Africa.

OTHER SPECIES Botanically related to the oregano family – see Botanical Classification section. Not to be mistaken for the so-called 'Spanish verbena' or 'verbena' oil (Spanish) *(Thymus hiamalis)*, nor confused with the herb 'vervain' *(Verbena officinalis)*. This is further confused since the French name for verbena is *verveine (Verveine citronelle, Verveine odorante)*.

HERBAL/FOLK TRADITION 'The uses of lemon verbena are similar to those of mint, orange flowers and melissa.'[108] It is indicated especially in nervous conditions which manifest as digestive complaints. The dried leaves are still used as a popular household tea especially on the Continent, both as a refreshing, uplifting 'pick-me-up' and to help restore the liver after a hang-over.

ACTIONS Antiseptic, antispasmodic, carminative, detoxifying, digestive, febrifuge, hepatobiliary stimulant, sedative (nervous), stomachic.

EXTRACTION Essential oil by steam distillation from the freshly harvested herb.

CHARACTERISTICS A pale olive or yellow mobile liquid with a sweet, fresh, lemony, fruity-floral fragrance. It blends well with neroli, palmarosa, olibanum, Tolu balsam, elemi, lemon and other citrus oils.

PRINCIPAL CONSTITUENTS Citral (30–35 per cent), nerol and geraniol, among others.

SAFETY DATA Possible sensitization; phototoxicity due to high citral levels. Other safety data is unavailable at present – however, true verbena oil is virtually non-existent. Most so-called 'verbena oil' is either from the Spanish verbena (an inferior oil), or a mix of lemongrass, lemon, citronella, etc.

AROMATHERAPY/HOME USE
DIGESTIVE SYSTEM: Cramps, indigestion, liver congestion.
NERVOUS SYSTEM: Anxiety, insomnia, nervous tension and stress-related conditions.

OTHER USES Used in perfumery and citrus colognes – 'eau de verveine' is still popular in France, Europe and America.

VETIVER
Vetiveria zizanoides

FAMILY Poaceae (Gramineae)

SYNONYMS *Andropogon muricatus*, vetivert, khus khus.

GENERAL DESCRIPTION A tall, tufted, perennial, scented grass, with a straight stem, long narrow leaves and an abundant complex lacework of undergound white rootlets.

DISTRIBUTION Native to south India, Indonesia and Sri Lanka. Also cultivated in Reunion, the Philippines, the Comoro Islands, Japan, West Africa and South America. The oil is mainly produced in Java, Haiti and Reunion; some is distilled in Europe and the USA.

OTHER SPECIES Botanically related to lemongrass, citronella, litsea cubeba and flouve oil (also from the roots of a tropical grass).

HERBAL/FOLK TRADITION The rootlets have been used in the East for their fine fragrance since antiquity. They are used by the locals to protect domestic animals from vermin, and the fibres of the grass are woven into aromatic matting. It is grown in India to protect against soil erosion during the tropical rainy season.
In India and Sri Lanka the essence is known as 'the oil of tranquillity'.

ACTIONS Antiseptic, antispasmodic, depurative, rubefacient, sedative (nervous system), stimulant (circulatory, production of red corpuscles), tonic, vermifuge.

EXTRACTION Essential oil by steam distillation from the roots and rootlets – washed, chopped, dried and soaked. (A resinoid is also produced by solvent extraction for perfumery work.)

CHARACTERISTICS A dark brown, olive or amber viscous oil with a deep smoky, earthy-woody odour with a sweet persistent undertone. The colour and scent can vary according to the source – Angola produces a very pale oil with a dry-woody odour. It blends well with sandalwood, rose, violet, jasmine, opopanax, patchouli, oakmoss, lavender, clary sage, mimosa, cassie and ylang ylang.

PRINCIPAL CONSTITUENTS Vetiverol, vitivone, terpenes, e.g. vetivenes, among others.

SAFETY DATA Non-toxic, non-irritant, non-sensitizing.

AROMATHERAPY/HOME USE
SKIN CARE: Acne, cuts, oily skin, wounds.
CIRCULATION, MUSCLES AND JOINTS: Arthritis, muscular aches and pains, rheumatism, sprains, stiffness.

NERVOUS SYSTEM: Debility, depression, insomnia, nervous tension – 'Vetiver is deeply relaxing, so valuable in massage and baths for anybody experiencing stress.'[109]

OTHER USES Employed as a fixative and fragrance ingredient in soaps, cosmetics and perfumes, especially oriental types. The oil is used in food preservatives, especially for asparagus.

VIOLET
Viola odorata

FAMILY Violaceae

SYNONYMS English violet, garden violet, blue violet, sweet-scented violet.

GENERAL DESCRIPTION A small, tender, perennial plant with dark green, heart-shaped leaves, fragrant violet-blue flowers and an oblique underground rhizome.

DISTRIBUTION Native to Europe and parts of Asia; cultivated in gardens worldwide. It is mainly grown in southern France (Grasse) and to a lesser extent in Italy and China for perfumery use.

OTHER SPECIES There are over 200 species of violet; the main types cultivated for aromatic extraction are the 'Parma' and the 'Victoria' violets.

HERBAL/FOLK TRADITION Both the leaf and flowers have a long tradition of use in herbal medicine, mainly for congestive pulmonary conditions and sensitive skin conditions, including capillary fragility. The leaf has also been used to treat cystitis and as a mouthwash for infections of the mouth and

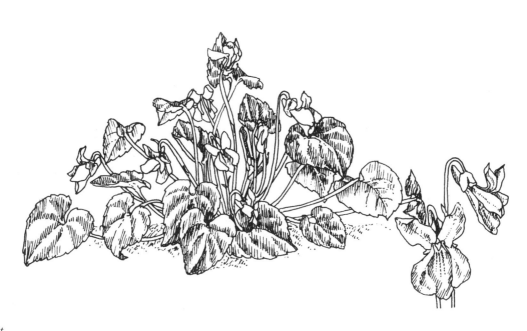

Violet

throat. It is reported to have mild pain-killing properties, probably due to the presence of salicylic acid (as in 'aspirin').

The flowers are still used to make a 'syrup of violet' which is used as a laxative and colouring agent. The dried leaf and flowers are current in the British Herbal Pharmacopoeia as a specific for 'eczema and skin eruptions with serious exudate, particularly when associated with rheumatic symptoms'.

ACTIONS Analgesic (mild), anti-inflammatory, antirheumatic, antiseptic, decongestant (liver), diuretic, expectorant, laxative, soporific, stimulant (circulation).

EXTRACTION A concrete and absolute from 1. fresh leaves, and 2. flowers.

CHARACTERISTICS 1. The leaf absolute is an intense dark green viscous liquid with a strong green-leaf odour and a delicate floral undertone. 2. The flower absolute is a yellowish-green viscous liquid with a sweet, rich, floral fragrance, characteristic of the fresh flowers. It blends well with tuberose, clary sage, boronia, tarragon, cumin, hop, basil, hyacinth and other florals.

PRINCIPAL CONSTITUENTS Both leaves and petals contain nonadienal, parmone, hexyl alcohol, benzyl alcohol, ionone and viola quercitin, among others.

SAFETY DATA Non-toxic, non-irritant, possible sensitization in some individuals.

AROMATHERAPY/HOME USE
SKIN CARE: Acne, eczema, refines the pores, thread veins, wounds.
CIRCULATION, MUSCLES AND JOINTS: Fibrosis, poor circulation, rheumatism.
RESPIRATORY SYSTEM: Bronchitis, catarrh, mouth and throat infections.
NERVOUS SYSTEM: Dizziness, headaches, insomnia, nervous exhaustion – the scent was believed to 'comfort and strengthen the heart'.

OTHER USES Used in high class perfumery work; occasionally used in flavouring, mainly confectionery.

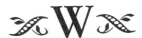

WINTERGREEN
Gaultheria procumbens

FAMILY Ericaceae

SYNONYMS Aromatic wintergreen, checkerberry, teaberry, gaultheria (oil).

GENERAL DESCRIPTION A small evergreen herb up to 15 cm high with slender creeping stems shooting forth erect twigs with leathery serrated leaves and drooping white flowers, which are followed by fleshy scarlet berries.

DISTRIBUTION Native to North America, especially the north eastern region and Canada. The oil is produced in the USA.

OTHER SPECIES There are several other *Gaultheria* species which are also used for oil production, sharing similar properties.

HERBAL/FOLK TRADITION The plant has been used for respiratory conditions such as chronic mucous discharge, but is mainly employed for joint and muscular problems such as lumbago, sciatica, neuralgia, myalgia, etc. The dried leaf and stem are current in the British Herbal Pharmacopoeia as a specific for rheumatoid arthritis.

The essential oil has been used interchangeably with sweet birch oil, both being made up almost exclusively of methyl salicylate.

ACTIONS Analgesic (mild), anti-inflammatory, antirheumatic, antitussive, astringent, carminative, diuretic, emmenagogue, galactagogue, stimulant.

EXTRACTION Essential oil by steam (or water) distillation from the leaf, previously macerated in warm water. The essential oil does not occur crudely in the plant, but is only produced during the process of decomposition in warm water.

CHARACTERISTICS A pale yellow or pinkish liquid with an intense sweet-woody, almost fruity odour. It blends well with oregano, mints, thyme, ylang ylang, narcissus and vanilla.

PRINCIPAL CONSTITUENTS Almost exclusively methyl salicylate (up to 98 per cent), with formaldehyde and gaultheriline.

SAFETY DATA Toxic, irritant and sensitizing – an environmental hazard or marine pollutant. The true oil is almost obsolete, having been replaced by synthetic methyl sallicylate. See also *sweet birch oil.*

AROMATHERAPY/HOME USE None. 'Avoid both internally and externally.'[112]

OTHER USES Some pharmaceutical use, such as 'Olbas' oil. Some perfumery applications especially in forest-type fragrances. Extensively used as a flavouring agent in the USA for toothpaste, chewing gum, root beer, Coca Cola, and other soft drinks.

WORMSEED
Chenopodium ambrosioides var. anthelminticum

FAMILY Chenopodiaceae

SYNONYMS *C. anthelminticum,* American wormseed, chenopodium, Californian spearmint, Jesuit's tea, Mexican tea, herb sancti mariae, Baltimore (oil).

GENERAL DESCRIPTION A hairy, coarse, perennial wayside herb up to 1 metre high with stout, erect stem, oblong-lanceolate leaves and numerous greenish-yellow flowers, the same colour as the leaves.

DISTRIBUTION Native to South America; cultivated mainly in the east and south east USA, also India, Hungary and the USSR.

OTHER SPECIES The parent plant, *C. ambrosioides,* is also used to produce an essential oil with similar properties. There are many different members in the *Chenopodium* or Goosefoot family, such as Good King Henry *(C. bonus-henricus),* a European variety whose leaves were eaten like spinach. See also Botanical Classification section.
   The so-called 'Russian wormseed oil' or wormseed Levant *(Artemisia cina)* is quite different from the American type, although it is also used as an anthelmintic and is extremely toxic, containing mainly cineol.

HERBAL/FOLK TRADITION 'Used for many years by the local Indians as an effective anthelmintic ... several Indian tribes of the eastern part of the United States use the whole of the herb decocted to help ease painful menstruation and other female complaints.'[113]
   Apart from being used to expel roundworm, hookworm and dwarf tapeworm, the herb has also been employed for asthma, catarrh and other chest complaints, and to treat nervous disease. In China it is used to treat articular rheumatism. Causes dizziness and vomiting in concentration.

ACTIONS Anthelmintic, antirheumatic, antispasmodic, expectorant, hypotensive.

EXTRACTION Essential oil by steam distillation from the whole herb, especially the fruit or seeds.

CHARACTERISTICS A colourless or pale yellow oil with a sweet-woody, camphoraceous, heavy and nauseating odour.

PRINCIPAL CONSTITUENTS Ascaridole (60–80 per cent), cymene, limonene, terpinene, myrcene.

SAFETY DATA A very toxic oil – cases of fatal poisoning have been reported even in low doses. Effects can be cumulative. Due to high ascaridole content, the oil may explode when heated or treated with acids.

AROMATHERAPY/HOME USE None. 'Should not be used in therapy either internally or externally. One of the most toxic essential oils.'[114]

OTHER USES In pharmaceuticals its anthelmintic applications have been replaced by synthetics. Used as a fragrance component in soaps, detergents, cosmetics and perfumes. Its use is not permitted in foods.

WORMWOOD
Artemisia absinthium

FAMILY Asteraceae (Compositae)

SYNONYMS Common wormwood, green ginger, armoise, absinthium (oil).

GENERAL DESCRIPTION A perennial herb up to 1.5 metres high with a whitish stem, silvery-green, divided leaves covered in silky fine hairs, and pale yellow flowers.

DISTRIBUTION Native to Europe, North Africa and western Asia; naturalized in North America. It is extensively cultivated in central and southern Europe, the USSR, North Africa and the USA, where the oil is mainly produced.

OTHER SPECIES There are many other *Artemisia* species such as davana and the Roman wormwood. See also entry on mugwort *(A. vulgaris)* also commonly called 'armoise'.

HERBAL/FOLK TRADITION Used as an aromatic-bitter for anorexia, as a digestive tonic and as a choleretic for liver and gall bladder disorders, usually in the form of a dilute extract. It is also used to promote menstruation, reduce fever and expel worms. It was once used as a remedy for epilepsy and as an aromatic strewing herb to banish fleas.

ACTIONS Anthelmintic, choleretic, deodorant, emmenagogue, febrifuge, insect repellent, narcotic, stimulant (digestive), tonic, vermifuge.

EXTRACTION Essential oil by steam distillation from the leaves and flowering tops. (An absolute is occasionally produced by solvent extraction.)

CHARACTERISTICS A dark green or bluish oil with a spicy, warm, bitter-green odour and a sharp, fresh topnote. The 'de-thujonized' oil blends well with oakmoss, jasmine, orange blossom, lavender and hyacinth.

PRINCIPAL CONSTITUENTS Thujone (up to 71 per cent), azulenes, terpenes.

SAFETY DATA Toxic. Abortifacient. Habitual use can cause restlessness, nightmares, convulsions, vomiting and, in extreme cases, brain damage. In 1915 the French banned the production of the drink Absinthe with this plant, due to its narcotic and habit-forming properties.

AROMATHERAPY/HOME USE None. 'Should not be used in therapy either internally or externally.'[115]

OTHER USES Occasionally used in rubefacient pharmaceutical preparations and as a fragrance component in toiletries, cosmetics and perfumes. Widely employed (at minute levels) as a flavouring agent in alcoholic bitters and vermouths; also to a lesser extent in soft drinks and some foods, especially confectionery and desserts.

YARROW
Achillea millefolium

FAMILY Asteraceae (Compositae)

SYNONYMS Milfoil, common yarrow, nosebleed, thousand leaf – and many other country names.

GENERAL DESCRIPTION A perennial herb with a simple stem up to 1 metre high, with finely dissected leaves giving a lacy appearance, bearing numerous pinky-white, dense flowerheads.

DISTRIBUTION Native to Eurasia; naturalized in North America. Now found in most temperate zones of the world. The oil is mainly distilled in Germany, Hungary, France and Yugoslavia, also the USA and Africa.

OTHER SPECIES A very extensive species. Other varieties include the Ligurian yarrow *(A. ligustica)* and the musk yarrow or iva *(A. moschata)*, which also produces an essential oil containing mainly cineol – used in the preparation of 'iva liquor', a medicinal aperitif.

HERBAL/FOLK TRADITION An age-old herbal medicine used for a wide variety of complaints including fever, respiratory infections, digestive problems, nervous tension and externally for sores, rashes and wounds. Its use in the treatment of wounds is said to go back to Achilles who used it for injuries inflicted by iron weapons.

It is used in China mainly for menstrual problems and haemorrhoids. In Norway it is also used for rheumatism. The stalks are traditionally used for divination in the *I Ching*, the Chinese classic.

It is current in the British Herbal Pharmacopoeia as a specific for thrombotic conditions with hypertension.

ACTIONS Anti-inflammatory, antipyretic, antirheumatic, antiseptic, antispasmodic, astringent, carminative, cicatrisant, diaphoretic, digestive, expectorant, haemostatic, hypotensive, stomachic, tonic.

EXTRACTION Essential oil by steam distillation from the dried herb.

CHARACTERISTICS A dark blue or greenish-olive liquid with a fresh, green, sweet-herbaceous, slightly camphoraceous odour. It blends well with cedarwood, pine, chamomile, valerian, vetiver and oakmoss.

PRINCIPAL CONSTITUENTS Azulene (up to 51 per cent), pinenes, caryophyllene, borneol, terpineol, cineol, bornyl acetate, camphor, sabinene and thujone, among others. Constituents, especially azulene levels, vary according to source.

SAFETY DATA Non-toxic, non-irritant, possible sensitization in some individuals.

AROMATHERAPY/HOME USE
SKIN CARE: Acne, burns, cuts, eczema, hair rinse (promotes hair growth), inflammations, rashes, scars, tones the skin, varicose veins, wounds.
CIRCULATION, MUSCLES AND JOINTS: Arteriosclerosis, high blood pressure, rheumatoid arthritis, thrombosis.
DIGESTIVE SYSTEM: Constipation, cramp, flatulence, haemorrhoids, indigestion.
GENITO-URINARY SYSTEM: Amenorrhoea,

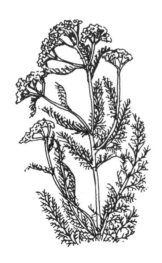

Yarrow

dysmenorrhoea, cystitis and other infections.
IMMUNE SYSTEM: Colds, fever, 'flu, etc.
NERVOUS SYSTEM: Hypertension, insomnia,
stress-related conditions.

OTHER USES Occasionally used in
pharmaceutical bath preparations for skin
conditions. Limited use in perfumes and
aftershaves. Employed as a flavour ingredient in
vermouths and bitters.

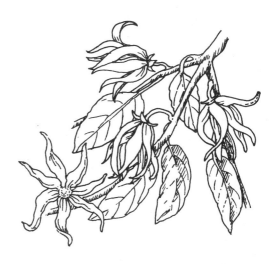

YLANG YLANG

Cananga odorata var. genuina

FAMILY Annonaceae

SYNONYMS *Unona odorantissimum,* flower
of flowers.

Ylang Ylang

GENERAL DESCRIPTION A tall tropical tree
up to 20 metres high with large, tender, fragrant
flowers, which can be pink, mauve or yellow.
The yellow flowers are considered best for the
extraction of essential oil.

DISTRIBUTION Native to tropical Asia,
especially Indonesia and the Philippines. Major
oil producers are Madagascar, Reunion and the
Comoro Islands.

OTHER SPECIES Very closely related to
cananga *(C. odoratum var. macrophylla),*
although the oil produced from the ylang ylang
is considered of superior quality for perfumery
work, having a more refined quality.

HERBAL/FOLK TRADITION In Indonesia,
the flowers are spread on the beds of newly
married couples on their wedding night. In the
Molucca Islands, an ointment is made from
ylang ylang and cucuma flowers in a coconut oil
base for cosmetic and hair care, skin diseases, to
prevent fever (including malaria) and fight
infections.

In the Victorian age, the oil was used in the
popular hair treatment Macassar oil, due to its

stimulating effect on the scalp, encouraging hair
growth. The oil was also used to soothe insect
bites, and is thought to have a regulating effect
on cardiac and respiratory rhythm.

ACTIONS Aphrodisiac, antidepressant, anti-
infectious, antiseborrhoeic, antiseptic, euphoric,
hypotensive, nervine, regulator, sedative
(nervous), stimulant (circulatory), tonic.

EXTRACTION Essential oil by water or steam
distillation from the freshly picked flowers. The
first distillate (about 40 per cent) is called ylang
ylang extra, which is the top grade. There are
then three further successive distillates, called
Grades 1, 2 and 3. A 'complete' oil is also
produced which represents the total or
'unfractionated' oil, but this is sometimes
constructed by blending ylang ylang 1 and 2
together, which are the two least popular
grades. (An absolute and concrete are also
produced by solvent extraction for their long-
lasting floral-balsamic effect.)

CHARACTERISTICS Ylang ylang extra is a
pale yellow, oily liquid with an intensely sweet,
soft, floral-balsamic, slightly spicy scent – a

good oil has a creamy rich topnote. A very intriguing perfume oil in its own right, it also blends well with rosewood, jasmine, vetiver, opopanax, bergamot, mimosa, cassie, Peru balsam, rose, tuberose, costus and others. It is an excellent fixative. The other grades lack the depth and richness of the ylang ylang extra.

PRINCIPAL CONSTITUENTS Methyl benzoate, methyl salicylate, methyl para-cretol, benzyl acetate, eugenol, geraniol, linalol and terpenes: pinene, cadinene, among others.

SAFETY DATA Non-toxic, non-irritant, a few cases of sensitization reported. Use in moderation, since its heady scent can cause headaches or nausea.

AROMATHERAPY/HOME USE
SKIN CARE: Acne, hair growth, hair rinse, insect bites, irritated and oily skin, general skin care.
CIRCULATION, MUSCLES AND JOINTS: High blood pressure, hyperpnoea (abnormally fast breathing), tachycardia, palpitations.
NERVOUS SYSTEM: Depression, frigidity, impotence, insomnia, nervous tension and stress-related disorders – 'The writer, working with odorous materials for more than twenty years, long ago noticed that ... ylang ylang soothes and inhibits anger born of frustration.'[116]

OTHER USES Extensively used as a fragrance component and fixative in soaps, cosmetics and perfumes, especially oriental and floral types; ylang ylang extra tends to be used in high class perfumes, ylang ylang 3 in soaps, detergents, etc. Used as a flavour ingredient, mainly in alcoholic and soft drinks, fruit flavours and desserts.

References

Part I

1. Naves, Y.R. *Natural Perfume Materials*, p.3.
2. Davis, P. *Aromatherapy An A-Z*, p.7.
3. Tisserand, R. *The Art of Aromatherapy*, p.21.
4. Naves, as above, p.5.
5. Chetwynd, T. *Dictionary of Symbols*, p.9.
6. *Yearbook of Pharmacy and Transactions of the British Pharmaceutical Conference, 1907*, p.217.
7. Maury, M. *Guide to Aromatherapy*, p.7.
8. Valnet, J. *The Practice of Aromatherapy*, p.44.
9. *Agbiotech News and Information,* 1990, Vol. II, No.2, p.211.
10. Baerheim & Scheffer, *Essential Oils and Aromatic Plants*.
11. Davis, as above, p.173.
12. Baerheim & Scheffer, as above.
13. Tisserand, R. Psychology of Perfumery, '91 Conference Report. *International Journal of Aromatherapy*, Vol. III, No.3, p.10.
14. Maury, as above, p.94.
15. Whitmont, E. *Psyche and Substance*, p.24.
16. Hoffman, D. *The New Holistic Herbal*, p.14.
17. Lavabre, M. *Aromatherapy Workbook*, p.98.
18. Steele, J. *International Journal of Aromatherapy*, Vol. II, No.2, p.8.

Part II

1. Davis, P. London School of Aromatherapy notes, 1983.
2. Tisserand, R. *The Essential Oil Safety Data Manual*, p.76.
3. Grieve, M. *A Modern Herbal*, p.63.
4. Davis, P. *Aromatherapy An A–Z*, p.221.
5. Hoffmann, D. *The Holistic Herbal*, p.168.
6. Tisserand, R. *The Essential Oil Safety Data Manual*, p.102.
7. Tisserand, R.*The Art of Aromatherapy*, p.183.
8. Ceres, *Herbs for Healthy Hair*, p.19.
9. Leung, A.Y. *Encyclopedia of Common Natural Ingredients*, p.62.
10. Maury, M. *Guide to Aromatherapy*, p.96.
11. Leung, as above, p.64.
12. Mills, S.Y. *The A-Z of Modern Herbalism*, p.36.
13. Tisserand, *The Essential Oil Safety Data Manual*, p.78.
14. Grieve, as above p.127.
15. Cribb, J.W. & A.B. *Useful Wild Plants in Australia*, p.36.
16. Grieve, as above, p.155.
17. *British Herbal Pharmocopoeia 1983*, p.14.
18. Tisserand, as above, p.79.
19. Tisserand, as above, p.81.
20. Mills , as above, p.59.
21. Arctander, S. *Perfume and Flavor Materials of Natural Origin*, p.157.
22. Lavabre, M. *Aromatherapy Workbook*, p.117.
23. Arctander, as above, p.170.
24. Culpeper. N. *Complete Herbal*, p.110.
25. Davis, as above, p.135.
26. Grieve, as above, p.426.
27. Culpeper, as above, p.202.
28. Tisserand, as above, p.81.
29. Parvati, J. *Hygieia, A Woman's Herbal*, p.105.
30. de Bairacli Levy, J. *The Illustrated Herbal Handbook*, p.54.
31. Tisserand, as above, p.82.
32. Leung , as above, p.149.
33. Leung as above, p.155.
34. Tisserand, as above , p.84.
35. Franchomme, P. *Phytoguide I*, p.35.
36. Maury, as above, p.104.
37. Leung, as above , p.166.
38. Lassak, E.V. & McCarthy, T. *Australian Medicinal Plants*, p.201.
39. Grieve, as above, p.79.
40. Lavabre, as above, p.123.
41. Maury, as above, p.104.
42. School of Herbal Medicine, *Materia Medica*, Part II, p.27.
43. Tisserand, as above, p.85.
44. Culpeper, as above, p.198.
45. Worwood, V.A. *The Fragrant Pharmacy*, p.107.
46. Grieve, as above, p.445.
47. Tisserand, R. *The Art of Aromatherapy*, p.238.
48. Culpeper, as above, p.211.
49. Grieve, as above, p.471.
50. Culpeper, as above, p.216.
51. Grieve, as above, p.517.
52. Davis, as above, p.214.
53. Culpeper, as above, p.227.
54. Grieve, as above, p.522.
55. School of Herbal Medicine, as above, p.25.
56. Culpeper , as above, p.234.
57. Grieve, as above, p.536.
58. Tisserand, *The Essential Oil Safety Data Manual*, p.86.
59. Tisserand, as above, p.86.
60. Culpeper, as above, p.247.
61. Davis, as above, p.233.

62. Grieve, as above, p.573.
63. *British Herbal Pharmacopoeia 1983,* p.148.
64. Younger, D. *Household Gods,* p.53.
65. Younger, as above, p.43.
66. Davis, as above, p.236.
67. Tisserand, as above, p.189.
68. Tisserand, R. *The Essential Oil Safety Data Manual,* p.88
69. Tisserand, as above, p.88.
70. Guenther, E. *The Essential Oils, Vol. IV,* p.5.
71. Maury, as above, p.89.
72. Grieve, as above, p.626.
73. Tisserand, as above, p.89.
74. Maury, as above, p.90.
75. Younger, as above, p.67.
76. Warren-Davis, D. The symbolism of the rose, *The Herbal Review,* Autumn 1989, p.2.
77. Maury, as above, p.87.
78. Culpeper, as above, p.298.
79. *British Herbal Pharmacopoeia 1983,* p.181.
80. Lavabre, as above, p.86.
81. Culpeper, as above, p.305.
82. Arctander, as above, p.563.
83. Tisserand, as above, p.107.
84. Culpeper, as above, p.211
85. Culpeper , as above, p.211
86. Grieve, as above, p.715
87. Tisserand, as above, p.90.
88. Arctander, as above, p.581.
89. Tisserand, as above, p.92.
90. Culpeper, as above, p.319.
91. Tisserand, as above, p.69.
92. Valnet, J. *The Practice of Aromatherapy,* p.186.
93. Tisserand, as above, p.69.
94. Le Strange, R. *A History of Herbal Plants,* p.44.
95. The Holy Bible; St John 12:3.
96. Lavabre, as above, p.64.
97. Arctander, as above, p.607.
98. Tisserand, as above, p.94.
99. Culpeper, as above, p.363.
100. Davis, as above, p.328.
101. Tisserand, as above, p.96.
102. Davis, as above, p.326.
103. Grieve, as above, p.819.
104. Guenther, E. *The Essential Oils, Vol. V,* p.348.
105. Lautie, R. & Passebecq, A. *Aromatherapy, The Use of Plant Essences in Healing,* p.86.
106. Valnet, as above, p.188.
107. *British Herbal Pharmacopoeia, 1983,* p.226
108. Grieve, as above, p.831.
109. Davis, as above, p.342.
110. *British Herbal Pharmacopoeia, 1983* p.233.
111. Grieve, as above, p.835.
112. Tisserand, as above, p.112
113. Le Strange , as above, p.72.
114. Tisserand, as above, p.96.
115. Tisserand, as above, p.98.
116. Moncrieff, R.W. *Odours,* 1970.

BIBLIOGRAPHY

Arber, A. *Herbals, Their Origin and Evolution,* Cambridge University Press, 1912.

Arctander, S. *Perfume and Flavor Materials of Natural Origin,* published by the author, Elizabeth, New Jersey, 1960.

de Bairacli, Levy, J. *The Illustrated Herbal Handbook,* Faber & Faber, 1982.

Baerheim, S.A. & Scheffer J.J.C. *Essential Oils and Aromatic Plants,* Dr. W. Junk Publications, 1989.

Beckett, S. *Herbs to Soothe Your Nerves,* Thorsons, 1977.

Beresford-Cooke, C. *Massage for Healing and Relaxation,* Arlington, 1986.

Bianchini, F. & Corbetta. F. *Health Plants of the World – Atlas of Medicinal Plants,* Newsweek Books, New York, 1977.

Blunt, W. *The Art of Botanical Illustration,* Collins, 1950.

Boulos, C. & Danin A. *Medicinal Plants of North Africa,* Reference Publications, 1983.

British Herbal Pharmacopoeia, British Herbal Medicine Association, 1983.

Buchman, D.D. *Feed Your Face,* Duckworth, 1980.

Buchman, D.D. *Herbal Medicine,* Rider, 1984.

Ceres, *Herbs for Healthy Hair,* Thorsons, 1977.

Chetwynd, T. *A Dictionary of Symbols,* Paladin, 1982.

Chiej, R. *The Macdonald Encyclopedia of Medicinal Plants,* Arnoldo Mondadori Editore, Milan, 1984.

Conway, D. *The Magic of Herbs,* Mayflower, 1973.

Coon, N. *The Dictionary of Useful Plants,* Rodale, Emmaus, Pa., 1974.

Cribb, A.B. & J.W. *Useful Wild Plants in Australia,* Fontana/Collins, 1982.

Culpeper, N. *Culpeper's Complete Herbal,* W. Foulsham & Co. Ltd, 1952.

Dastur, J.F. *Useful Plants of India and Pakistan*, D.B. Taraporevala Sons & Co. Ltd, India, 1985.

Davies, W.C. *New Zealand Native Plant Studies*, A.H. & A.W. Reed, Wellington, 1961.

Davis, P. *Aromatherapy An A-Z* , C.W.Daniel, 1988.

Day, I. *Perfumery with Herbs*, Darton, Longman and Todd, 1979.

Douglas, J.S. *Making Your Own Cosmetics*, Pelham Books, 1979.

Downing,G. *The Massage Book*, Penguin, 1974.

Franchomme, P. *Phytoguide I*, International Phytomedical Foundation, La Courtête, France, 1985.

Furia, T.E. & Bellanca. N. *Fenaroli's Handbook of Flavour Ingredients Vol. I*, 2nd ed., CRC Press, Cleveland, Ohio, 1975.

Gardner, J. *Healing Yourself During Pregnancy*, The Crossing Press, California,1987.

Grieve, M. *A Modern Herbal*, Penguin, 1982.

Griggs, B. *The Home Herbal*, Pan, 1983.

Guenther, E. *The Essential Oils*, Van Nostrand, New York, 1948.

Hall, R., Klemme D.& Nienhaus J. *The H & R Book: Guide to Fragrance Ingredients*, Johnson Publishing, 1985.

Hepper, C. *Herbal Cosmetics*, Thorsons, 1987.

Heriteau, J. *Potpourris and other Fragrant Delights*, Penguin, 1975.

Hoffmann, D. *The New Holistic Herbal*, Element Books, 1990.

Huxley, A. *Natural Beauty With Herbs*, Darton, Longman and Todd, 1977.

Jessee, J.E. *Perfume Album*, Robert E. Krieger, 1974.

Khan, I. *The Development of Spiritual Healing*, Sufi Publishing Co., 1974.

Krochmal A. & C. *A Guide to the Medicinal Plants of the United States*, Quadrangle, The New York Times Book Co., 1973.

Lassak, E.V. & McCarthy, T. *Australian Medicinal Plants*, Methuen, Australia, 1983.

Launert, E. *Edible and Medicinal Plants of Britain and Northern Europe*, Hamlyn, 1981.

Lautie, R. & Passebecq, A. *Aromatherapy: the Use of Plant Essences in Healing*, Thorsons, 1982.

Lavabre, M. *Aromatherapy Workbook*, Healing Arts Press, Vermont, 1990.

Lawrence, B.M. *Essential Oils*, Allured Publishing Co., Wheaton, USA, 1978.

Leung, A.Y. *Encyclopedia of Common Natural Ingredients*, John Wiley, New York, 1980.

Little, K. *Kitty Little's Book of Herbal Beauty*, Penguin, 1980.

Maury, M. *Marguerite Maury's Guide to Aromatherapy*, C.W.Daniel, 1989.

Mabey, R. *The Complete New Herbal*, Elm Tree Books, 1988.

McIntyre, A. *Herbs for Pregnancy and Childbirth*,

Sheldon Press, 1988.

Metcalfe, J. *Herbs and Aromatherapy*, Webb & Bower, 1989.

Meunier,C. *Lavandes et Lavandins*, Charle-Yves Chaudoreille, Edisud, Aix-en-Provence, France, 1985.

Mills, S.Y. *The A-Z of Modern Herbalism*, Thorsons, 1989.

Naves, Y.R. & Mazuyer, G. *Natural Perfume Materials*, Reinhold Publishing, New York, 1947.

Page, M. *The Observers Book of Herbs*, Frederick Warne, 1980.

Parvati. J. *Hygieia, A Womans Herbal*, Wildwood House, 1979.

Phillips, R. *Wild Flowers of Britain*, Pan, 1977.

Poucher, W.A. *Perfumes, Cosmetics and Soaps Vol II*, Chapman and Hall, 1932.

Price, S. *Practical Aromatherapy*, Thorsons, 1983.

Rapgay, L. *Tibetan Therapeutic Massage*, published by the author, India, 1985.

Ranson, F. *British Herbs*, Penguin 1949.

Rose, F. *The Wild Flower Key*, Frederick Warne, 1981.

Ryman, D. *The Aromatherapy Handbook*, Century, 1984.

Stead, C. *The Power of Holistic Aromatherapy*, Javelin Books, 1986.

Stobart, T. *Herbs, Spices and Flavourings*, Penguin, 1979.

Le Strange, R. *A History of Herbal Plants*, Angus and Robertson, 1977.

Temple, A.A. *Flowers and Trees of Palestine*, SPCK, Macmillan, 1929

Thomson, W.A.R. *Healing Plants - A Modern Herbal*, Macmillan, 1978.

Tisserand, M. *Aromatherapy for Women*, Thorsons, 1985.

Tisserand, R. *The Essential Oil Safety Data Manual*, The Association of Tisserand Aromatherapists, 1985.

Tisserand, R. *The Art of Aromatherapy*, C.W. Daniel, 1985.

Valnet, J. *The Practice of Aromatherapy*, C.W. Daniel, (English translation), 1982.

Weiss, R.F. *Herbal Medicine*, Arcanum, 1988.

Whitmont, E.C. *Psyche and Substance*, North Atlantic Books, 1980.

Williams, D. *Lecture Notes on Essential Oils*, Eve Taylor Ltd, 1989.

Worwood, V.A. *The Fragrant Pharmacy*, Macmillan, 1990.

Wren, R.C. *Potters New Cyclopaedia of Botanical Drugs and Preparations*, C.W. Daniel, 1988.

Yearbook of Pharmacy and Transactions of the British Pharmaceutical Conference, The Pharmaceutical Press, Bloomsbury, London, 1907.

Younger, D. *Household Gods*, E.W.Allen, 1898.

Useful Addresses

A *wide selection of essential oils, base oils and aromatic products is available from:*

Aqua Oleum
Unit 3, Lower Wharf
Wallbridge
Stroud
Glos GL5 3JA
T: +44 (0)1453 753555
F: +44 (0)1453 752179
www.aqua-oleum.co.uk
info@aqua-oleum.co.uk

and distributed in the following countries by:

Canada & USA
Natura Trading
Box 263
1857 West 4th Avenue
Vancouver B.C.
Canada

Hong Kong
7 Old Bailey Street
Central
Hong Kong

Norway
Terapi Consultas
Frysjaveien 27
0883 Oslo

Taiwan
Grace and Pearl Corporation
6 Lane 97
Tung An Street
Taipei 100

Finland
Luonnonruokkatakku Aduki Oy
Kirvesmiehenkatu 10
00810 Helsinki

Ireland
Wholefoods Wholesale
Unit 2D
Kylemore Industrial Estate
Dublin 10

Kenya
Armaan Ltd
PO Box 614
The Village Market
Nairobi 00621

Information regarding qualified aromatherapists and training programmes in the UK can be obtained from:

International Federation of Aromatherapists
182 Chiswick High Road
London W4 1PP
T: +44 (0)20 8742 2605

and in America from:

The American Aromatherapy Association
PO Box 3679
South Pasadena
CA 91031
T: +1 (818) 457 1742

Information regarding qualified medical herbalists and training programmes can be obtained from:

College of Phytotherapy (Herbal Medicine)
Bucksteep Manor
Bodle Street
Hailsham BN27 4RJ
T: +44 (0)1323 834800

National Institute of Medical Herbalists
56 Longbrook Street
Exeter EX4 6AH
T: +44 (0)1392 426022

and in America from:

American Botanical Council and Herb Research
Foundation
PO Box 201660
Austin
TX 78720
T: +1 (512) 331 8868
F: +1 (512) 331 1924

and

Californian School of Herbal Studies
9309 HWY 116
Forestville
CA 95436

General information on holistic forms of treatment can be obtained from:

Natural Medicine Society
PO Box 134
Chessington
Surrey KT9 1HP
T/F: +44 (0)20 8974 1166

THERAPEUTIC INDEX

Essential oils can be used to treat a wide range of common complaints, including those listed below. Special care must be taken regarding the use of oils which can cause irritation in concentration, and those oils which are known to be phototoxic, such as bergamot, lemon and orange. Before using a particular oil, the **Safety Data** information on the individual oils should be consulted.

Many of the conditions mentioned here could benefit from combining an aromatherapy approach with other forms of treatment, such as dietary measures, exercise, herbal medicines, osteopathy or counselling, among others.

The most useful and commonly available oils for a particular condition are shown in italics.

A guide to abbreviated terms of suggested application as outlined in the chapters 'How to Use Essential Oils at Home' and 'Creative Blending', is as follows:

M: Massage   **S:** Skin oil/lotion   **C:** Compress
H: Hair care   **F:** Flower Water   **B:** Bath
V: Vaporization   **I:** Inhalation (Steam)
D: Douche   **N:** Neat Application

Skin Care:

Acne (M,S,F,B,I,N): *Bergamot,* camphor (white), cananga, cedarwood (Atlas, Texas & Virginian), *chamomile (German & Roman),* clove bud, galbanum, *geranium,* grapefruit, helichrysum, juniper, lavandin, *lavender (spike & true), lemon,* lemongrass, lime, linaloe, litsea cubeba, mandarin, mint (peppermint & spearmint), myrtle, niaouli, *palmarosa,* patchouli, petitgrain, *rosemary,* rosewood, sage (clary & Spanish), sandalwood, *tea tree,* thyme, vetiver, violet, yarrow, ylang ylang.

Allergies (M,S,F,B,I): *Lemon balm , chamomile (German & Roman),* helichrysum, *true lavender ,* spikenard.

Athlete's foot (S): Clove bud, eucalyptus, *lavender (true & spike),* lemon, lemongrass, *myrrh,* patchouli, *tea tree.*

Baldness & hair care (S,H): *West Indian bay,* white birch, cedarwood (Atlas, Texas & Virginian), *chamomile (German & Roman),* grapefruit, juniper, patchouli, *rosemary,* sage (clary & Spanish), *yarrow,* ylang ylang.

Boils, abscesses & blisters (S,C,B): *Bergamot, chamomile (German & Roman),* eucalyptus blue gum, galbanum, helichrysum, lavandin, *lavender (spike & true),* lemon, mastic, niaouli, clary sage, *tea tree,* thyme, turpentine.

Bruises (S,C): *Arnica* (cream), borneol, clove bud, *fennel,* geranium, *hyssop,* sweet marjoram, *lavender,* thyme.

Burns (C,N): Canadian balsam, chamomile (German & Roman), clove bud, eucalyptus blue gum, geranium, helichrysum, lavandin, *lavender (spike & true),* marigold, niaouli, tea tree, yarrow.

Chapped & cracked skin (S,F,B): Peru balsam, *Tolu balsam, benzoin, myrrh, patchouli,* sandalwood.

Chilblains (S,N): Chamomile (German & Roman), *lemon,* lime, *sweet marjoram, black pepper.*

Cold sores/herpes (S): *Bergamot, eucalyptus blue gum,* lemon, *tea tree.*

Congested & dull skin (M,S,F,B,I): *Angelica,* white birch, sweet fennel, *geranium, grapefruit,* lavandin, *lavender (spike & true),* lemon, lime, mandarin, mint (peppermint & spearmint), myrtle, niaouli, orange (bitter & sweet), palmarosa, rose (cabbage & damask), *rosemary,* rosewood, ylang ylang.

Cuts/sores (S,C): Canadian balsam, benzoin, borneol, cabreuva, cade, *chamomile (German & Roman),* clove bud, elemi, eucalyptus (blue gum, lemon & peppermint), galbanum, geranium, helichrysum, hyssop, lavandin, *lavender (spike & true),* lemon, lime, linaloe, *marigold,* mastic, myrrh, niaouli, Scotch pine, Spanish sage, Levant styrax, *tea tree,* thyme, turpentine, vetiver, *yarrow.*

Dandruff (S,H): *West Indian bay,* cade, cedarwood (Atlas, Texas & Virginian), eucalyptus, *spike lavender,* lemon, patchouli, *rosemary,* sage (clary & Spanish), tea tree.

Dermatitis (M,S,C,F,B): White birch, cade, cananga, carrot seed, cedarwood (Atlas, Texas & Virginian), *chamomile (German & Roman),* geranium, *helichrysum,* hops, hyssop, juniper, *true lavender,* linaloe, litsea cubeba, mint (peppermint & spearmint), *palmarosa,* patchouli, rosemary, sage (clary & Spanish), thyme.

Dry & sensitive skin (M,S,F,B): Peru balsam, Tolu balsam, cassie, *chamomile (German & Roman)*, frankincense, *jasmine*, lavandin, lavender (spike & true), rosewood, *sandalwood*, violet.

Eczema (M,S,F,B): Lemon balm, Peru balsam, Tolu balsam, *bergamot*, white birch, cade, carrot seed, cedarwood (Atlas, Texas & Virginian), *chamomile (German & Roman)*, geranium, *helichrysum*, hyssop, juniper, lavandin, *lavender (spike & true)*, marigold, myrrh, *patchouli*, *rose (cabbage & damask)*, rosemary, Spanish sage, thyme, violet, yarrow.

Excessive perspiration (S,B): Citronella, *cypress*, lemongrass, litsea cubeba, petitgrain, Scotch pine, Spanish sage.

Greasy or oily skin/scalp (M,S,H,F,B): West Indian bay, *bergamot*, cajeput, camphor (white), cananga, carrot seed, citronella, *cypress*, sweet fennel, *geranium*, jasmine, juniper, *lavender*, lemon, lemongrass, litsea cubeba, mandarin, marigold, mimosa, myrtle, niaouli, palmarosa, patchouli, petitgrain, rosemary, rosewood, *sandalwood*, clary sage, *tea tree*, thyme, vetiver, ylang ylang.

Haemorrhoids/piles (S,C,B): Canadian balsam, Copaiba balsam, coriander, cubebs, *cypress*, geranium, *juniper*, *myrrh*, myrtle, parsley, *yarrow*.

Insect bites (S,N): *Lemon balm*, French basil, bergamot, cajeput, cananga, *chamomile (German & Roman)*, cinnamon leaf, eucalyptus blue gum, lavandin, *lavender (spike & true)*, lemon, marigold, niaouli, *tea tree*, thyme, ylang ylang.

Insect repellent (S,V): Lemon balm, French basil, bergamot, borneol, camphor (white), *Virginian cedarwood*, *citronella*, clove bud, cypress, eucalyptus (blue gum & lemon), geranium, *lavender*, lemongrass, litsea cubeba, mastic, patchouli, rosemary, turpentine.

Irritated & inflamed skin (S,C,F,B): Angelica, benzoin, camphor (white), Atlas cedarwood, *chamomile (German & Roman)*, elemi, helichrysum, hyssop, *jasmine*, lavandin, *true lavender*, *marigold*, *myrrh*, *patchouli*, *rose (cabbage & damask)*, clary sage, spikenard, tea tree, yarrow.

Lice (S,H): Cinnamon leaf, eucalyptus blue gum, galbanum, geranium, lavandin, *spike lavender* , parsley, Scotch pine, rosemary, thyme, turpentine.

Mouth & gum infections/ulcers (S,C): Bergamot,

cinnamon leaf, cypress, *sweet fennel*, lemon, mastic, *myrrh*, orange (bitter & sweet), sage (clary & Spanish), thyme.

Psoriasis (M,S,F,B): *Angelica*, *bergamot*, white birch, carrot seed, chamomile (German & Roman), *true lavender*.

Rashes (M,S,C,F,B): Peru balsam, *Tolu balsam*, carrot seed, *chamomile (German & Roman)*, hops, *true lavender*, *marigold*, sandalwood, spikenard, tea tree, yarrow.

Ringworm (S,H): Geranium, *spike lavender*, mastic, mint (peppermint & spearmint), *myrrh*, Levant styrax, *tea tree*, turpentine.

Scabies (S): Tolu balsam, bergamot, *cinnamon leaf*, lavandin, *lavender (spike & true)*, lemongrass, mastic, *mint (peppermint & spearmint)*, Scotch pine, rosemary, Levant styrax, thyme, turpentine.

Scars & stretch marks (M,S): Cabreuva, elemi, *frankincense*, galbanum, *true lavender*, mandarin, *orange blossom*, palmarosa, patchouli, rosewood, *sandalwood*, spikenard, violet, yarrow.

Slack tissue (M,S,B): Geranium, *grapefruit*, juniper, lemongrass, lime, mandarin, *sweet marjoram*, orange blossom, *black pepper*, petitgrain, rosemary, yarrow.

Spots (S,N): Bergamot, cade, cajeput, camphor (white), eucalyptus (lemon), helichrysum, lavandin, *lavender (spike & true)*, *lemon*, lime, litsea cubeba, mandarin, niaouli, *tea tree*.

Ticks (S,N): *Sweet marjoram*.

Toothache & teething pain (S,C,N): *Chamomile (German & Roman)*, *clove bud*, mastic, mint (peppermint & spearmint), *myrrh*.

Varicose veins (S,C): *Cypress*, lemon, lime, orange blossom, *yarrow*.

Veruccae (S,N): *Tagetes, tea tree*.

Warts & corns (S,N): Cinnamon leaf, *lemon*, lime, *tagetes, tea tree*.

Wounds (S,C,B): Canadian balsam, Peru balsam, Tolu balsam, bergamot, cabreuva, *chamomile (German & Roman)*, clove bud, cypress, elemi, *eucalyptus (blue gum & lemon)*, frankincense, galbanum, geranium, helichrysum, hyssop, juniper, lavandin, *lavender (spike & true)*, linaloe, marigold, mastic, *myrrh*, niaouli, patchouli, rosewood, Levant styrax, *tea tree*, turpentine, vetiver, *yarrow*.

Wrinkles & mature skin (M,S,F,B): Carrot seed, *elemi*, sweet fennel, *frankincense*, g*albanum*, geranium, jasmine, labdanum, true lavender, mandarin, mimosa, myrrh, *orange blossom*, palmarosa, patchouli, *rose (cabbage & damask)*, rosewood, clary sage, sandalwood, spikenard, ylang ylang.

Circulation, Muscles and Joints:

Accumulation of toxins (M,S,B): *Angelica, white birch, carrot seed*, celery seed, coriander, cumin, *sweet fennel, grapefruit, juniper*, lovage, parsley.

Aches and pains (M,C,B): Ambrette, star anise, aniseed, French basil, West Indian bay, cajeput, calamintha, camphor (white), *chamomile (German & Roman), coriander, eucalyptus (blue gum & peppermint)*, silver fir, galbanum, *ginger*, helichrysum, lavandin, *lavender (spike & true)*, lemongrass, *sweet marjoram*, mastic, mint (peppermint & spearmint), niaouli, nutmeg, *black pepper*, pine (longleaf & Scotch), *rosemary*, sage (clary & Spanish), hemlock spruce, thyme, turmeric, turpentine, vetiver.

Arthritis (M,S,C,B): Allspice, angelica, *benzoin*, white birch, cajeput, camphor (white), carrot seed, cedarwood (Atlas, Texas & Virginian), celery seed, *chamomile (German & Roman)*, clove bud, coriander, *eucalyptus (blue gum & peppermint)*, silver fir, *ginger*, guaiacwood, juniper, lemon, *sweet marjoram*, mastic, myrrh, nutmeg, parsley, *black pepper*, pine (longleaf & Scotch), *rosemary*, Spanish sage, thyme, tumeric, turpentine, vetiver, yarrow.

Cellulitis (M,S,B): *White birch*, cypress, *sweet fennel, geranium, grapefruit, juniper*, lemon, parsley, rosemary, thyme.

Debility/poor muscle tone (M,S,B): Allspice, ambrette, borneol, ginger, *grapefruit, sweet marjoram, black pepper*, pine (longleaf & Scotch), *rosemary*, Spanish sage.

Gout (M,S,B): *Angelica*, French basil, *benzoin, carrot seed*, celery seed, coriander, guaiacwood, *juniper*, lovage, mastic, pine (longleaf & Scotch), *rosemary*, thyme, turpentine.

High blood pressure & hypertension (M,B,V): Lemon balm, cananga, *garlic, true lavender*, lemon, *sweet marjoram*, clary sage, *yarrow, ylang ylang*.

Muscular cramp & stiffness (M,C,B): *Allspice*, ambrette, coriander, cypress, grapefruit, jasmine, lavandin, *lavender (spike & true), sweet marjoram, black pepper*, pine (longleaf & Scotch), *rosemary*, thyme, vetiver.

Obesity (M,B): *White birch, sweet fennel*, juniper, lemon, mandarin, orange (bitter & sweet).

Oedema & water retention (M,B): *Angelica, white birch, carrot seed*, cypress, *sweet fennel*, geranium, *grapefruit*, juniper, *lovage*, mandarin, orange (bitter & sweet), rosemary, Spanish sage.

Palpitations (M): Orange (bitter & sweet), orange blossom, rose (cabbage & damask), *ylang ylang*.

Poor circulation & low blood pressure (M,B): Ambrette, Peru balsam, West Indian bay, benzoin, white birch, borneol, cinnamon leaf, *coriander*, cumin, cypress, *eucalyptus blue gum*, galbanum, geranium, *ginger*, lemon, lemongrass, lovage, niaouli, nutmeg, orange blossom, *black pepper*, pine (longleaf & Scotch), rose (cabbage & damask), *rosemary, Spanish sage*, hemlock spruce, thyme, violet.

Rheumatism (M,C,B): Allspice, angelica, star anise, aniseed, Peru balsam, French basil, West Indian bay, benzoin, *white birch*, borneol, cajeput, calamintha, camphor (white), carrot seed, cedarwood (Atlas, Texas & Virginian), celery seed, *chamomile (German & Roman)*, cinnamon leaf, clove bud, coriander, *cypress, eucalyptus (blue gum & peppermint)*, sweet fennel, silver fir, galbanum, ginger, helichrysum, *juniper*, lavandin, *lavender (spike & true)*, lemon, lovage, *sweet marjoram*, mastic, niaouli, nutmeg, parsley, black pepper, *pine (longleaf & Scotch), rosemary*, Spanish sage, hemlock spruce, thyme, turmeric, turpentine, vetiver, violet, yarrow.

Sprains & strains (C): West Indian bay, borneol, camphor (white), *chamomile (German & Roman)*, clove bud, eucalyptus (blue gum & peppermint), ginger, helichrysum, jasmine, lavandin, *lavender (spike & true), sweet marjoram*, black pepper, pine (longleaf & Scotch), rosemary, thyme, turmeric, vetiver.

Respiratory System:

Asthma (M,V,I): Asafetida, lemon balm, Canadian balsam, Peru balsam, benzoin, cajeput, clove bud, costus, cypress, *elecampane*, eucalyptus (blue gum, lemon & peppermint), *frankincense*, galbanum, helichrysum, hops, hyssop, lavandin, *lavender (spike & true)*, lemon, lime, sweet marjoram, *mint (peppermint & spearmint)*, myrrh, myrtle, niaouli, pine (longleaf & Scotch), rose (cabbage & damask), rosemary, *sage (clary & Spanish)*, hemlock spruce, tea tree, thyme.

Bronchitis (M,V,I): Angelica, star anise, aniseed, asafetida, lemon balm, *Canadian balsam*, copaiba balsam, Peru balsam, Tolu balsam, French basil, *benzoin, borneol*, cajeput, camphor (white), caraway, cascarilla bark, cedarwood (Atlas, Texas & Virginian), clove bud, costus, cubebs, cypress, *elecampane*, elemi, *eucalyptus (blue gum & peppermint)*, silver fir, *frankincense*, galbanum, helichrysum, hyssop, labdanum, lavandin, lavender (spike & true), lemon, *sweet marjoram*, mastic, mint (peppermint & spearmint), *myrrh, myrtle*, niaouli, orange (bitter & sweet), pine (longleaf & Scotch), rosemary, *sandalwood*, hemlock spruce, Levant styrax, tea tree, thyme, turpentine, violet.

Catarrh (M,V,I): Canadian balsam, Tolu balsam, cajeput, cedarwood (Atlas, Texas & Virginian), cubebs, elecampane, elemi, *eucalyptus (blue gum & peppermint)*, frankincense, galbanum, ginger, hyssop, jasmine, lavandin, *lavender (spike & true)*, lemon, lime, mastic, *mint (peppermint & spearmint)*, myrrh, myrtle, niaouli, black pepper, *pine (longleaf & Scotch)*, sandalwood, Levant styrax, *tea tree, thyme*, turpentine, violet.

Chill (M,B): Copaiba balsam, benzoin, cabreuva, calamintha, camphor (white), *cinnamon leaf, ginger*, grapefruit, orange (bitter & sweet), *black pepper*.

Chronic coughs (M,V,I): Lemon balm, *Canadian balsam*, costus, cubebs, cypress, *elecampane*, elemi, *frankincense*, galbanum, helichrysum, hops, *hyssop*, jasmine, mint (peppermint & spearmint), *myrtle*, sandalwood, Levant styrax.

Coughs (M,V,I): Angelica, star anise, aniseed, *copaiba balsam, Peru balsam*, Tolu balsam, French basil, *benzoin*, borneol, cabreuva, cajeput, camphor (white), caraway, cascarilla bark, *Atlas cedarwood, eucalyptus (blue gum & peppermint)*, silver fir, ginger, *hyssop*, labdanum, *sweet marjoram*, myrrh, niaouli, black pepper, *pine (longleaf & Scotch)*, rose (cabbage & damask), rosemary, *sage (clary & Spanish), hemlock spruce*, tea tree.

Croup (M,I): *Tolu balsam*.

Earache (C): French basil, *chamomile (German & Roman), lavender (spike & true)*.

Halitosis/offensive breath (S): Bergamot, *cardomon, sweet fennel*, lavandin, lavender (spike & true), mint

(peppermint & spearmint), *myrrh*.

Laryngitis/hoarseness (I): *Tolu balsam, benzoin*, caraway, cubebs, lemon eucalyptus, frankincense, jasmine, lavandin, *lavender (spike & true)*, myrrh, sage (clary & Spanish), *sandalwood, thyme*.

Sinusitis (I): French basil, cajeput, cubebs, *eucalyptus blue gum*, silver fir, ginger, labdanum, *peppermint*, niaouli, *pine (longleaf & Scotch)*, tea tree.

Sore throat & throat infections (V,I): Canadian balsam, bergamot, cajeput, eucalyptus (blue gum, lemon & peppermint), geranium, ginger, *hyssop*, lavandin, lavender (spike & true), myrrh, myrtle, niaouli, pine (longleaf & Scotch), *sage (clary & Spanish)*, sandalwood, tea tree, *thyme*, violet.

Tonsillitis (I): Bay laurel, bergamot, geranium, hyssop, myrtle, sage (clary & Spanish), *thyme*.

Whooping cough (M,I): Asafetida, helichrysum, hyssop, *true lavender*, mastic, *niaouli*, rosemary, sage (clary & Spanish), *tea tree*, turpentine.

Digestive System:

Colic (M): Star anise, aniseed, lemon balm, calamintha, caraway, cardomon, carrot seed, *chamomile (German & Roman)*, clove bud, coriander, cumin, dill, sweet fennel, ginger, hyssop, lavandin, *lavender (spike & true)*, *sweet marjoram*, *mint (peppermint & spearmint)*, orange blossom, parsley, black pepper, rosemary, clary sage.

Constipation & sluggish digestion (M,B): Cinnamon leaf, cubebs, sweet fennel, lovage, sweet marjoram, nutmeg, orange (bitter & sweet), palmarosa, *black pepper*, tarragon, turmeric, yarrow.

Cramp/gastric spasm (M,C): *Allspice*, star anise, aniseed, caraway, cardomon, cinnamon leaf, coriander, costus, cumin, galbanum, *ginger*, lavandin, *lavender (spike & true)*, lovage, mint (peppermint & spearmint), orange (bitter & sweet), orange blossom, black pepper, *clary sage*, tarragon, lemon verbena, yarrow.

Griping pains (M): *Cardomon, dill, sweet fennel*, parsley.

Heartburn (M): *Cardomon*, black pepper.

Indigestion/flatulence (M): *Allspice*, angelica, *star anise, aniseed*, lemon balm, French basil, bay laurel, calamintha, *caraway, cardomon*, carrot seed, cascarilla bark, celery seed, *chamomile (German & Roman)*, cinnamon leaf, clove bud, coriander, costus, cubebs, cumin, dill, *sweet fennel*, galbanum, ginger, hops, hyssop, lavandin, *lavender (spike & true)*, lemongrass, linden, litsea cubeba, lovage, mandarin, *sweet marjoram, mint (peppermint & spearmint)*, myrrh, nutmeg, *orange (bitter & sweet)*, orange blossom, parsley, black pepper, petitgrain, rosemary, clary sage, tarragon, thyme, valerian, lemon verbena, yarrow.

Liver congestion (M): Carrot seed, celery seed, helichrysum, linden, rose (cabbage & damask), *rosemary*, Spanish sage, turmeric, lemon verbena.

Loss of appitite (M): Bay laurel, *bergamot*, caraway, cardomon, ginger, myrrh, black pepper.

Nausea/vomiting (M,V): Allspice, lemon balm, French basil, cardomom, cascarilla bark, *chamomile (German & Roman)*, clove bud, coriander, *sweet fennel*, ginger, lavandin, *lavender (spike & true), mint (peppermint & spearmint)*, nutmeg, black pepper, rose (cabbage & damask), rosewood, sandalwood.

Genito-urinary and Endocrine Systems:

Amenorrhoea/lack of menstruation (M,B): French basil, bay laurel, carrot seed, celery seed, cinnamon leaf, dill, sweet fennel, hops, hyssop, juniper, lovage, *sweet marjoram, myrrh*, parsley, rose (cabbage & damask), *sage (clary & Spanish)*, tarragon, yarrow.

Dysmenorrhoea/cramp, painful or difficult menstruation (M,C,B): Lemon balm, French basil, carrot seed, *chamomile (German & Roman)*, cypress, frankincense, hops, jasmine, juniper, lavandin, *lavender (spike & true)*, lovage, *sweet marjoram*, rose (cabbage & damask), rosemary, *sage (clary & Spanish)*, tarragon, yarrow.

Cystitis (C,B,D): Canadian balsam, copaiba balsam, *bergamot*, cedarwood (Atlas, Texas & Virginian), celery seed, *chamomile (German & Roman)*, cubebs, eucalyptus blue gum, frankincense, juniper, lavandin, *lavender (spike & true)*, lovage, mastic, niaouli, parsley, Scotch pine, *sandalwood*, tea tree, thyme, turpentine, yarrow.

Frigidity (M,S,B,V): Cassie, cinnamon leaf, *jasmine*, nutmeg, *orange blossom*, parsley, *patchouli*, black pepper, *cabbage rose*, rosewood, clary sage, sandalwood, *ylang ylang*.

Lack of nursing milk (M): Celery seed, dill, *sweet fennel*, hops.

Labour pain & childbirth aid (M,C,B): Cinnamon leaf, *jasmine, true lavender, nutmeg*, parsley, *rose (cabbage & damask)*, clary sage.

Leucorrhoea/white discharge from the vagina (B,D): *Bergamot*, cedarwood (Atlas, Texas & Virginian), cinnamon leaf, cubebs, eucalyptus blue gum, frankincense, hyssop, lavandin, *lavender (spike & true)*, sweet marjoram, mastic, *myrrh*, rosemary, clary sage, *sandalwood*, tea tree, turpentine.

Menopausal problems (M,B,V): Cypress, sweet fennel, *geranium*, jasmine, *rose (cabbage & damask)*.

Menorrhagia/excessive menstruation (M,B): Chamomile (German & Roman), *cypress, rose (cabbage & damask)*.

Premenstrual tension /PMT (M,B,V): Carrot seed, *chamomile (German & Roman)*, geranium, *true lavender*, sweet marjoram, orange blossom, tarragon.

Pruritis/itching (D): *Bergamot*, Atlas cedarwood, juniper, *lavender, myrrh, tea tree*.

Sexual overactivity (M,B): Hops, *sweet marjoram*.

Thrush/candida (B,D): Bergamot, geranium, myrrh, *tea tree*.

Urethritis (B,D): Bergamot, cubebs, mastic, *tea tree*, turpentine.

Immune System:

Chickenpox (C,S,B): Bergamot, chamomile (German & Roman), eucalyptus (blue gum & lemon), *true lavender, tea tree*.

Colds/'flu (M,B,V,I): Angelica, star anise, aniseed, copaiba balsam, Peru balsam, French basil, bay laurel, West Indian bay, bergamot, *borneol*, cabreuva, cajeput, camphor (white), caraway, cinnamon leaf, citronella, clove bud, coriander, *eucalyptus (blue gum, lemon & peppermint)*, silver fir, frankincense, ginger, grapefruit, helichrysum, juniper, lemon, lime, sweet marjoram, mastic, mint (peppermint & spearmint), myrtle, *niaouli*, orange (bitter & sweet), *pine (longleaf & Scotch)*, rosemary, rosewood, *Spanish sage*, hemlock spruce, *tea tree, thyme*, turpentine, yarrow.

Fever (C,B): French basil, bergamot, borneol, camphor (white), *eucalyptus (blue gum, lemon & peppermint)*, silver fir, ginger, helichrysum, juniper, lemon, lemongrass, lime, *mint (peppermint & spearmint)*, myrtle, niaouli, *rosemary*, rosewood, Spanish sage, hemlock spruce, *tea tree*, thyme, *yarrow*.

Measles (S,B,I,V): Bergamot, *eucalyptus blue gum*, lavender (spike & true), *tea tree*.

Nervous System:

Anxiety (M,B,V): Ambrette, *lemon balm*, French basil, *bergamot*, cananga, *frankincense*, hyssop, *jasmine*, juniper, *true lavender*, mimosa, orange blossom, hemlock spruce, Levant styrax, lemon verbena, *ylang ylang*.

Depression (M,B,V): Allspice, ambrette, lemon balm, Canadian balsam, French basil, *bergamot*, cassie, grapefruit, helichrysum, *jasmine*, *true lavender*, *orange blossom*, *rose (cabbage & damask)*, clary sage, *sandalwood*, hemlock spruce, vetiver, *ylang ylang*.

Headache (M,C,V): *Chamomile (German & Roman)*, citronella, cumin, eucalyptus (blue gum & peppermint), grapefruit, hops, lavandin, *lavender (spike & true)*, lemongrass, linden, sweet marjoram, *mint (peppermint & spearmint)*, rose (cabbage & damask), rosemary, rosewood, sage (clary & Spanish), thyme, violet.

Insomnia (M,B,V): *Lemon balm*, French basil, calamintha, *chamomile (German & Roman)*, *hops*, *true lavender*, *linden*, mandarin, sweet marjoram, *orange blossom*, petitgrain, rose (cabbage & damask), sandalwood, thyme, *valerian*, lemon verbena, vetiver, violet, yarrow, ylang ylang.

Migraine (C): Angelica, lemon balm, French basil, chamomile (German & Roman), citronella, coriander, *true lavender*, linden, sweet marjoram, mint (peppermint & spearmint), clary sage, valerian, yarrow.

Nervous exhaustion or fatigue/debility (M,B,V): Allspice, *angelica*, asafetida, *French basil*, *borneol*, cardomon, cassie, cinnamon leaf, citronella, coriander, costus, cumin, elemi, eucalyptus (blue gum & peppermint), ginger, grapefruit, helichrysum, hyacinth, hyssop, *jasmine*, lavandin, spike lavender, lemongrass, *mint (peppermint & spearmint)*, nutmeg, palmarosa, patchouli, petitgrain, Scotch pine, *rosemary*, *sage (clary & Spanish)*, thyme, *vetiver*, violet, ylang ylang.

Neuralgia/sciatica (M,B): Allspice, West Indian bay, borneol, celery seed, *chamomile (German & Roman)*, citronella, coriander, eucalyptus (blue gum & peppermint), geranium, helichrysum, hops, *spike lavender*, *sweet marjoram*, mastic, mint (peppermint & spearmint), nutmeg, pine (longleaf & Scotch), *rosemary*, turpentine.

Nervous tension and stress (M,B,V): Allspice, ambrette, angelica, asafetida, *lemon balm*, Canadian balsam, copaiba balsam, Peru balsam, French basil, *benzoin*, *bergamot*, borneol, calamintha, cananga, cardomon, cassie, *cedarwood (Atlas, Texas & Virginian)*, *chamomile (German & Roman)*, cinnamon leaf, costus, *cypress*, elemi, *frankincense*, galbanum, geranium, helichrysum, *hops*, hyacinth, hyssop, *jasmine*, juniper, *true lavender*, lemongrass, linaloe, *linden*, mandarin, *sweet marjoram*, mimosa, mint (peppermint & spearmint), orange (bitter & sweet), *orange blossom*, palmarosa, *patchouli*, petitgrain, Scotch pine, *rose (cabbage & damask)*, rosemary, rosewood, *clary sage*, *sandalwood*, hemlock spruce, thyme, valerian, lemon verbena, *vetiver*, violet, yarrow, *ylang ylang*.

Shock (M,B,V): *Lemon balm*, lavandin, lavender (spike & true), *orange blossom*.

Vertigo (V,I): Lemon balm, lavandin, *lavender (spike & true)*, *mint (peppermint & spearmint)*, violet.

General Glossary

Abortifacient: capable of inducing abortion.

Absolute: a highly concentrated viscous, semi-solid or solid perfume material, usually obtained by alcohol extraction from the concrete.

Acrid: leaving a burning sensation in the mouth.

Aerophagy: swallowing of air.

Allergy: hypersensitivity caused by a foreign substance, small doses of which produce a violent bodily reaction.

Alliaceous: garlic or onionlike.

Alopecia: baldness, loss of hair.

Alterative: corrects disordered bodily function.

Amenorrhoea: absence of menstruation.

Amoebicidal: a substance with the power of destroying amoebae.

Anaemia: deficiency in either quality or quantity of red corpuscles in the blood.

Anaemic: relating to anaemia, caused by or suffering from anaemia.

Anaesthetic: loss of feeling or sensation; substance which causes such a loss.

Analgesic: remedy or agent which deadens pain.

Anaphrodisiac: reduces sexual desire.

Annual: refers to a plant which completes its life cycle in one year.

Anodyne: stills pain and quiets disturbed feelings.

Anorexia: condition of being without, or having lost the appetite for food.

Anthelmintic: a vermifuge, destroying or expelling intestinal worms.

Anti-anaemic: an agent which combats anaemia.

Anti-arthritic: an agent which combats arthritis.

Antibilious: an agent which helps remove excess bile from the body.

Antibiotic: prevents the growth of, or destroys, bacteria.

Anticatarrhal: an agent which helps remove excess catarrh from the body.

Anticonvulsant: helps arrest or prevent convulsions.

Antidepressant: helps alleviate depression.

Antidiarrhoeal: efficacious against diarrhoea.

Anti-emetic: an agent which reduces the incidence and severity of nausea or vomiting.

Antihaemorrhagic: an agent which prevents or combats haemorrhage or bleeding.

Antihistamine: treats allergic conditions; counteracts effects of histamine (which produces capillary dilation and, in larger doses, haemoconcentration).

Anti-inflammatory: alleviates inflammation.

Antilithic: prevents the formation of a calculus or stone.

Antimicrobial: an agent which resists or destroys pathogenic micro-organisms.

Antineuralgic: relieves or reduces nerve pain.

Anti-oxidant: a substance used to prevent or delay oxidation or deterioration, especially with exposure to air.

Antiphlogistic: checks or counteracts inflammation.

Antipruritic: relieves sensation of itching or prevents its occurrence.

Antiputrescent: an agent which prevents and combats decay or putrefaction.

Antipyretic: reduces fever; *see also* febrifuge.

Antirheumatic: helps prevent and relieve rheumatism.

Antisclerotic: helps prevent the hardening of tissue.

Antiscorbutic: a remedy for scurvy.

Antiscrofula: combats the development of tuberculosis of lymph nodes (scrofula).

Antiseborrhoeic: helps control the production of sebum, the oily secretion from sweat glands.

Antiseptic: destroys and prevents the development of microbes.

Antispasmodic: prevents and eases spasms or convulsions.

Antitoxic: an antidote or treatment that counteracts the effects of poison.

Antitussive: relieves coughs.

Antiviral: substance which inhibits the growth of a virus.

Aperient: a mild laxative.

Aphonia: loss of voice.

Aperitif: a stimulant of the appetite.

Aphrodisiac: increases or stimulates sexual desire.

Apoplexy: sudden loss of consciousness, a stroke or sudden severe haemorrhage.

Aril: the husk or membrane covering the seed of a plant.

Aromatherapy: the therapeutic use of essential oils.

Aromatic: a substance with a strong aroma or smell.

Arteriosclerosis: loss of elasticity in the walls of the arteries due to thickening and calcification.

Arthritis: inflammation of a joint or joints.

Asthenia: *see* debility.

Astringent: causes contraction of organic tissues.

Atony: lessening or lack of muscular tone or tension.

Axil: upper angle between a stem and leaf or bract.

Bactericidal: an agent that destroys bacteria (a type of microbe or organism).

Balsam: a resinous semi-solid mass or viscous liquid exuded from a plant, which can be either a pathological or physiological product. A 'true' balsam is characterized by its high content of benzoic acid, benzoates, cinnamic acid or cinnamates.

Balsamic: a soothing medicine or application having the qualities of a balsam.

Bechic: anything which relieves or cures coughs; or referring to cough.

Biennial: a plant which completes its life cycle in two years, without flowering in the first year.

Bilious: a condition caused by an excessive secretion of bile.

Bitter: a tonic component which stimulates the appetite and promotes the secretion of saliva and gastric juices by exciting the taste buds.

Blenorrhoea: abnormally free secretion and discharge of mucus, sometimes from the genitals (as in gonorrhoea).

Blepharitis: inflammation of the eyelids.

Calculus: a solid pathological concentration (or 'stone'), usually of inorganic matter in a matrix of protein and pigment, formed in any part of the body.

Calmative: a sedative.

Calyx: the sepals or outer layer of floral leaves.

Capsule: a dry fruit, opening when ripe, composed of more than one carpel.

Cardiac: pertaining to the heart.

Cardiotonic: having a stimulating effect on the heart.

Carminative: settles the digestive system, relieves flatulence.

Catarrh: inflammation of mucous membranes, usually associated with an increase in secretion of mucus.

Cathartic: purgative, capable of causing a violent purging or catharsis of the body.

Cellulite: accumulation of toxic matter in the form of fat in the tissue.

Cephalic: remedy for disorders of the head; referring or directed towards the head.

Cerebral: pertaining to the largest part of the brain, the cerebrum.

Chemotype: the same botanical species occurring in other forms due to different conditions of growth, such as climate, soil, altitude, etc.

Chlorosis: a form of anaemia rarely encountered nowadays.

Cholagogue: stimulates the secretion and flow of bile into the duodenum.

Cholecystokinetic: agent which stimulates the contraction of the gall bladder.

Choleretic: aids excretion of bile by the liver, so there is a greater flow of bile.

Cholesterol: a steroid alcohol found in nervous tissue, red blood cells, animal fat and bile. Excess can lead to gallstones.

Cicatrisant: an agent which promotes healing by the formation of scar tissue.

Cirrhosis: degenerative change in any organ (especially liver), caused by various poisons, bacteria or other agents, resulting in fibrous tissue overgrowth.

Colic: pain due to contraction of the involuntary muscle of the abdominal organs.

Colitis: inflammation of the colon.

Compress: a lint or substance applied hot or cold to an area of the body, for relief of swelling and pain, or to produce localized pressure.

Concrete: a concentrated, waxy, solid or semi-solid perfume material prepared from previously live plant matter, usually using a hydrocarbon type of solvent.

Constipation: congestion of the bowels; incomplete or infrequent action of bowels.

Contagious disease: a disease spreading from person to person by direct contact.

Cordial: a stimulant and tonic.

Corolla: the petals of a flower considered as a whole.

Counter-irritant: applications to the skin which relieve deep-seated pain, usually applied in the form of heat; *see also* rubefacient.

Cutaneous: pertaining to the skin.

Cystitis: bladder inflammation, usually characterized by pain on urinating.

Cytophylactic: referring to cytophylaxis – the process of increasing the activity of leucocytes in defence of the body against infection.

Cytotoxic: toxic to all cells.

Debility: weakness, lack of tone.

Decoction: a herbal preparation, where the plant material (usually hard or woody) is boiled in water and reduced to make a concentrated extract.

Decongestive: an agent for the relief or reduction of congestion, e.g. mucous.

Demulcent: a substance which protects mucous membranes and allays irritation.

Depurative: helps combat impurity in the blood and organs; detoxifying.

Deodorant: an agent which corrects, masks or removes unpleasant odours.

Dermal: pertaining to the skin.

Dermatitis: inflammation of the skin; many causes.

Diaphoretic: *see* sudorific.

Diarrhoea: frequent passage of unformed liquid stools.

Digestive: substance which promotes or aids the digestion of food.

Disinfectant: prevents and combats the spread of germs.

Diuretic: aids production of urine, promotes urination, increases flow.

Dropsy: excess of fluid in the tissues; *see also* oedema.

Drupe: a fleshy fruit, with one or more seeds, each surrounded bt a stony layer.

Dysmenorrhoea: painful and difficult menstruation.

Dyspepsia: difficulty with digestion associated with pain, flatulence, heartburn and nausea.

Elliptical: shaped like an ellipse, or regular curve.

Emetic: induces vomiting.

Emmenagogue: induces or assists menstruation.

Emollient: softens and soothes the skin.

Emphysema: condition in which the alveoli of the lungs are dilated, or an abnormal amount of air is present in tissues of body cavities.

Engorgement: congestion of a part of the tissues, or fullness (as in the breasts).

Enteritis: inflammation of the mucous membrane of the intestine.

Enzyme: complex proteins that are produced by living cells, and catalyse specific biochemical reactions.

Erythema: a superficial redness of the skin due to excess of blood.

Essential oil: a volatile and aromatic liquid (sometimes semi-solid) which generally constitutes the odorous principles of a plant. It is obtained by a process of expression or distillation from a single botanical form or species.

Expectorant: helps promote the removal of mucous from the respiratory system.

Febrifuge: combats fever.

Fixative: a material which slows down the rate of evaporation of the more volatile components in a perfume composition.

Fixed oil: a name given to vegetable oils obtained from plants which, in contradistinction to essential oils, are fatty, dense and non-volatile, such as olive or sweet almond oil.

Florets: the small individual flowers in the flowerheads of the Compositae family.

Follicle: a dry, one celled, many-seeded fruit.

Fungicidal: prevents and combats fungal infection.

Galactagogue: increases secretion of milk.

Gastritis: inflammation of stomach lining.

Genito-urinary: referring to both the genital and reproductive systems.

Germicidal: destroys germs or micro-organisms such as bacteria, etc.

Gingivitis: inflammation of the gums, manifested by swelling and bleeding.

Gout: a disease which involves excess uric acid in the blood.

Gums: 'true' gums are little used in perfumery, being virtually odourless. However, the term 'gum' is often applied to 'resins', especially with relation to turpentines, as in the Australian 'gum tree'. Strictly speaking, gums are natural or synthetic water-soluble materials, such as gum arabic.

Haematuria: blood in the urine.

Halitosis: offensive breath.

Hallucinogenic: causes visions or delusions.

Haemorrhoids: piles, dilated rectal veins.

Haemostatic: arrests bleeding.

Heartwood: the central portion of a tree trunk.

Hepatic: relating to the liver (tones and aids its fuction).

Herpes: inflammation of the skin or mucous membrane with clusters of deep-seated vesicles.

Hormone: a product of living cells which produces a specific effect on the activity of cells remote from its point of origin.

Hybrid: a plant originating by fertilization of one species or subspecies by another.

Hypertension: raised blood pressure.

Hypertensive: agent which raises blood pressure.

Hypnotic: causing sleep.

Hypocholesterolaemia: lowering the cholesterol content of the blood.

Hypoglycaemia: lowered blood sugar levels or concentration.

Hypotension: low blood pressure, or a fall in blood pressure below the normal range.

Hypotensive: agent which lowers blood pressure.

Hysteria: a psychoneurosis manifesting itself in various disorders of the mind or body.

Inflorescence: flowering structure above the last stem leaves (including bracts and flowers).

Infusion: a herbal remedy prepared by steeping the plant material in water.

Insecticide: repels insects.

Insomnia: inability to sleep.

Lanceolate: lance-shaped, oval and pointed at both ends (usually a leaf shape).

Larvicidal: an agent which prevents and kills larvae.

Laxative: promotes evacuation of the bowels.

Legume: a fruit consisting of one carpel, opening on one side, such as a pea.

Leucocyte: white blood cells responsible for fighting disease.

Leucocytosis: an increase in the number of white blood cells above the normal limit.

Leucorrhoea: white discharge from the vagina.

Ligulet: a narrow projection from the top of a leaf sheath in grasses.

Linear: of leaves, narrow and more or less parallel-sided.

Lipolytic: causing lipolysis, the chemical disintegration or splitting of fats.

Lithuria: a morbid condition marked by the presence of excessive amounts of uric acid in the urine.

Lumbago: a painful rheumatic affliction of the muscles and fibrous tissue of the lumbar region of the back.

Lymphatic: pertaining to the lymph system.

Macerate: soak until soft.

Menopause: the normal cessation of menstruation, a life change for women.

Menorrhagia: excessive menstruation.

Metrorrhagia: uterine bleeding outside the menstrual cycle.

Microbe: a minute living organism, especially pathogenic bacteria, viruses, etc.

Mucilage: a substance containing gelatinous constituents which are demulcent.

Mucolytic: dissolving or breaking down mucous.

Narcotic: a substance which induces sleep; intoxicating or poisonous in large doses.

Nervine: strengthening and toning to the nerves and nervous system.

Nephritis: inflammation of the kidneys.

Neuralgia: a stabbing pain along a nerve pathway.

Neurasthenia: nervous exhaustion.

Oedema: a painless swelling caused by fluid retention beneath the skin's surface.

Oestrogen: a hormone produced by the ovary, necessary for the development of female secondary sexual characteristics.

Oleo gum resin: a natural exudation from trees and plants that consists mainly of essential oil, gum and resin.

Oleoresin: a natural resinous exudation from plants, or an aromatic liquid preparation, extracted from botanical matter using solvents. They consist almost entirely of a mixture of essential oil and resin.

Olfaction: the sense of smell.

Ophthalmia: inflammation of the eye, a term usually applied to conjunctivitis.

Otitis: inflammation of the ear.

Ovate: egg-shaped.

Palpitation: undue awareness of the heartbeat, occasioned by anxiety. Rapid heart beats or abnormal rhythm.

Panacea: a cure-all.

Pappus: the calyx in a composite flower having feathery hairs, scales or bristles.

Parasiticide: prevents and destroys parasites such as fleas, lice, etc.

Parturient: aiding childbirth.

Pathogenic: causing or producing disease.

Pathological: unnatural or destructive process on living tissue.

Pediculicide: an agent which destroys lice.

Peptic: applied to gastric secretions and areas affected by them.

Perennial: a plant which lives for more than two years, normally flowering every year.

Petiole: the stalk of a leaf.

Pharmacology: medical science of drugs which deals with their actions, properties and characteristics.

Pharmacopoeia: an official publication of drugs in common use, in a given country.

Physiological: describes the natural biological processes of a living organism.

Phytohormones: plant substances that mimic the action of human hormones.

Phytotherapy: the treatment of disease by plants; herbal medicine.

Pinnate: a leaf composed of more than three leaflets arranged in two rows along a common stalk.

Pomade: a prepared perfume material obtained by the enfleurage process.

Poultice: the therapeutic application of a soft moist mass (such as fresh herbs) to the skin, to encourage local circulation and to relieve pain.

Prophylactic: preventive of disease or infection.

Prostatitis: any inflammatory condition of the prostate gland.

Prurigo: chronic skin disease with irritation, itching and papular eruption.

Pruritis: itching.

Psoriasis: a skin disease characterized by red patches and silver scaling.

Psychosomatic: the manifestation of physical symptoms resulting from a mental state.

Pulmonary: pertaining to the lungs.

Purgative: a substance stimulating an evacuation of the bowels.

Pyelitis: inflammation of the kidney.

Pyorrhoea: bleeding or a discharge of pus.

Raceme: an inflorescence, usually conical in outline in which the lowest flowers open first.

Receptacle: the upper part of the stem from which the floral parts arise.

Rectification: the process of redistillation applied to essential oils to rid them of certain constituents.

Refrigerant: cooling – reduces fever.

Regulator: an agent that helps balance and regulate the functions of the body.

Relaxant: soothing, causing relaxation, relieving strain or tension.

Renal: pertaining to the kidney.

Resins: a natural or prepared product, either solid or semi-solid in nature. Natural resins are exudations from trees, such as mastic; prepared resins are oleoresins from which the essential oil has been removed.

Resinoids: a perfumery material prepared from natural resinous mattter, such as balsams, gum resins, etc., by extraction with a hydrocarbon type of solvent.

Resolvent: an agent which disperses swelling, or effects absorption of a new growth.

Restorative: an agent that helps strengthen and revive the body systems.

Revulsive: relieves pain by means of the diversion of blood or disease from one part of the body to another; *see also* counter-irritant.

Rhinitis: inflammation of the mucous membrane of the nose.

Rhizome: an underground stem lasting more than one season.

Rosette: leaves which are closely arranged in a spiral.

Rubefacient: a substance which causes redness of the skin, possibly irritation.

Sciatica: pain down the back of the legs, in the area supplied by the sciatic nerve, due to various causes including pressure on the nerve roots.

Sclerosis: hardening of tissue due to inflammation.

Scrofula: an outdated name for tuberculosis.

Seborrhoea: increased secretion of sebum, usually associated with excessive oily secretion from the sweat glands.

Sedative: an agent which reduces functional activity; calming.

Sessile: without a stalk.

Sialogogue: an agent that stimulates the secretion of saliva.

Soporific: a substance which induces sleep.

Spasmolytic: *see* antispasmodic.

Spike: an inflorescence in which the sessile flowers are arranged in a raceme.

Splenic: relating to the spleen, the largest endocrine gland.

Splenitis: inflammation of the spleen.

Stimulant: an agent which quickens the physiological functions of the body.

Stomachic: digestive aid and tonic; improving appetite.

Styptic: an astringent agent which stops or reduces external bleeding.

Sudorific: an agent which causes sweating.

Synergy: agents working together harmoniously; coordination in the action of muscles, organs or substances such as drugs.

Tachycardia: abnormally increased heartbeat and pulse rate.

Tannin: a substance which has an astringent action, and helps seal the tissue.

Thrombosis: formation of a thrombus or blood clot.

Thrush: an infection of the mouth or vaginal region caused by a fungus (candida).

Tincture: a herbal remedy, or perfumery material prepared in an alcohol base.

Tonic: strengthens and enlivens the whole or specific parts of the body.

Tracheitis: inflammation of the windpipe.

Trifoliate: a plant having three distinct leaflets.

Tuber: a swollen part of an underground stem of one year's duration, capable of new growth.

Umbel: umbrella-like; a flower where the petioles all arise from the top of the stem

Uterine: pertaining to the uterus.

Urticaria: hives, nettle rash, acute or chronic affection of the skin characterized by the formation of weals, attended by itching, stinging or burning.

Vasoconstrictor: an agent which causes narrowing of the blood vessels.

Vasodilator: an agent which dilates the blood vessels.

Vermifuge: expels intestinal worms.

Vesicant: causing blistering to the skin; a counter-irritant.

Vesicle: a small blister or sac containing fluid.

Volatile: unstable, evaporates easily, as in 'volatile oil'; *see* essential oil.

Vulnerary: an agent which helps heal wounds and sores by external application.

Whorl: a circle of leaves around a node.

Botanical Classification

The following list is based on the work of Arthur O. Tucker and Brian M. Lawrence published in *Herbs, Spices and Medicinal Plants Vol II*, Oryx Press, 1987, as the 'Botanical Nomenclature of Commercial Sources of Essential Oils, Concretes and Absolutes'. It represents an up-to-date survey of aromatic materials currently produced commercially, in which the botanical names are in accordance with the recent guidelines set out by the International Organization for Standardization.

Parmeliaceae
Parmelia cirrhata (P. nepalensis): Indian moss.

Usneaceae
Evernia furfuraceae: Tree moss.
Evernia prunastri: Oakmoss.
Ramalina fastigiata: Chinese moss.
Ramalina subcomplanata: Indian moss.
Usnea barbata is harvested with *Evernia furfurcea* as Tree moss.
Usnea lucea is harvested with *Ramalina subcomplanata* as Haraphool.

Pinaceae
Abies alba (A. pectinata): Silver fir, white fir, silver spruce, European silver fir, white spruce.
Abies balsamea (A. balsamifera, Pinus balsamea): Balsam fir, Canadian balsam, balsam tree, American silver fir, balm of gilead fir, Canada turpentine (oil)
Abies sachalinensis: Sachalin fir, Japanese fir needle (oil).
Abies mayriana: Mayr Sakhalin fir, Japanese fir needle (oil).
Abies sibirica: Siberian fir, Siberian 'pine' (oil).
Cedrus atlantica: Atlantic cedar, Atlas cedar, African cedar, Moroccan cedarwood (oil), libanol (oil).
Cedrus deodara (C. deodorata): Deodar cedar, Himalayan cedar.
Cedrus libani: Cedar of Lebanon.
Picea abies (P. excelsa): Norway spruce, common spruce, burgundy pitch (oil), Jura turpentine (oil).
Picea glauca (P. alba, P. canadensis): White spruce, Canadian spruce.
Picea jezoensis: Yeddo spruce, Yezo spruce.
Picea mariana (P. nigra): Black spruce, Canadian black 'pine'.
Pinus ayacahuite: Mexican white pine, turpentine (oil).
Pinus contorta var. latifolia: Lodgepole pine, turpentine (oil); other subspecies exist.

Pinus elliottii (P. caribaea): Slash pine, turpentine (oil); other subspecies exist.
Pinus halepensis: Aleppo pine, Jerusalem pine.
Pinus insularis (P. khasya, P. kesiya, P. khasyana, P. langbianensis): Khasi pine, Benguet pine, Indian turpentine (oil).
Pinus koraiensis: Korean pine.
Pinus massoniana: Masson pine, southern red pine, turpentine (oil).
Pinus merkusii (P. latteri): Merkus pine.
Pinus mugo (P. montana): Mountain pine, Swiss mountain pine; other subspecies exist including
   var. mughus (P. mughus): Mugho pine
   var. pumilio (P. pumilio): Dwarf pine, pine needle (oil)
Pinus nigra: Austrian pine, black pine; other subspecies exist.
Pinus palustris: Longleaf pine, longleaf yellow pine, southern yellow pine, pitch pine, gum turpentine (oil).
Pinus pinaster: Sea pine, turpentine (oil).
Pinus ponderosa: Ponderosa pine, western yellow pine; other subspecies exist.
Pinus radiata: Monterey pine, New Zealand turpentine (oil).
Pinus roxburghii: Chir pine, Indian turpentine (oil).
Pinus strobus: White pine, Canadian white pine; many subspecies exist.
Pinus sylvestris: Scotch pine, turpentine (oil); many subspecies and cultivars exist.
Pinus tabulaeformis: Chinese pine.
Pinus yunnanensis: Yunnan pine, Chinese pine.
Pseudotsuga menziesii (P. taxifolia): Douglas fir, Oregon balsam (oil); two main subspecies exist *var. menziesii:* Coast Douglas fir.
   var. glauca: Rocky Mountain Douglas fir.
Tsuga canadensis (Pinus canadensis, Abies canadensis): Hemlock, eastern hemlock, common hemlock, spruce (oil); many cultivars exist.

Taxodiaceae
Cryptomeria japonica: Cryptomeria, Japanese cedar, sugi; many cultivars exist.

Cupressaceae
Chamaecyparis funebris (Cupressus funebris): Mourning cypress, Chinese weeping cypress, Chinese cedarwood (oil).
Chamaecyparis lawsoniana: Port Orford cedar, Oregon cedar, Lawson false cypress; numerous cultivars exist.

Chamaecyparis nootkatensis: Alaska cedar, Alaska yellow cedar, yellow cedar.

Chamaecyparis obtusa exists in two varieties:
    var. obtusa: Hinoki false cypress
    var. formosana (C. taiwanensis): Formosan hinoki.

Cupressus lusitanica: Kenya cypress

Cupressus sempervirens: Mediterranean cypress; many cultivars exist, the most common being 'Stricta', the Italian cypress.

Cupressus torulosa: Himalayan cypress.

Juniperus ashei (J. mexicana): Mountain cedar, rock cedar, Mexican cedar, Mexican juniper.

Juniperus communis: Juniper, common juniper; many cultivars exist such as
    var. depressa: Canadian juniper
    var. communis (var. erecta).

Juniperus oxycedrus: Prickly juniper, cade juniper, juniper tar, cade (oil), prickly cedar, medlar tree.

Juniperus phoenicea: Phoenician juniper, Phoenician savin (oil).

Juniperus sabina (Sabina cacumina): Savin juniper, savin (oil); many cultivars exist.

Juniperus smerka: Yugoslavian juniper.

Juniperus squamata (J. recurva var. squamata): Single-seed juniper, scaly-leaved Nepal juniper; several cultivars exist.

Juniperus virginiana: Eastern red cedar, red cedar, southern red cedar, Bedford cedarwood (oil),Virginian cedarwood (oil); many cultivars exist.

Neocallitropsis pancheri (N. araucarioides, Callitropsis araucarioides): Pancher neocallitropsis, araucaria (oil).

Thuja occidentalis: Northern white cedar, white cedar, eastern white cedar, American arborvitae, thuja, swamp cedar, cedarleaf (oil); many cultivars exist.

Thuja orientalis (Biota orientalis): Chinese or Japanese cedar

Thuja plicata: Western red cedar, western arborvitae, Washington cedar.

Thujopsis dolobrata: Hiba; two varieties exist:
    var. dolobrata: Azunaro
    var. hondae: Hinoki-asunaro.

Widdringtonia cupressoides (W. dracomontana, W. whytei): Mountain widdringtonia, mlange cedar.

Podocarpaceae

Dacrydium franklinii: Huon pine, huon dacrydium.

Araucariaceae

Agathis australis: Kauri, kauri pine, New Zealand kauri.

Pandanaceae

Pandanus fascicularis (P. odoratissimus): Padang, attar of kewda (oil), attar of keora (oil).

Poaceae (Gramineae)

Anthoxanthum odoratum: Sweet vernalgrass, flouve (oil).

Cymbopogon citratus (Andropogon citratus, A. schoenathus): West Indian lemongrass, Madagascar lemongrass, Guatemala lemongrass.

Cymbopogon flexuosus (Andropogon flexuosus): East Indian lemongrass.

Cymbopogon martinii (Andropogon martinii): Rosha; this species occurs in two eco-chemotypes:
    var. martinii (var. motia): Palmarosa, motia, East Indian geranium, Turkish geranium, Indian rosha
    var. sofia: Gingergrass, sofia.

Cymbopogon nardus (Andropogon nardus): Citronella; this exists in two varieties:
    var. nardus: Ceylon citronella, Lenabatu citronella.
    var. confertiflorus.

Cymbopogon pendulus (Andropogon pendulus): Jammu lemongrass.

Cymbopogon winterianus: Java citronella.

Vetiveria zizanoides (Andropogon muricatus): Vetiver, khus khus, vetivert (oil).

Cyperaceae

Cyperus mitis (C. scariosus sensu): Nagar motha.

Cyperus rotundus: Nut-grass, coco-grass.

Araceae

Acorus calamus var. angustatus (Calamus aromaticus): Sweet flag, calamus, sweet sedge, sweet root, sweet rush, sweet cane, sweet myrtle, myrtle grass, myrtle sedge, cinnamon sedge; several varieties exist.

Liliaceae

Allium cepa: Onion; numerous cultivars exist.

Allium fistulosum: Welsh onion, cibol, stone leek.

Allium kurrat (A. porrum var. aegyptiacum): kurrat.

Allium sativum: Garlic, allium, poor man's treacle; three varieties exist:
    var. sativum: Cultivated garlic
    var. ophioscorodon: Serpent garlic, giant garlic, rocambole
    var. pekinense: Peking garlic.

Allium schoenoprasum: Chives, cive; two varieties exist:
    var. schoenoprasum: Cultivated chives
    var. alpinum (A. sibiricum): Large chives.

Allium scorodoprasum: Sand leek; several subspecies exist.

Allium tricoccum: Ramps, wild leek.

Allium tuberosum (A. odorum): Chinese chives, garlic chives, oriental garlic.

Hyacinthus orientalis (Scilla nutans): Hyacinth, bluebell.

Smilaceae
Smilax medica (S. aristolochiaefolia): Mexican
    sarsaparilla; several subspecies exist.

Amaryllidaceae
Narcissus jonquilla: Jonquil.
Narcissus poeticus: Poet's narcissus, pheasant's eye;
    two subspecies exist:
    var. poeticus
    var. radiiflorus.

Agavaceae
Polianthes tuberosa (Polyanthes tuberosa): Tuberose.

Iridaceae
Iris florentina: Florentine orris, orris root.
Iris germanica: German iris, flag iris, orris root.
Iris pallida: Pale iris, orris root.

Zingiberaceae
*Alpinia officinarum (Languas officinarum, Radix
    galanga minoris):* Galanga, lesser galangal, Chinese
    ginger, small ginger, East Indian ginger, colic root,
    ginger root.
*Curcuma longa (C. domestica, Amomoum
    curcuma):* Turmeric, curcuma, Indian saffron, Indian
    yellow root.
Elettaria cardamomum: Cardomom, cardomum,
    cardomon; there are two main varieties:
    var. cardamomum (var. minus, var. minuscula):
    Mysore cardamom
    var. major: Wild cardamom.
Hedychium flavescens (H. flavum): Longoze.
Hedychium spicatum: Sanna, ekangi.
Zingiber officinale: Ginger, common ginger, Jamaica
    ginger.

Orchidaceae
Vanilla planifolia (V. fragrans): Vanilla, Bourbon
    vanilla, Mexican vanilla, common vanilla, Reunion
    vanilla.
Vanilla pompona: West Indian vanilla, vanillon,
    Pompona vanilla, Guadeloupe vanilla.
Vanilla tahitensis: Tahiti vanilla.

Piperaceae
Piper cubeba (Cubeba officinalis): Cubebs, cubeba,
    tailed pepper, cubeb pepper.
Piper nigrum: Pepper, black pepper, white pepper, piper.

Betulaceae
*Betula alba (B. odorata, B. alba var. pubescens, B.
    pendula):* White birch, silver birch, European white
    birch.

Betula alleghaniensis: Yellow birch.
Betula lenta (B. capinefolia): Sweet birch, southern
    birch, cherry birch, mountain mahogany, mahogany
    birch.
Betula nigra: Black birch.
Betula papyrifera: Paper birch, birch bud (oil); several
    subspecies exist.
Betula verrucosa: Birch bud (oil), birch tar (oil); many
    cultivars exist.

Salicaceae
Populus balsamifera (P. tacamahacca): Poplar,
    tacamahac, hackmatack; two subspecies exist.

Moraceae
Ficus carica: Fig.
Humulus lupulus: Hops, common hop, European hop,
    lupulus.

Santalaceae
Santalum album: East Indian sandalwood, white
    sandalwood, white saunders, yellow sandalwood,
    yellow saunders, sanderswood, Mysore sandalwood,
    yellow sandalwood.
Santalum spicatum (Eucarya spicata): Australian
    sandalwood.

Aristolochiaceae
Aristolochia serpentaria: Virginian snakeroot,
    serpentaria (oil).
Asarum canadense: Canadian snakeroot, wild ginger,
    Indian ginger.

Chenopodiaceae
Chenopodium album: Lamb's quarters.
*Chenopodium ambrosioides (var.
    anthelminticum):* Wormseed, American wormseed,
    chenopodium, Californian spearmint, Jesuit's tea,
    Mexican tea, herb sancti mariae, Baltimore (oil).
Chenopodium bonus-henricus: Allgood, Good King
    Henry.

Caryophyllaceae
Dianthus caryophyllus: Carnation, clove pink.
Dianthus plumarius: Pink.

Magnoliaceae
Michelia champaca: Champaca.
Michelia figo.

Illiciaceae
Illicium verum: Star anise, Chinese anise, illicium,
    Chinese star anise.

Annonaceae
Cananga odorata (Canangium odoratum): two forms exist:
var. odorata (var. genuina, Unona odorantissimum): Ylang ylang
var. macrophylla: Cananga.

Myristicaceae
Myristica fragrans (M. officinalis, M. moschana, M. aromatica, M. amboinensis): Nutmeg and mace.

Monimiaceae
Peumus boldus (Boldu boldus, Boldoa fragrans): Boldo, boldus, boldu.

Lauraceae
Aniba duckei: Brazilian rosewood, bois de rose.
Aniba parviflora: Brazilian rosewood, bois de rose.
Aniba rosaeodora var. amazonica: Brazilian rosewood, bois de rose.
Cinnamomum burmanii (C. pedunculata): Indonesian cassia, padang cassia, padang cinnamon, Batavia cassia, Java cassia, Korintje cassia.
Cinnamomum camphora (Laurus camphora): Camphor tree, true camphor, laurel camphor, gum camphor, Japanese camphor, Formosa camphor; several subvarieties exist.
Cinnamomum cassia (C. aromaticum, Laurus cassia): Cassia, Chinese cinnamon, false cinnamon, cassia cinnamon, cassia lignea.
Cinnamomum cecidodaphne: Nepalese tejpat.
Cinnamomum culiliban (C. culiliwan): Lawang.
Cinnamomum loueirii: Saigon cinnamon
Cinnamomum micranthum: Chinese sassafras.
Cinnamomum tamala: Indian cassia.
Cinnamomum zeylanicum (C. verum, Laurus cinnamomum): Cinnamon, Ceylon cinnamon, Seychelles cinnamon, Madagascar cinnamon, true cinnamon.
Cryptocarya massoy (Massoia aromatica): Massoi.
Laurus nobilis; Grecian laurel, sweet bay, laurel, true bay, Mediterranean bay, Roman laurel, noble laurel, laurel leaf (oil); three subspecies exist.
Lindera umbellata var. umbellata: Kuru-moji; several other subspecies exist.
Litsea cubeba (L. citrata): May-chang, exotic verbena, tropical verbena.
Nectandra elaiophora: Louro nhamuy.
Ocotea caudata (Licaria guianensis): Cayenne rosewood.
Ocotea cymbarum (Mespilodaphne sassafras): Amazonian sassafras.
Ocotea pretiosa: Brazilian sassafras.
Phoebe nanmu.

Sassafras albidum (S. officinale, Laurus sassafras, S. variifolium): Common sassafras, North American sassafras, sassafrax.

Brassicaceae (Cruciferae)
Armoracia rusticana (A. lapathifolia, Cochlearia armoracia): Horseradish, red cole, raifort.
Brassica juncea: Indian mustard, brown mustard.
Brassica nigra: Black mustard.
Cheiranthus cheiri: Wallflower.

Resedaceae
Reseda odorata: Reseda, common mignonette.

Grossulariaceae
Ribes nigrum: Blackcurrant, niribine (oil); several cultivars exist.

Hamamelidaceae
Liquidambar orientalis: Oriental sweetgum, Levant styrax, Asiatic styrax, storax, Turkish sweetgum, liquid storax.
Liquidambar styraciflua: Sweetgum, American styrax, storax, red gum.

Rosaceae
Prunus dulcis (P. communis, P. amygdalus, Amygdalus communis, A. dulcis):
Almond; there are two varieties:
var. dulcis: Sweet almond
var. amara: Bitter almond.
Rosa alba (R. damascena var. alba): White rose ; the main cultivar is called 'Semiplena', similar to the Bulgarian 'Suaveolens'.
Rosa canina: Dogrose, doghip.
Rosa centifolia: Cabbage rose, Provence rose, French rose, rose de mai, hundred-leaved rose.
Rosa damascena: Summer damask rose, Turkish rose, Bulgarian rose; the main cultivar is 'Trigintipetala' or 'Kazanlik rose'. There are also several other subspecies including:
var. semperflorens: Autumn damask rose.
Rosa gallica: French rose, Provins rose; the two main cultivars were once 'Conditorum' or the Hungarian rose, and 'Officinalis', 'Apothecary' rose or the red damask rose.
Rosa indica: Tea rose, oriental rose.
Rosa muscatta: Musk rose
Rosa rubiginosa (R. eglanteria): Eglantine, sweet briar.
Rosa rugosa: Rugosa rose, ramanas rose, Japanese rose, Chinese rose.

Mimosaceae
Acacia caven (A. cavenia): Roman cassie.

Acacia dealbata (A. decurrens var. dealbata): Mimosa, Sydney black wattle.

Acacia farnesiana (Cassia ancienne): Sweet acacia, cassie, huisache, popinac, opopanax.

Fabaceae (Leguminosae)

Copaifera coricea: Copaiba.

Copaifera guyanensis: Copaiba.

Copaifera lansdorffinii: Copaiba.

Copaifera martii: Copaiba.

Copaifera multijuga: Copaiba.

Copaifera officinalis: Copaiba, copahu balsam, copaiva, Jesuit's balsam, para balsam, Maracaibo balsam, balsam copaiba (oil).

Copaifera reticulata: Copaiba.

Daniellia thurifera: Ogea gum, illorin gum, balsam Sierra Leone, 'frankincense'.

Dipteryx odorata (Coumarouna odorata): Tonka, Dutch tonka bean, tonquin bean.

Glycyrrhiza glabra: Liquorice, licorice.

Melilotus officinalis: Yellow melilot, common melilot, white melilot, corn melilot, melilot trefoil, sweet clover, plaster clover, sweet lucerne, wild laburnum, king's clover, melilotin (oleoresin).

Myrocarpus fastigiatus: Cabreuva, cabureicica.

Myrocarpus frondosus: Cabreuva.

Myroxylon balsamum: this group is divided into three main sub-species:
  var. *balsamum (var. genuinum, Myrospermum toluiferum, Toluiferum balsamum, Balsamum americanum, Balsamum tolutanum:* Opobalsam, Tolu balsam, Thomas balsam, resin tolu
  var. *pereirae (Myrospermum pereirae, Toluifera pereirae, Myroxylon pereirae):*
  Peru Balsam, Peruvian balsam, Indian balsam, black balsam
  var. *punctatum (Myroxylon punctatum).*

Robinia pseudo-acacia: Black locust, false acacia.

Spartium junceum (Genista juncea): Spanish broom, weaver's broom, genista, genet.

Trifolium pratense: Red clover; several varieties exist.

Trigonella foenum-graecum: Fenugreek.

Geraniaceae

Geranium macrorrhizum: Bulgarian geranium.

Pelargonium graveolens: Rose geranium, geranium; numerous other varieties and cultivars exist such as: *P. odoratissimum, P. radens, P. capitatum* and *P.x asperum.*

Zygophyllaceae

Bulnesia sarmienti: Guaiacwood, champaca wood (oil).

Rutaceae

Agathosma betulina (Barosma betulina): Buchu, mountain buchu, short buchu, bookoo, buku, bucco.

Agathosma crenulata (Barosma crenulata): Oval buchu, crenate buchu.

Amyris balsamifera (Schimmelia oleifera): Amyris, West Indian sandalwood, West Indian rosewood.

Boronia megastigma: Boronia, brown boronia.

Citrus aurantifolia (C. latifolia, C. medica var. acida): Lime, Mexican lime, West Indian lime, sour lime.

Citrus aurantium var. amara (C. vulgaris, C. bigaradia): Bitter orange, sour orange, Seville orange, bigarade (oil), neroli bigarade (oil), orange flower (oil), petitgrain orange (oil).

Citrus bergamia (C. aurantium subsp.bergamia): Bergamot; the two main cultivars are 'Castagnaro' and 'Femmenillo'.

Citrus hystrix: Leech-lime, Mauritius papeda, combava (oil).

Citrus jambhiri: Rough lemon (Java lemon); the two main cultivars are 'Estes' and 'Milam'.

Citrus limetta: Italian lime, limette (oil).

Citrus limon (C. limonum): Lemon, cedro (oil); there are many cultivars notably 'Berna', 'Eureka', 'Lisbon', 'Femminello Ovale' and 'Femminello Sfusato'.

Citrus medica: Citron, cedrat; the main cultivar is 'Diamante'.

Citrus x paradisi (C. maxima var. racemosa, C. racemosa): Grapefruit; there are many cultivars.

Citrus reticulata (C. deliciosa, C. nobilis, C. unshiu): Mandarin, tangerine, satsuma; there are many cultivars, the most common being 'Crava'.

Citrus sinensis (C. aurantium var. sinensis, C. aurantium var. dulcis): Sweet orange, Portugal orange, China orange; there are many cultivars notably 'Valencia'; also produces neroli Portugal or neroli petalae (oil).

Citrus jambhiri x C. aurantifolia: Lemon n'lime.

Citrus limon x C. sinensis: Lemonange.

Citrus reticulata x C. x paradisi: Tangelo.

Dictamus albus: Dittany, fraxinella, burning bush, gas plant.

Galipea trifoliata (G. officinalis, G. cusparia, Cusparia trifoliata): Angustora.

Luvunga scandens: Sugandh kokila.

Pilocarpus jaborandi (Pernambuco jaborandi, P. pennatifolius): Jaborandi, Iaborandi, jamborandi.

Ruta angustifolia: Sardinian rue, North African rue.

Ruta chalepensis (R. bracteosa): Winter rue, Sicilian rue, North African rue.

Ruta graveolens: Rue, garden rue, herb-of-grace, herbygrass.

Ruta montana: Summer rue, Spanish rue, North African rue.

Skimmia laureola.
Zanthoxylum alatum: Tomarseed.
Zanthoxylum piperitum: Prickly ash, 'san-sho'.
Zanthoxylum rhetsa (Z. bodrunga): Mulilam.
Zanthoxylum schinifolium (Z. mantchuricum):
   Pepperbush.
Zanthoxylum simulans (z. bungei): Chinese pepper,
   Szechuan pepper.

Burseraceae
Boswellia bhau-dajiana: Frankincense.
Boswellia carteri: Frankincense, olibanum, gum thus.
Boswellia frereana: African elemi, elemi frankincense.
Boswellia papyrifera: Sudanese frankincense.
Boswellia sacra (B. thurifera sensu): Saudi frankincense.
Boswellia serrata: Indian frankincense, Indian olibanum.
Bursera aloexylon: Linaloe.
Bursera fagaroides: Linaloe.
Bursera glabrifolia (B. delpechiana): Linaloe, Mexican
   linaloe, 'copal lemon'.
Bursera penicillata: Linaloe.
Bursera simaruba (Elaphrium simaruba): West Indian
   birch, West Indian elemi, gumbo limbo, incense tree.
Canarium luzonicum (C. commune): Elemi, Manila
   elemi, elemi gum, elemi resin.
Commiphora erythraea: Opopanax, bisabol myrrh.
Commiphora madagascariensis (C. abyssinica,
   Balsamodendron habessinica): Abyssinian myrrh.
Commiphora molmol: Somalian myrrh.
Commiphora myrrha: Common myrrh, hirabol myrrh.

Meliaceae
Aglaia odorata.
Cabralea cangerana: Cangerana.
Cedrela odorata: West Indian cedar, Spanish cedar,
   cigar-box cedar, Barbados cedar.

Euphorbiaceae
Croton eluteria: Cascarilla, sweetwood bark, sweet
   bark, Bahama cascarilla, aromatic quinquina, false
   quinquina, cascarilla bark (oil).

Anacardiaceae
Pistacia lenticus: Mastic, mastick tree, mastix, mastich,
   lentisk.
Schinus molle: Peruvian pepper tree, Peruvian mastic,
   California pepper tree.

Tiliaceae
Tilia vulgaris (T. europaea): Lime tree, linden, common
   lime, lyne, tillet, tilea.

Aquifoliaceae
Ilex paraguayensis: Paraguay tea.

Malvaceae
Abelmoschus moschatus (Hibiscus abelmoschus):
   Ambrette, seed musk seed, Egyptian alcee, target-
   leaved hibiscus, muskmallow.

Byttneriaceae
Theobroma cacoa: Cocoa, chocolate; several cultivars
   exist.

Theaceae
Camellia sinensis: Tea; there are two varieties:
   var. sinensis: China tea
   var. assamica: Assam tea.

Dipterocarpaceae
Dipterocarpus alatus: Gurjun.
Dipterocarpus jourdainii: Gurjun.
Dipterocarpus tuberculatus: Gurjun.
Dipterocarpus turbinatus: Gurjun, East Indian copaiba
   balsam.
Dryobalanops aromatica (D. camphora): Borneo
   camphor, East Indian camphor, Baros camphor,
   Sumatra camphor, Malayan camphor, Borneol (oil).

Cistaceae
Cistus ladaniferus: Labdanum, cistus, ciste, cyste,
   ambreine, European rock rose.
Cistus incanus (C. villosus, C. polymorphus):
   Labdanum; three subspecies exist:
   C. polymorphus, C. corsicus and *C. creticus.*

Violaceae
Viola alba: Parma violet; there are three subspecies.
Viola odorata: Sweet violet, English violet, garden
   violet, blue violet.
Viola suavis: Russian violet.

Thymelaeaceae
Aquilaria agallocha: Agarwood, aloes wood, agar.
Aquilaria malaccensis: Indonesian agarwood.

Myrtaceae
Eucalyptus citriodora: Lemon-scented gum, citron-
   scented gum, spotted gum.
Eucalyptus cneorifolia: Kangaroo Island narrow-leaved
   mallee.
Eucalyptus dives: Broad-leaved peppermint, blue
   peppermint, peppermint.
Eucalyptus dumosa: Mallee, Congo mallee.
Eucalyptus elata (E. andreana, E. lindleyana, E.
   longifolia, E. numerosa): River peppermint, river
   white gum.
Eucalyptus globulus (var. globulus): Blue gum,
   Tasmanian blue gum, southern blue gum, fever tree,

gum tree, eucalyptus, stringy bark.

Eucalyptus goniocalyx (E. elaeophora): Long-leaved box, bundy, apple jack, olive-barked box.

Eucalyptus leucoxylon: Yellow gum, white ironbark, white gum; three subspecies exist.

Eucalyptus macarthurii: Camden woolybut, Paddy's river box.

Eucalyptus oleosa: Red mallee, glossy-leaved red mallee.

Eucalyptus piperita: Peppermint eucalyptus.

Eucalyptrus polybractea: Blue-leaved mallee.

Eucalyptus radiata (E. australiana, E. phellandra): Narrow-leaved peppermint, grey peppermint; two subspecies exist.

Eucalyptus sideroxylon: Red ironbark, ironbark, mugga; two subspecies exist.

Eucalyptus smithii: Gully gum, gully peppermint, blackbutt peppermint.

Eucalyptus staigerana.

Eucalyptus viminalis; two subspecies exist.

Eucalyptus viridis: Green mallee.

Melaleuca alternifolia (M. linariifolia var. alternifolia): Tea tree, narrow-leaved paperbark tea tree, ti-tree, ti-trol, melasol.

Melaleuca bracteata: Tea tree.

Melaleuca cajeputi: Cajuput, cajeput, white tea tree, white wood, swamp tea tree, punk tree, paperbark tree.

Melaleuca leucadendra (Myrtus leucodendra): Cajeput, cajuput, river tea tree, weeping tea tree.

Melaleuca linariifolia: Tea tree.

Melaleuca minor: Cajuput, cajeput.

Melaleuca quinquenervia: Cajeput, cajuput.

Melaleuca viridiflora: Niaouli.

Myrtus communis: Myrtle; at least two subspecies exist.

Pimenta dioica (P. officinalis): Allspice, pimento, pimenta, Jamaica pepper.

Pimenta racemosa (P. acris, Myrcia acris): Bay, West Indian bay, bay rum tree, wild cinnamon, bayberry, myrcia.

Syzygium aromaticum (Eugenia aromatica, E. caryophyllata, E. caryophyllus): Clove.

Turneraceae

Turnera diffusa (T. aphrodisiaca): Damiana.

Apiaceae (Umbelliferae)

Ammi visnaga: Khella seed, visnaga.

Anethum graveolens (Peucedanum graveolens, Fructus anethi): Dill, European dill, American dill.

Anethum sowa: Indian dill.

Angelica archangelica (A. officinalis): Angelica, European angelica, garden angelica; two

subspecies exist.

Angelica atropurpurea: Purple angelica, American angelica.

Angelica keiskei: Japanese angelica.

Angelica ursina: Japanese angelica.

Anthricus cerefolium (A. longirostris): Chervil, garden chervil, salad chervil.

Apium graveolens: Celery; there are at least four varieties, including:

var. dulce: Sweet celery

var. rapaceum: Celeriac.

Carum carvi (Apium carvi): Caraway, carum.

Carum roxburghianum: Ajmud (Indian).

Coriandrum maritimum: Samphire, rock samphire.

Coriandrum sativum: Coriander, Chinese parsley.

Cuminum cyminum (C. odorum): Cumin, cummin, Roman caraway.

Daucus carota: Carrot, wild carrot, Queen Anne's lace, bird's nest, carrot seed (oil); there are at least twelve subspecies.

Dorema ammoniacum: Ammoniac, Bombay sumbul, boi.

Ferula asa-foetida: Asafetida, asafoetida, gum asafetida, devil's dung, food of the gods, giant fennel.

Ferula diversittata (F. suavolens): Sumbul, muskroot.

Ferula foetida: Asafetida.

Ferula galbaniflua (F. gummosa): Galbanum, 'bubonion'.

Ferula jaeschkeana; four varieties exist.

Ferula moschata (F. sumbul): Sumbul, muskroot.

Foeniculum vulgare (F. officinale, F. cappilaceum, Anethum foeniculum): Fennel, fenkel; its subspecies include:

var. azoricum: Florence fennel

var. dulce: Sweet fennel

var. amara: Bitter fennel

Levisticum officinale (Angelica levisticum, Ligusticum levisticum): Lovage, garden lovage, common lovage, old English lovage, Italian lovage, maggi herb, smellage, Cornish lovage.

Levisticum mutellina: Alpine lovage.

Ligusticum scoticum: Sea lovage.

Pastinaca sativa: Parsnip; there are four subspecies.

Petroselinum sativum (P. hortense, Apium petroselinum, Carum petroselinum): Parsley; there are four varieties including:

Petroselinum crispum: Curly-leaved parsley.

Pimpinella anisum (Anisum officinalis, A. vulgare): Aniseed, anise, sweet cumin.

Pimpinella major: Great burnet, saxifrage.

Pimpinella saxifraga: Burnet saxifrage, black caraway.

Trachyspermum copticum (T. ammi, Carum copticum, Carum ajowan, Ptychotis ajowan, Ammi copticum): Ajowan, ajuan, omum.

Ericaceae

Gaultheria procumbens: Wintergreen, tea berry, checkerberry, aromatic wintergreen, gaultheria (oil).

Styracaceae

Styrax benzoin: Gum benzoin, styrax benzoin, gum benjamin, Sumatra benzoin.

Styrax macrothyrsus: Vietnam styrax.

Styrax paralleloneurus: Haminjon toba (Indonesian), Sumatra benzoin.

Styrax tonkinensis: Siam styrax, Siam benzoin

Oleaceae

Jasminum auriculatum: Indian jasmine.

Jasminum grandiflorum (J. officinale var. grandiflorum): Catalonian jasmine, Royal jasmine, jasmin, Spanish jasmine, Italian jasmine.

Jasminum officinale: Jasmine, common jasmine, poet's jessamine, jessamine.

Jasminum sambac: Arabian jasmine, sambac; there are two cultivars: 'Grand Duke' and 'Maid of Orleans'.

Osmanthus fragrans: Sweet olive, fragrant olive, tea olive.

Syringa vulgaris: Common lilac; numerous cultivars exist.

Boraginaceae

Heliotropium arborescens (H. peruvianum): Heliotrope.

Verbenaceae

Aloysia triphylla (A. citriodora, Lippia citriodora, L. triphylla, Verbena triphylla): Lemon verbena, verbena, herb Louisa.

Lippia abyssinica (L. adoensis): Gambian tea bush.

Lippia affinis: Oregano.

Lippia cardiostegia: Oregano.

Lippia formosa: Oregano.

Lippia fragrans: Oregano.

Lippia graveolens (L. berlandieri): Mexican oregano.

Lippia micromeria: False thyme.

Lippia origanoides: Oregano.

Lippia palmeri: Mexican oregano.

Lippia pseudo-thea: Brazilian tea.

Lippia umbellata: Oregano.

Lamiaceae (Labiatae)

Aeollanthus gamwelliae (A. graveolens): Ninde.

Calamintha officinalis (C. clinopodium, Melissa calminta): Calamintha, calamint, common calamint, mill mountain, mountain balm, mountain mint, basil thyme.

Hedeoma floribundum: Oregano.

Hedeoma patens: Oregano.

Hedeoma pulegioides: North American pennyroyal, squaw mint, stinking balm, tickweed, mosquito plant.

Hyssopus officinalis: Hyssop, 'azob'; four subspecies exist, including *var. decumbens*.

Lavandula angustifolia (L. officinalis, L. vera): Common lavender, true lavender, garden lavender; this variety is divided into two subspecies: *L. delphinensis* and *L. fragrans*. In addition many cultivars exist.

Lavandula x intermedia (L. hybrida, L. hortensis): Lavandin; several cultivars exist.

Lavandula latifolia (L. spica): Spike lavender, spike, aspic, broad-leaved lavender, lesser lavender.

Lavandula stoechas: French lavender, stoechas lavender; six subspecies exist.

Melissa officinalis: Lemon balm, balm, melissa, common balm, bee balm, sweet balm, heart's delight, honeyplant; two subspecies exist.

Mentha aquatica: Water mint, bergamot mint.

Mentha canadensis (M. arvensis var. villosa, M. arvensis var. glabrata, M. arvensis var. piperascens): Corn mint, Japanese peppermint, North American field mint.

Mentha x gracilis (M. gentilis): Scotch spearmint, red mint.

Mentha x piperita: Peppermint.

Mentha pulegium: Pennyroyal, European pennyroyal, pudding plant, pulegium.

Mentha spicata (M. viridis, M. longifolia): Spearmint.

Mentha suaveolens (M. rotundifolia): Pineapple mint.

Mentha x villosa var. alopecuroides: Woolly mint, apple mint, Bowles' mint, Egyptian mint.

Monarda citriodora: Lemon bee balm, lemon bergamot; two varieties exist.

Monarda clinopodia: Bee balm, wild bergamot.

Monarda didyma: Oswego tea, oswego bee balm, bergamot.

Monarda fistulosa: Wild bergamot, horsemint, bee balm; four varieties exist including *var. menthifolia*.

Monarda x media: several cultivars exist.

Monarda pectinata: Pony bee balm.

Nepeta cataria: Catnip, catmint.

Ocimum basilicum: Basil, sweet basil; numerous cultivars and chemotypes exist, including 'Comoran' basil (exotic or Reunion Basil) and the 'true' sweet basil (French, European or common Basil).

Ocimum canum (O. americanum): Hoary basil, hairy basil.

Ocimum gratissimum (O. viride): East Indian basil, tree basil, shrubby basil.

Ocimum kilimanjaricum: Camphor basil.

Ocimum sanctum: Holy basil, sacred basil.

Origanum x applii: Oregano.

Origanum marjorana (Marjorana hortensis): Sweet

marjoram, knotted marjoram.

Origanum x marjorana: Oregano, marjoram.

Origanum onites: Pot marjoram, French marjoram.

Origanum syriacum (O. maru): Syrian oregano.

Origanum vulgare: Common oregano; this is divided into six subspecies:

subsp.vulgare: Wild marjoram, oreganum (oil); several cultivars exist.

subsp.glandulosum: Oregano.

subsp.gracile (O. tytthanthum, O. kopetdaghense): Russian oregano.

subsp.hirtum (O. hirtum, O. heracleoticum): Winter, Greek or Italian oregano.

subsp.virens (O. virens): Wild marjoram.

subsp.viride (O. heracleoticum): Wild marjoram.

Perilla frutescens (P. ocymoides): Perilla, beefsteak plant; numerous varieties exist.

Pogostemon cablin (P. patchouly): Patchouli, patchouly, puchaput.

Pogostemon heyneanus (P. patchouli): False patchouly.

Rosmarinus officinalis: Rosemary; other varieties exist including:

var. officinalis: Common rosemary; numerous cultivars and forms exist.

var. angustifolia (R. tenuifolius): Pine-scented rosemary, pine-needled rosemary.

var. lavendulaceus (R. officinalis f. humulis, f. procumbens): Prostrate rosemary; numerous cultivars exist.

Salvia clevelandii: Blue sage.

Salvia dorisiana: Peach-scented sage, British Honduran sage.

Salvia elegans (S. rutilans): Pineapple-scented sage.

Salvia fruticosa (S. triloba): Greek sage.

Salvia lavendulidefolia: Spanish sage, lavender-leaved sage.

Salvia leucophylla: Grey sage, purple sage.

Salvia officinalis: Common sage, dalmatian sage, garden sage; many cultivars exist.

Salvia pomifera (S. calycina): Apple sage.

Salvia sclarea: Clary, clary sage, muscatel sage, clary wort, clear eye, see bright, common clary, clarry, eye bright.

Salvia verbenacea (S. clandestina, S. horminoides): Vervain sage, wild clary.

Salvia viridis (S. horminum): Bluebeard sage, Joseph sage, red-topped sage.

Satureja douglasii (Micromeria chamissonis, M. douglasii): Yerba buena (Spanish).

Satureja hortensis (Satureia hortensis, Calamintha hortensis): Summer savory, garden savory.

Satureja montana (S. obovata, Calamintha montana): Winter savory; at least five subspecies exist.

Satureja thymbra: Za'atar rumi (Arabic).

Thymus caespititius (T. micans, T. serpyllum): Tiny thyme, tufted thyme.

Thymus capitatus (Satureja capitata, Thymbra capitata, Coridothymus capitatus): Conehead thyme, corido thyme, Cretan thyme, thyme of the ancients, headed savory, Spanish oreganum (oil), Israeli oreganum (oil).

Thymus cephalatos.

Thymus x citriodorus (T. lanuginosus var. citriodorum, T. serpyllum var. citriodorus, T. 'Limoneum'): Lemon thyme

Thymus herba-barona: Caraway thyme.

Thymus hirtus.

Thymus hyemalis: often wrongly cited as the source of Spanish verbena oil.

Thymus loscosii; two subspecies exist.

Thymus mastichina: Mastic thyme, Spanish marjoram.

Thymus praecox: Creeping thyme; five subspecies exist and several cultivars.

Thymus pulegoides: Wild thyme, Dutch tea thyme; several subspecies and cultivars exist.

Thymus quinquecostatus: Japanese thyme; two forms are known.

Thymus serpyllum: Wild thyme, mother-of-thyme; two subspecies exist.

Thymus vulgaris (T. aestivus, T. ilerdensis, T. webbianus, T. valentianus): garden thyme, common thyme, French Thyme, red thyme (oil), white thyme (oil).

Thymus zygis (T. sabulicola, T. sylvestris): Spanish sauce thyme, red thyme (oil).

Other lesser known species and cultivars also exist in the *Thymus* group.

Solanaceae

Nicotiana tabacum: Tobacco.

Rubiaceae

Anthocephalus indicus (A. cadamba): Cadamba, kadamba.

Coffea arabica: Coffee, common coffee, Arabian coffee; many cultivars exist.

Coffea canephora (C. robusta): Robusta coffee; many cultivars exist.

Gardenia jasminoides (G. florida, G. grandiflora, G. radicans): Common gardenia, Cape jasmine, gardinia.

Leptactina senegambica: Karo-karounde.

Caprifoliaceae

Lonicera etrusca (L. gigantea): Honeysuckle.

Lonicera periclymenum: Common honeysuckle.

Sambucus nigra: Elderberry, elderflower.

Valerianaceae

Nardostachys chinensis: Chinese spikenard.

Nardostachys jatamansi: Nard, spikenard, 'false' Indian valerian root.

Valeriana fauriei (V. officinalis, V. officinalis var. angustifolia, V. officinalis var. latifolia): Common valerian, European valerian, Belgian valerian, fragrant valerian, garden valerian; other chemotypes exist such as:
Japanese valerian, 'kesso root'.

Valeriana wallichii: Indian valerian.

Asteraceae (Compositae)

Achillea erba-rotta (A. moschata): Iva, musk yarrow.

Achillea ligustica: Ligurian yarrow.

Achillea millefolium: Common yarrow, milfoil, nosebleed, thousand leaf; at least two subspecies exist.

Arnica montana (A. fulgens, A. sororia): Arnica, leopard's bane, wolf's bane; two subspecies exist.

Artemisia abrotanum: Southern wood, old man, lad's love.

Artemisia absinthium: Wormwood, common wormwood, green ginger, armoise, absinthium (oil).

Artemisia afra: African wormwood, lanyana, wildeals.

Artemisia annua: Annual wormwood, sweet Annie.

Artemisia dracunculus: French tarragon, Russian tarragon, estragon (oil).

Artemisia genipi (A. spicata, A. laxa, A. mutellina, A. glacialis): Genipi.

Artemisia herba-alba (A. sieversiana): Armoise.

Artemisia judaica: Semen contra.

Artemisia maritima (A. cina): Levant wormseed.

Artemisia pallens: Davana.

Artemisia pontica: Roman wormwood, small absinthe.

Artemisia princeps: Japanese mugwort.

Artemisia vestita.

Artemisia vulgaris: Mugwort, Indian wormwood.

Atractylodes lancea: Atractylis; two varieties exist.

Baccharis dracunculifolia: Vassoura.

Baccharis gennistelloides: Carquueja.

Balsamita major (Chrysanthemum balsamita, Pyrethrum majus): Costmary, mint geranium, sweet Mary, Bible leaf, balsamite.

Blumea balsamifera: Ngai camphor.

Blumea chinensis: Tombak-tombak.

Blumea lacera.

Blumea myriocephala (B. lanceolaria).

Brachylaena hutchinsii: Muhuhu.

Calendula officinalis: Poet's marigold, pot marigold, calendula, marygold, gold-bloom, hollygold, common marigold, marybud.

Carphephorus odoratissimus, Trilisa odoratissima, Liatris odoratissima, Frasera speciosa: Deertongue, hound's tongue, deer's tongue, Carolina vanilla, vanilla leaf, wild vanilla, vanilla trilisa, whart's tongue, liatris (oil).

Chamaemelum nobile (Anthemis nobilis): Roman chamomile, camomile, English chamomile, garden chamomile, sweet chamomile, true chamomile.

Chamaemelum suaveolens (Matricaria matricarioides): Pineapple weed.

Conyza canadensis (Erigeron canadensis): Fleabane, horseweed.

Eriocephalus punctulatus: Eriocephalee.

Helichrysum angustifolium: Immortelle, everlasting, helichrysum.

Helichrysum italicum: Curry plant, white-leaved everlasting.

Helichrysum stoechas: Everlasting, immortelle; at least two subspecies exist.

Helichrysum orientale: Everlasting, immortelle.

Inula helenium (Helenium grandiflorum, Aster officinalis, A. helenium): Elecampane, scabwort, alant, horseheal, yellow starwort, elf dock, wild sunflower, velvet dock.

Matricaria recutita, (M. chamomilla): German chamomile, Hungarian chamomile, sweet false chamomile, camomile, blue chamomile, single chamomile, wild chamomile.

Ormentis mixta (Anthemis mixta): Moroccan chamomile.

Ormentis multicaulis: Moroccan chamomile.

Pteronia incana: Pteronia, blue dog.

Santolina chamaecyparissus (Lavendula taemina): Santolina, cotton lavender.

Saussurea costus (S. lappa, Aucklandia costus, Aplotaxis lappa, A. auriculata): Costus.

Solidago odora: Sweet goldenrod, fragrant goldenrod.

Tagetes lucida: Sweet marigold, sweet mace, Mexican tarragon.

Tagetes erecta: African marigold, Aztec marigold,

Tagetes minuta (T. glandulifera): Taget (oil), tagetes, tagette.

Tagetes patula: French marigold, taget (oil).

Tanacetum vulgare (Chrysanthemum vulgare, C. tanacetum): Tansy, bitter buttons, bachelor's buttons, cheese, scented fern.

BOTANICAL INDEX